Yoga for Children

200+ Yoga Poses, Breathing Exercises, and Meditations for *Healthier, Happier, More Resilient* Children

Lisa Flynn, E-RYT, RCYT
Founder of ChildLight Yoga® and Yoga 4 Classrooms®

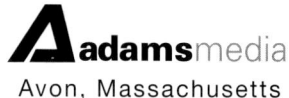

A adamsmedia

Avon, Massachusetts

Published by
Adams Media, a division of F+W Media, Inc.
57 Littlefield Street, Avon, MA 02322. U.S.A.
www.adamsmedia.com

ISBN 10: 1-4405-5463-3
ISBN 13: 978-1-4405-5463-6
eISBN 10: 1-4405-5464-1
eISBN 13: 978-1-4405-5464-3

Printed in the United States of America.

10   9   8   7

Photographs by Home Town Photo.

This book is available at quantity discounts for bulk purchases.
For information, please call 1-800-289-0963.

Praise for *Yoga for Children*

"[*Yoga for Children*] is a very comprehensive book for teaching yoga to children . . . . As it should be for children, the heart of the instruction is aimed at making the yoga experience fun and joyful. At the same time the goals are simple and holistic: encouraging the skills of focus, mindful reflection, and mind/body awareness; inspiring confidence, self-regulation, and self-efficacy; and teaching gratitude and optimism. There is no better place to start yoga than in childhood. Universal yoga instruction to our children will ease the growing mental and physical health problems they face in today's society. Importantly, it will also ultimately produce competent, resilient adults that are happy and healthy in mind, body, and spirit, and therefore nothing less than a better society overall. I highly recommend this book to anyone, be it a yoga instructor, parent, guardian, mentor, caretaker, or teacher, seeking to introduce the many benefits of yoga to children."

—Sat Bir S. Khalsa, PhD, Assistant Professor of Medicine,
Harvard Medical School; Yoga Researcher

"Lisa Flynn has mastered the art of bringing yoga to children, and her new book exudes this mastery. It is absolutely packed with clear and practical guidance for any of us who want to bring the healing grace of yoga to the kids in our lives. A whole generation of teachers and parents (and kids!) will be enormously grateful for Flynn's contribution. Indeed, it is the book we have been waiting for!"

—Stephen Cope, Director of the Kripalu Institute for Extraordinary Living;
Author of *Yoga and the Quest for the True Self*

"In this practical how-to guide, Lisa Flynn shares the secrets of empowering kids and families to connect with one another while learning positive, productive skills for managing the stresses of everyday life. Every parent should have a copy of this book!"

—Amy McCready, Founder of Positive Parenting Solutions; Author of
*If I Have to Tell You One More Time . . . The Revolutionary Program
That Gets Your Kids to Listen Without Nagging, Reminding, or Yelling*

"Truly, *Yoga for Children* is as much a parenting guide as a yoga guide. Far more than a collection of poses, the practices presented offer creative ways to connect physically, mentally, and spiritually with your child while nurturing his self-confidence, focus, and emotional well-being. Highly recommended!"

—Kelly McGonigal, PhD, Author of *The WillPower Instinct*;
Yoga for Pain Relief; and *The Neuroscience of Change*

"Lisa Flynn's *Yoga for Children* isn't a book so much as it is a means to connect to your child. This is a grounded, science-based, dogma-free guide to making yoga fun, challenging, and accessible. It gives children the tools to leave behind bullying, insecurity, ADHD, obesity, diabetes . . . and learn to appreciate themselves and the present moment; it offers a chance to breathe, play, relax, and regain their childhood; to live for the benefit of others, enjoy healthy food, focus at school, and cherish this planet."

—Waylon Lewis, Founder and Editor-in-Chief, *Elephant Journal*

"Lisa Flynn really understands children—and parents—and that's what makes this book so great. Instead of just watering down yoga in order to make it kid-friendly, she brings yoga right to where children live, the world of play and the delight they have in exploring what their bodies can do."

—Lawrence Cohen, PhD, Author of *Playful Parenting*

"If you have an interest in sharing yoga with children, this beautiful book will provide everything you need to fulfill that intention. The gentle, inviting, encouraging style is itself a demonstration of the essence of Yoga. I enthusiastically recommend *Yoga for Children!*"

—Amy Saltzman, MD, Director of Association for Mindfulness in Education; Author of *A Still Quiet Place: A Mindfulness Program for Teaching Children and Adolescents to Manage Stress and Difficult Emotions* (forthcoming 2014)

"If you are a parent, educator, or health professional concerned about your child's optimum mental health, *Yoga for Children* doesn't just belong on your bookshelf but in your hands every day. Written with a caring parent and yoga educator's deep understanding of a child's stress, this compassionate book is a Godsend—a manual of easy-to-lead practices that can bring children and the adults who love them moments of ease and deep connection. Play with the practices in this book and bolster your child's resilience and self-esteem as you enhance your relationship."

—Amy Weintraub, Author of *Yoga Skills for Therapists* and *Yoga for Depression*

"In *Yoga for Children*, [Lisa] Flynn simply and clearly addresses the questions of why and how to share yoga with children. Better yet, she gifts the reader with hundreds of practical applications in an accessible, user-friendly presentation. This is truly a gift to the next generation."

—John Kepner, MA, MBA, Executive Director, International Association of Yoga Therapists

"Lisa's book is like attending a top rate kids' yoga course. Including everything from mindfulness techniques to yoga games all in a very practical and approachable way, Lisa demystifies yoga for children and shows parents just how easy yoga is to do with your kids."

—Donna Freeman, Founder of Yoga in My School and Kids Yoga Academy; Author of *Once Upon a Pose: A Guide to Yoga Adventure Stories for Children*

"In this gem of a book, Lisa Flynn combines her extensive expertise in kids' yoga with her firsthand experience in parenting a child with special needs. *Yoga for Children* provides a wealth of well-balanced, research-based information in an easy-to-understand format that will be a wonderful resource for any parent, teacher, or therapist who wants to help the kids in their life experience the power of yoga to promote whole child wellness!"

—Angela Moorad, MS, CCC-SLP, IAYT, RCYP-2, Founder of OMazing Kids, LLC

"Lisa Flynn has created an easy-to-understand guide for fully engaging children in an age-appropriate yoga experience. With this book, both parent and child are sure to begin their journey for a lifelong practice and love for yoga together. I recommend this book to anyone who has kids and loves yoga."

—Shari Vilchez-Blatt, Founder & Director of Karma Kids Yoga

To my family, my inspiration,
John, Brooke, and Jack.

I am grateful to so many who have directly or indirectly contributed to this book. I'd first like to thank the editors and art team at Adams Media. A special thanks to my editor, Victoria Sandbrook, for encouraging and guiding this newbie through the process. To Brianne—apparently nothing is impossible, thanks to you.

My heartfelt gratitude to my teachers and mentors, Bob Butera, Julie Rost, and Carrie Tyler, among so many others with whom I've learned and grown.

To the many passionate and wise teachers, colleagues, and researchers leading the field of yoga and mindfulness education for youth and other experts with whom I've either trained or been otherwise blessed to connect with and learn from over the years: Marsha Therese Danzig, Helen Garabedian, Leah Kalish, Donna Freeman, Abby Wills, Craig Hanauer, Shakta Khalsa, Erin Maile O'Keefe, Christy Brock, Allison Morgan, Shari Vilchez-Blatt, Jodi Komitor, Anne Desmond, Charlotte Reznick, Amy McGready, B.K. Bose, Sat Bir Khalsa, and Danielle Day, among others.

Big hugs to the beautiful, talented children, including some of my students, friends, and family, pictured throughout this book: Lilyanna, Bella, Judah, Shivani, Daniel, Tierney, Sophia, Grace, Malkias, Maia, Samantha, Wade, Izzy, Liam, Brooke, Jack, Hannah, Meghan, Shannen, Bridget, Taylor Ann, Ella, Luke, Madeleine, Erin, Bryn, Liam, Megan, Cullen, Maura, Emilie, Tyler, Delaney, and David, as well as to some of their parents, also pictured.

Thank you my team at ChildLight Yoga® and Yoga 4 Classrooms®, especially Stacey, Julie, Marina, Sharon, Heather, and Sally for their enduring commitment to this work and continuous encouragement and support, and also to former team members, Lisa Burk-McCoy and Heather Warr.

To my friends and extended family—for the advice, the carpooling and childcare, supportive e-mails, calls and Facebook messages, patience and love, I am grateful.

To my mom, husband, and children—thank you for not only putting up with many days and nights of neglect as I wrote, but for also being my inspiration and personal cheerleading section throughout. I love you.

And finally, to the many children, families, and educators I've been blessed to share with and learn from over the years—*Namaste*.

Contents

An Invitation

Do you remember playing outside when you were a kid? Starting pickup games of kickball or softball? Creating something to do, all by yourself? Walking or biking to a friend's house across town? Do you remember sitting down to dinner with your family, at least occasionally? Playing board games together? I do! Though our backgrounds and upbringing may not be the same, one cannot argue the fact that our children are living in a very different age.

In today's busy world, our levels of stress and anxiety have skyrocketed. Demanding days of school, overscheduled extracurricular activities, competitive sports, and ever-increasing homework have replaced most opportunities for natural antidotes to stress like unstructured free play and playing outside. And despite our best intentions, our kids feed off our stressed states of being, eat overprocessed foods, and endure inappropriate child-directed media and an increasingly technological world. Phew! With few coping mechanisms for managing all that is coming in, a child's mind and body can easily become overwhelmed. Not surprisingly, increasing numbers of children are being diagnosed with anxiety, anger issues, and attention disorders.

Over the past twenty-five years, much has been written about the negative effects of stress on adult health. However, research on the effects of stress on children did not start until the past ten years or so. Now, published articles, books, and other materials related to stress in children are coming out every day, a sign we have a crisis on our hands.

A stressed child may present with symptoms such as night terrors, hyperactivity, lethargy, fearfulness, headaches, bed-wetting, and emotional problems such as overeating, low self-esteem, lack of compassion, anger, and violent outbursts. In addition, numerous studies have illustrated how children are unable to focus and learn when their bodies and minds are in a stressed, disconnected state.

My own son was diagnosed with Sensory Processing Disorder and Attention Deficit Disorder when he was six years old. The irony that his mother teaches yoga and mindfulness to children has not escaped me. We yogis are apparently not exempt from having children with attention challenges (an exaggerated inability to be present). But, I like to think Jack was born to me because I am a children's yoga teacher. In so many ways, on so many levels, he is my teacher as well. He has helped inspire this work to a deeper and more personal level.

I have seen firsthand the negative effects of too much TV or computer time versus outdoor, creative play: general crankiness, desire for constant entertainment, focus and attention issues, hyperactivity or lethargy, anxiety, and inappropriate behavior. For my son, and for many other children, a predisposition to anxiety and trouble focusing is only exaggerated by the demands of our current culture. However, all children can be negatively affected by stress and overstimulation.

No child wants to feel uncomfortable, cranky, or anxious, or to get in trouble because of hyperactive or inappropriate behavior. Children are intrinsically joyful, peaceful, and compassionate. But oftentimes, as the stimuli from their external world increases, it can become challenging for many children to connect with their authentic, peaceful selves. In fact, it is my belief, and one of the cornerstones of the ChildLight Yoga® and Yoga 4 Classrooms® programs, that without having the time and space for reflection and connection, children (and adults) can "forget" that they have the ability to do so at all.

To be successful, creative learners and compassionate, respectful, and self-aware human beings, children must be given opportunities to draw their awareness away from our overwhelming, chaotic world. In doing so, they are brought into the present moment, a place where they can pause, truly hear and feel, and reflect and learn. A few deep breaths, mindful movement or stretching, opportunities to connect and share with our family or classroom community, and moments for quiet introspection are quick and easy ways to reset the mind/body system to a calm, focused, connected state. It is also in this place that children develop the ability to know, understand, and appreciate their true nature. Children can be empowered to go within and know the gifts of inner wisdom: confidence, joy, compassion, and contentedness.

In 2007, the first Symposium on Yoga Therapy and Research was held in Los Angeles. Nearly a quarter of the studies submitted for the symposium focused on children and adolescents. Since then, an increasing number of studies focusing on yoga for children and youth have been conducted, with many more on the way. Evidence is mounting in support of what many of us have known to be true from our own experience working with children: The practice of yoga is beneficial for all, particularly for children.

I want to personally congratulate you on your decision to learn more about sharing yoga with your child. Perhaps you are new to yoga or maybe you have experienced the benefits of yoga in your own life but have been unsure about how to get started sharing the practice with your child. To begin a yoga and mindfulness practice with your child, you do not need to be an expert. This book will show you how to quickly, easily, and effectively bring the gifts of yoga to the child/ren in your care. Though the activities shared in this book are steeped in research and tested for efficacy through my own personal experience working with children, I have kept the content of this book practical in hopes of inspiring and empowering you and your children to jump right in.

I hope this guide will prove helpful to you as you begin the joyful journey of sharing yoga with your child. Ultimately, connectedness is what yoga is all about. Let "yoga time" with your child be an opportunity for bonding and connection. Have fun experimenting with the material and feel free to make it your own. I look forward to hearing about your stories and experiences using this book!

PART I

Yoga
with Your
Child

Welcome! In this first part of the book, you will find most of the information you need to get started building your yoga sessions with your child. There is general information on the background and history of the yoga practice; a chapter on the many benefits of yoga for you, your child, and your family; and all of the information you need to set up your practice with your child in your home. You'll learn about "yoga through the ages"—special considerations for each age group, the best place to set up your home yoga practice, the basic materials you need, and fun "props" that are especially useful and engaging for children's yoga. Also provided are ten tips for success, and ideas about when to practice yoga (virtually any time!). You'll learn about the yoga principles (yoga's ethical guidelines) that are applicable to children—and how to incorporate them into your practice, planting the seeds for fruitful discussions that can bring you and your child closer, while inspiring an early introduction to healthy living. Let's begin!

CHAPTER 1

An Introduction to Yoga

WHAT IS YOGA?

Chances are, if you've chosen this book, you already have an inkling about what yoga is about. Perhaps you have a practice of your own, and now wish to bring the joys of yoga to your child. Whether you are a yogi or not, entertaining the question "What is yoga?" is an important precursor to setting up and introducing this wonderful practice to your child. So just what *is* yoga and how does it work?

Yoga is everywhere—in television ads, in gyms, on your Wii Fit—and for good reason. The 5,000-year-old discipline was designed to empower health, happiness, and a greater sense of self. Originating in ancient India, yoga is one of the longest surviving practices of holistic health care in the world. It has been passed down through generations and was first introduced in America in the late 1800s. It is now practiced worldwide by all cultures and religions. Scientific research has confirmed what ancient yogis learned through personal observation thousands of years ago—that yoga is good for the body, mind, and soul.

HOW DOES YOGA WORK?

Translated from Sanskrit, *yoga* means "to yoke" or "to unite." Yoga is a system of connecting the whole self: body, mind, and spirit. The term "spirit" is derived from the Greek word *spirare*, which means "to breathe," so you might also think of the union of the mind, body, and breath (in fact, that is how we describe yoga to children). By practicing yoga postures, bones are brought into alignment and muscles are strengthened, stretched, and relaxed. In turn, blood is oxygenated, helping to tone the nervous system, improve circulation and other bodily functions, promote flexibility, and release tension. Focusing on the breath on its own or while doing yoga-based stretches and balancing postures brings the physical body into balance with the mind. Continued practice supports and develops this connection, counteracting the effects of stress and eventually bringing us to a more centered place—a place where we are "yoked," body, mind, and spirit. As a result, we become more integrated, focused, and relaxed.

The science behind yoga is really fairly simple. When we're frustrated, anxious, angry, sad, etc., our bodies respond by producing stress hormones, specifically adrenaline and cortisol. This causes our heart rate to speed up, our breathing to become shallow, and our neck and back muscles to tighten. Blood gets diverted away from the brain and organs to the large muscles of the body, the "take off and run" ones. Our eye muscles expand to an extent that they literally cannot focus. (Remember the first time you had to stand up in front of the class to do a presentation and couldn't read your note cards?) These instinctive responses to stress are necessary if we're in serious danger and need to fight or flee a situation . . . but most of the time we are not. With no outlet for these built-up hormones, we can become chronically stressed. Chronic stress, of course, is the cause of countless health problems, diseases, and disorders.

To counteract stress, adults might choose to go for a run, have a massage, or call a friend. But what do children do with their stress? Where are their outlets? Today, they have even fewer constructive mechanisms to cope with stress than we do.

The good news is that yoga overrides the stress response, short-circuiting the fight-or-flight hormones. That's true for both adults and children. When we do yoga, we develop mental and physical focus, strength, balance, flexibility, and overall health. When we are focused and balanced, everything else becomes easier—from concentrating and learning, to sleeping, to being less reactive and making better decisions. Yoga facilitates connection. We become more self-aware as we increase our ability to self-regulate. Our abilities to manage our emotions and reactions, to focus and concentrate, and to calm and center ourselves are significantly improved. In this improved state of balance, we are better able to tap into our innate joy, love, and peace—for ourselves, others, and the world as a whole. It is this state of connectedness, from the inside out, that is the essence of yoga.

With children, we may start with yoga poses, breathing exercises, and other mindfulness-building activities to settle the mind, in combination with some discussion and reflection on yoga principles such as honesty, nonviolence, and cleanliness (such as eating nutritious foods). All of these components of a "yoga lifestyle" work synergistically to help children achieve a more peaceful existence in both body and mind.

THE TRUTH ABOUT YOGA—SOME COMMON MYTHS DEBUNKED

Now that yoga is everywhere in Western culture, inevitably, myths have sprung up. You probably have heard a few, and maybe wondered about them yourself. Below you'll find explanations for the most common yoga myths. This should help debunk misinformation, offer a deeper understanding of yoga, and ease any doubts or lingering fears you may have about the practice itself.

Myth #1: Yoga is a religion. I must have Buddhist or Hindu beliefs to practice yoga.

Yoga is a *discipline*, not a religion. You can be a practicing Christian, Jew, Muslim, or adhere to no belief system at all—and still do yoga.

Yoga is a way of life, for adults and children alike. The guidelines to a yogic lifestyle set forth by Pantajali include universal principles providing us with tools for living a life of purity in body and mind (Chapter 3); yoga postures (Chapters 6 and 10) to purify the physical body through structured movement, stretching, strengthening, and balance work; and conscious breath work (Chapter 5) and meditation practices (Chapter 4) to calm the body/mind system. Together, these practices pave the way toward spiritual exploration. So, rather than enforcing a doctrine, yoga gives kids a tool for spiritual exploration. Indeed, yoga nurtures the hearts, minds, and bodies of children (and adults) without violating the individual beliefs of their families, and may even deepen children's connections to their families' beliefs.

Myth #2: You must be a vegetarian or eat all raw foods to be a yogi.

You can eat anything you want and still be a yogi. Be warned, though: Being a practicing yogi, you may eventually gravitate toward vegetarianism, since yoga encourages peaceful living.

Even though you don't need to follow any special diet to practice yoga, healthy eating *is* an important aspect of the yoga lifestyle. In yoga, *sattva* is defined as the quality of purity or goodness. A recommended yoga diet is *sattvic*, made up of whole, fresh foods that are minimally processed. Foods with a high sugar content and caffeinated beverages are considered *rajasic*, or agitating, and shelf-stable foods that are highly processed are considered *tamasic*, or energy-draining.

Within the United States, foods are also sorted into categories, based on their nutritional makeup and value. The USDA categorizes foods into five food groups, and sets guidelines for how much to each from each category. In 2005, the U.S. National Heart, Lung, and Blood Institute created new categories for foods that are even easier for kids to understand: "Go Foods," "Slow Foods," and "Whoa Foods." Log on to *www.nhlbi.nih.gov* to learn more.

Whichever food guidelines your family follows, always remember: "You are what you eat." Food has an enormous effect on the body. What you feed your child will affect his ability to regulate his body and moods, sleep well, stay fit, and learn. While it's not necessary to follow any special eating regimen to practice yoga, eating healthfully is an integral part of *supporting* your child's yoga practice and the many wonderful and beneficial effects that will emerge as you and your child build a practice together.

For more great nutrition and overall health information for kids, visit the website *www.kidshealth.org*.

Eating Mindfully

Being "mindful" means to pay close attention to what we are doing at any given moment. Eating mindfully means paying attention to what we eat and to the process of eating. Mindful eaters sit down, appreciate their food, and eat slowly and deliberately. Thorough chewing ensures food is digested properly and necessary nutrients are delivered effectively throughout the body.

You can encourage your child to be a mindful eater. Help him record everything he eats for one week, thinking about how his choices compare with recommendations in this section. Repeat the process in a month to see if anything has changed. If no improvements are noted, encourage your child to keep trying! Small changes add up to big changes over time. Bring him to the market and read labels together, discuss options, and make better choices together. Sit down with your child during meals, and make dinner a ritual of slow, mindful eating!

Myth #3: You need to be super flexible and in great physical shape to practice yoga.

Anyone can practice yoga. *Asana,* or physical posture, is the focus of just one of the eight limbs of yoga, yet it is probably the most recognized aspect of yoga in our Western culture. Essentially, if you can breathe, you can do yoga. Our individual yoga practices will vary based on our unique physical abilities, and there are acceptable modifications for just about every pose. There is chair yoga, beginner yoga, wheelchair yoga, yoga for the bedridden, yoga for sports injuries, prenatal yoga, and yoga for a variety of special needs and medical conditions. Yoga is for every*body*!

(**Note:** *If your child has a specific medical condition, a doctor should be consulted before involving him in any type of yoga practice.*)

Myth #4: To meditate, you need to chant "Om" for hours in a quiet room.

There are *many* ways to meditate. In fact, the physical yoga practice itself is considered a "moving meditation." Om or no om, if you're practicing yoga, you're meditating on some level.

Meditation refers to a set of practices and techniques designed to bring the mind into a state of stillness. It sounds easy enough, but if you've tried it, you know it is not quite as simple as it sounds. Our minds tend to be quite active and our attention darts here and there. This is especially true for children! The word "meditation" can bring many stereotypical images to mind. You may think of a person sitting in Lotus Pose chanting a mantra, such as "Om" (A-U-M). This is the media's favorite depiction of meditation and why it is the most recognized. In fact, there are several types of meditation practices available to help us train the body and mind and to come into the present moment. Some people sit in silence with their eyes closed, using a mantra or repeated phrase as a point of focus. This can be an effective way to focus and begin to settle their active minds. For others, simply focusing on the breath, a visual image, a phrase, or a concept works well. Even mindful walking, running, swimming, and other physical activities can serve as forms of meditation. Your personality type may be drawn to different types of meditation practices. No one approach is superior to another. In fact, focusing on just about anything can help quiet and clear the mind.

With that said, most child-friendly meditation practices are in fact practices in mindful awareness. Children can "meditate," but the word has a different meaning for them than it does for adults. In fact, with children we primarily focus on helping them and bring their awareness inward (*pratyhara*), a precursor to meditation on the eight-limbed path of classical yoga. Since young children are sensing their environment rather than projecting out onto it, it's most important for *parents* to be practicing meditation, modeling, and carrying that energy into the home for children to see and sense.

Now that we've explored the basics of yoga and the most common myths associated with it, you should have a solid understanding of the practice itself. In the next chapter, we'll explore the many benefits associated with the practice— and how they apply to your child and to your family. Truly, bringing yoga into your home is one of the best gifts you can give to yourself and your child!

CHAPTER 2

Benefits of Yoga for Children and Families

STRENGTHEN YOUR CHILD'S BODY, MIND, AND SPIRIT

Your child might feel overwhelmed on a daily basis. Many children today are suffering from a lack of connection to their bodies, to their environment, and to themselves. Our information-saturated, hectic, and stimulus-rich culture pulls kids in many directions, splitting their attention. For many children, it has become too much for their young, developing minds to absorb and process.

More and more American children from all walks of life are overweight, have stress and anger issues, and have attention and learning problems. There is a real separation of mind and body—your child's attention might be pulled outward toward the ever-increasing distractions of the external world. Overworked parents and overscheduled children often face isolation from their families and their communities. Rather than sitting down to dinner together, it is now quite common for children and parents to communicate mainly via text messaging and e-mail. Does any of this sound familiar?

As mindful parents and adults, we must give our children every tool possible to assist them in counteracting a culture and environment that is potentially hazardous to their health and well-being. Through the use of yoga tools, stories, and play, we can provide children with opportunities to grow physically, mentally, emotionally, and spiritually, helping them connect with themselves and others with compassion, understanding, and clarity.

Healthy Bodies

In 2012, the CDC reported that childhood obesity had more than tripled in the past thirty years. Children are simply spending more time indoors and less time moving. Even if your child is active, she can still benefit from yoga-based movement. With regular practice, her muscles, bones, and joints will lengthen and strengthen as her overall flexibility is improved. In addition, all of your child's major bodily systems are supported by movement and improved circulation, including the digestive, endocrine, immune, and respiratory systems. Yoga strengthens your child's *entire* body!

Here are some recognized benefits that yoga can provide for your child's body:

- Assists neuromuscular development
- Promotes development of the vestibular system
- Increases circulation, uptake of oxygen, and functioning of hormones
- Encourages motor development on both sides of the body
- Increases balance, coordination, and overall body awareness
- Develops core strength, essential for posture and alignment
- Reduces the risk of injury; improves performance in sports
- Improves digestion and elimination
- Strengthens the immune system
- Helps manage chronic illness
- Relaxes the body, promoting better sleep
- Improves brainpower

Research suggests that when behaviors are sustained over time, they become part of the brain's permanent neurological wiring. This is called *neuroplasticity*— meaning that the brain is malleable, or capable of change. Each time your child performs a new action, the neurons in her brain form new connections to help her learn and remember that action. With consistency, these actions and thought patterns become habits. As previously stated, "you are what you eat"— neuroplasticity means "you are what you do." Consistently repeating positive behaviors, movements, and thought patterns with your child can literally help rewire the way our bodies and brains behave, ultimately leading to positive life habits. What a gift for your child!

When you practice yoga with your child, you'll help create a strong, healthy mind. Studies show that yoga:

- Calms and clears the mind
- Brings your child into the present moment
- Relieves tension and stress
- Increases concentration, focus, and attention span
- Promotes thinking and boosts memory
- Stimulates auditory processing and responsiveness
- Expands imagination and creativity
- Improves ability to be less reactive, more mindful of thoughts, speech, and action
- Reduces stress and anxiety
- Balances low/high energy levels

- Improves attention and emotional control
- Positively influences neurotransmitter function *(G)*

Exercise for the Spirit

A 2010 report published in the *Journal of Happiness Studies* showed that children aged eight to twelve who were more spiritual were also happier. Spirituality in this case was defined not by a child's religious practices, such as attending church, but by a child's ability to find meaning and value in his life, and engage in deep interpersonal relationships. Your child's spirit connects him with others and is essential to a healthy, well-adjusted child. Yoga practices will help foster your child's spiritual growth by helping him see the beauty and light within himself, boosting confidence, and allowing him to feel more comfortable in his body. Yoga will help him get in touch with who he is inside, and in turn will help your child connect with himself, others, and the world in a richer, more positive, and peaceful way.

By establishing a yoga routine, your child will gain many of the recognized benefits of yoga for a child's spirit. He'll build confidence and self-esteem, support character development and emotional intelligence, and enhance team skills and social interaction. Yoga helps develop self-control, supports individuality and self-expression, and encourages a sense of civic obligation. With regular practice, your child will gain a sense of connectedness, inspiring respect for himself and others.

Nourish Your Child's Spirituality

Yoga research is now shifting to include perspectives on young children. In a 2008 study, Patricia Jennings, PhD, of Penn State University found that contemplative practices such as yoga begun in early childhood "may support children's quest for meaning and promote positive experiences of wonder and awe that motivate learning." Jennings also explains that contemplative knowing—often fostered through yoga—connects children to others, to shared human values, and to life's meaning.

Building Solid Life Values

Yoga helps foster important life values in children. By developing a consistent practice with your child, you will help your child cultivate discipline, self-control, patience, gratitude, respect, and contentment, among other positive qualities and life skills. The yoga principles (Chapter 3) that you promote in and out of yoga sessions with your child will be increasingly adopted the more you practice together. Donna Freeman, in her 2010 book, *Once Upon a Pose: A Guide to Yoga Adventure Stories for Children,* writes: "Teaching children these ethics helps them learn respect for themselves and others, as well as an appreciation for the world in which they live." Don't be surprised if after a few weeks, you notice your child cleaning up his room, actively taking part in chores without being told to, and generally being more respectful and aware of the people, belongings, and environment surrounding him—these are the yoga principles at work!

IMPROVING SCHOOL LIFE

Anti-bullying, health and wellness, and character education are all popular topics in American education today. As standardized testing has become more common, so has performance anxiety and stress in students (and teachers). It is not surprising to note that across the world, yoga and mindfulness education are increasingly being incorporated into the classroom day to help address these concerns, and with great results.

Yoga, by nature, supports and maximizes the learning process. Students experience improved concentration and creative thinking, and due to improvement in executive functions, they are better able to prioritize and organize. By doing yoga with your child, you will help him build better relationships with other students by promoting a sense of connectedness. If your child is athletic, a yoga lifestyle will help him maximize his performance by improving his focus, strengthening his muscles, improving his flexibility, and fostering team cooperation. If your child experiences social anxiety, yoga can help instill a greater sense of self-knowing, self-worth, and confidence.

Here's how yoga can benefit your child's life at school. Yoga:

- Brings students into the present moment, ready for learning
- Encourages community and connectedness in the classroom
- Helps create a feeling of confidence instead of competitiveness
- Eases anxiety before test taking
- Enhances focus, concentration, comprehension, and memory
- Supports social and emotional learning
- Wakes up sluggish minds and promotes creativity
- Enhances organizational and communication skills
- Improves posture, assisting with breathing, writing, and sitting for long periods
- Enhances team skills and social interaction
- Promotes the development of executive function skills

Movement and Learning

Yoga facilitates all kinds of movement, including cross-lateral movement, which is crucial for learning. Cross-lateral movements are those in which arms and legs cross over the midline of the body. The left side of the brain controls the right side of the body, and the right side of the brain controls the left side. When arms and legs cross the body's midline, both sides are forced to communicate. This integration of both sides of the brain enhances learning.

YOGA FOR SPEECH DEVELOPMENT

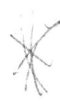

While yoga is becoming wildly popular with kids everywhere, one significant benefit often overlooked by parents and educators is the aspect of speech development. "Yoga," "yogurt," or "woga" classes can help advance a young child's speech development through slow, repetitive verbal instructions, songs, and the imitation of simple sounds found in nature.

Children with speech delays are often more physical in nature, especially boys. A movement class like yoga can pair physical motion with repetitive sounds, which will likely catch their attention more so than a simple, quiet conversation. For example, a preschooler who has not yet mastered sounding out letters like S and Z might enjoy slithering like a snake, not only attempting to "hiss" but also watching your mouth as you hiss and lower yourself to the ground in Cobra Pose. After repeating this pose in subsequent sessions, he will immediately recognize the word and sound that go along with the pose, and hopefully gain the confidence to try to say it himself.

Fun with Pose Practice!

Here's an idea for supporting your child's speech development. According to Heather Warr, SLP, "Poses that start with the same sound are excellent for speech development. The child can hear the beginning sound of a pose and group them as such. For example, boat, butterfly, and bee all start with B! The child can practice this sound as he is doing the pose." To maximize your child's speech development, develop a sequence of poses that begin with the same letter, and have your child say the name of the pose before he does each pose.

group "B" "S" "G" sounds in poses

Children who need extra support in learning speech patterns benefit from slow, exaggerated, repetitive speech demonstration. To an adult, this type of instruction may seem silly, but if you think about popular children's characters like Barney, Elmo, and Dora the Explorer, you'll note that these characters speak this way to their audience and, not surprisingly, kids respond favorably.

Heather Warr, a kids' yoga instructor and twenty-year pediatric speech pathologist, says breathing is key, because we speak on the exhale. "If a child doesn't have enough breath support, he'll not have enough air to formulate speech sounds, which require sustained airflow like /s/, /z/, and /th/," says Warr. "We work on correct postures for maximum rib expansion for volume and length of expression."

STRONG CHILDREN, STRONG FAMILIES

Sharing yoga as a family is not only fun but also has the power to strengthen the family unit. A strong family breeds well-adjusted children who are positively connected to those who love them and are empowered to reflect that love out into the world.

Understandably, it can be difficult to find downtime in a hectic family schedule. Fortunately, the practice of yoga is adaptable. You don't have a full half hour to dedicate to "yoga time"? Try taking a few deep breaths together in the car on the way to the play audition, practicing a couple of simple stretching poses paired with a calming breath before heading out onto the soccer field, letting off steam together with a Lion's Breath, or sharing a visual imagery exercise before bed. Adapting yoga sessions for your family—even 1 to 5 minutes here and there throughout the day—can be beneficial. These yoga breaks provide wonderful opportunities to connect as a family while providing your children an opportunity to experience how yoga can be used as a helpful tool any time!

Your family can benefit from "connecting moments" in yoga, moments found in partner poses, games, family activities and projects, family performances, or a quiet discussion of a yoga principle or following a visualization exercise. In these moments, you'll learn more about one another, build trust, engage in teamwork, and deepen bonds. Family communication and interaction becomes fun yet meaningful, enhancing connectedness between yourself and your children, and the family as a whole.

The weeks after a new school year begins, the holidays, the days leading up to an important test or a sports competition, or a traumatic family event are all examples of times when you and your child may experience increased anxiety, stress, and pressure. Taking a few minutes to practice yoga together will give you a safe "respite from the storm," remind you of what is most important, and teach skills to manage uncomfortable feelings. Practicing these skills will support your family members throughout their lives.

The following sections highlight just how yoga practice can benefit your family.

Promote Positive Communication

The kind of positive, playful communication and interactions found in yoga, when practiced together as a family, set the stage for improving intimacy, leading to more rewarding family relationships. Through partner poses, you will experience positive touch. Breathing together will connect you energetically. Encouraging one another when attempting new yoga postures provides a sense of appreciation and community. Through the discussion of the yoga principles, you'll be finding common ground and new language by which to communicate. With this newfound set of verbal and nonverbal communication skills, you'll find a new level of connection that ultimately supports the overall family system.

Promote Respect

Yoga is a practice in self-regulation. Through a regular yoga practice, your family will benefit from learning to pause, reflect, and think before acting or speaking. During times when tempers are hot and the potential for hurtful comments is high, having the language of yoga at your fingertips will offer your family an opportunity to pause together, choose and practice an appropriate calming yoga breath or activity, and then reconvene from a more peaceful, positive place. Armed with the knowledge of the yoga principles (Chapter 3), your family can learn to act respectfully both in and out of the home.

Reduce Family Stress

It's important to remember that for the most part, stress is a state of mind, and we can choose to be stressed or not. Families who learn and practice this concept together find their stress level decreases. No, many times we can't remove stressors from our family life. What we *can* do is learn to be less reactive to them, and we can teach that important skill to our children as well. Ultimately, being okay with the way things are is the goal of yoga (Chapter 3). Modeling nonreactivity is a powerful way to share this concept with your children. Alert your kids when you are feeling overwhelmed. "I'm looking around at a messy house, you would like my help with homework, and I still haven't made dinner. I'm feeling overwhelmed . . . will you sit and breathe with me?" This approach not only provides you with a moment to calm and regroup, but it also models positive coping skills for your child while giving you an opportunity to connect. Your children may enjoy reminding you when you need to "Count Down to Calm" (Chapter 5)—and you should let them! It can be fun to feign not remembering how to do it and to ask for their assistance in leading in the breath. They will feel valued and helpful, and everyone benefits.

During especially stressful moments, try calling your family to a "yoga rescue." Create a quiet corner of one room dedicated to yoga and other peaceful activities. Gather your family there, and have all members share their current feelings and thoughts. Based on what those are, choose a relevant, simple breath and yoga sequence to practice together. When finished, again share your current feelings and thoughts, noting any changes experienced in your minds and bodies. Have a family hug and move on with the day with a greater sense of peace and connectedness.

Promote Better Family Bonds

A family that spends time together is a well-bonded family. Having said that, practicing yoga with your child will give you an opportunity to bond in a way that is very different than making dinner together or playing ball. Yoga time is playful yet focused. It's a time to give your children your undivided attention, something hard to come by today. It opens the door to deep discussions about feelings—about fears, concerns, current challenges, and what brings us joy. It provides families with a unique language of wellness and a toolbox for living, improving bonds, and communication.

Provide a Source of Joy and Peace

Let's face it—families can get so busy; it's often all work and no play. Family yoga provides an opportunity to have fun as a family. You'll have plenty of opportunities for laughs moving your bodies into poses. Yoga is about finding joy in the body, and sharing this understanding with your child will add to the experience.

Though you are focusing on bringing yoga to your child, family yoga will bring you many gifts as well. The sense of play that naturally arises when you do yoga with your loved ones will inevitably have you reconnecting with your own "inner child," perhaps brining a new awareness and discovery of your true, authentic self!

Doing yoga at home as a family also encourages a greater sense of peace. As you create a quiet space together during mindful, focusing activities, and at the end of your practice during relaxation, you'll generate a sense of calm and peace in your hearts and home. Bedtimes will go much more smoothly after a yoga session!

Inspire Play!

Do you play as much as you work? Is play a part of your self-care regimen? According to the National Institute for Play, play is the gateway to vitality. Playfulness is a big contributor to overall wellness and happiness, for adults and children alike. Family yoga is an opportunity to bring beneficial play into your family life at home.

If you're a serious yoga practitioner, you can let that go at home. Doing yoga as a family automatically gives you permission to take it less seriously and have more fun. In a studio, you might focus on perfect alignment, being quiet, and listening to the instructor's every word. At home, while practicing with your family, you'll rediscover the joy in the experience as you laugh together trying a pose, falling, and getting back up again. You'll "ribbit" in Frog Pose, listen like a rabbit, wag your tail like a dog, and breathe into your balloon belly along with your child. How can that be anything but joyful? The joy experienced in your yoga sessions together will soon begin to permeate your home.

CHAPTER 3

Sharing Yoga with Children: What to Know

THE BASICS

In this chapter you will find the basics to get you started sharing yoga with your child at home. Here you'll discover the special challenges presented through the age ranges, ways to create yoga sessions tailored to your child's age and maturity level, and what you need to know about creating the setting for sessions. You'll also find information on materials needed, ideas of when to share yoga with your child, and ten tips for success. And finally, one of the most important components of your yoga practice—the Yoga Principles—is included here as well. These are essential guidelines upon which the practice of yoga is based, the wisdom that "exercises" your child's spirituality as the *asanas* exercise your child's body through poses. Lets get started!

YOGA FOR YOUR CHILD'S AGE

The yoga time you create for and with your child will provide a special and safe place for the two of you, encouraging compassion and connectedness. It might also be one of the few opportunities the two of you have to be together in such a mutually beneficial way. Having said that, it's important to understand your child in order to present the yoga concepts and activities in this book in both a chronologically and a developmentally appropriate manner.

You are likely quite attuned to your child's unique personality, needs, abilities, and learning style. Remember to take this into consideration with your expectations when sharing yoga with your child. Some children learn by doing, trying out all the poses as soon as they are presented, happily following along with each activity as it is introduced. Other children will sit back and just observe, some even seeming downright disinterested. Don't despair! These children may be the visual and/or auditory learners who will later demonstrate what they learned after time for processing, perhaps while playing around the house.

Following are typical characteristics of the various age ranges of children and related tips for keeping them engaged in the learning process. You are invited to keep these in mind as you begin sharing yoga with your child. Note that you may find some crossover in the age grouping information, so it's best to read through the entire section. Depending on your child's maturity level, she may fit into a higher or lower age group, or more than one group.

2- to 4-Year-Olds

Your 2- to 4-year-old may . . .

- Be highly inquisitive and curious
- Have a short attention span
- Respond best to simple, encouraging instruction

As you know, your 2- to 4-year-old is curious about everything! Children this age love to explore, move, roam, and ask lots of questions. Because of this, you may be skeptical about teaching yoga to your child/ren at this age. "But how will I get my child to sit still and listen?" you wonder. In general, yoga sessions with this age group look less like adult yoga and are more playful and active. Keeping some basic tips in mind will ensure success.

- **This age group learns best with lots of structure, repetition, and consistency.** Don't be afraid to repeat games, poses, and songs several times during a given session, and again at later sessions. Use the same basic sequencing, establishing a ritual beginning, middle, and end activity that you share together each time.
- **Plan to keep yoga sessions between 5 and 20 minutes.** Two- to 4-year-olds have a limited attention span. Move fairly quickly from one activity to the next and end on a positive note when your child cues you that she's had enough. Be sure to utilize the additional ideas provided with each activity for extra fun and engagement.
- **Use the simple songs referenced with some of the poses.** One- to two-verse songs, repeated several times, will not only engage your child but will also help her learn. Be playful, using an expressive voice, animated facial

expressions, and body movements to draw your child's attention. After all, if you are interested in and excited about what you are sharing, your child will automatically want to know more about it!

- **Use simple instructions.** It is important to guide your 2- to 4-year-old using simple language and as few words as possible. Instead of saying, "Take a big step back with your left leg. Keep your right knee aligned over your right ankle, weight evenly distributed between your feet," you might try, "Watch Mommy take a *great big* step back . . . now, you try! That's it, Jocelyn." It doesn't matter so much that she does it exactly right.

- **Be sure to recognize your child's accomplishments.** Children in this age group want to succeed and impress! Rather than using general praise such as "Good job," try to be specific using simple, encouraging words that also include the name of the pose or specific activity. Comments such as "You're doing Down Dog, Sarah!" or "Jack's in Tree Pose!" are incredibly effective, building self-esteem while helping your child associate his efforts with the particular activity.

- **Be prepared to adapt the session to your child's needs.** Of course, 2- to 4-year-olds are notorious for wanting to do what they want to do when they want to do it, a sign of their developing independence. Though you may have a specific plan for your yoga time with your child, it may just serve as a guideline in the end. Be prepared to change your agenda at a moment's notice, following the needs and interests of your child. This will become easier over time as you both become more familiar with the activities in this book.

4- to 6-Year-Olds

Your 4- to 6-year-old probably . . .

Has a strong desire to learn new things

Loves to pretend play, tell stories, and use his imagination

Is just developing a conscience

Four- to 6-year-olds are very eager to learn new things! The imagination that started developing in your child's toddler years now really begins to expand. Pretend play, including "being" animals, objects, etc., is especially appealing to your child in this age group and developmentally beneficial as well. Four- to 6-year-olds love to talk, tell stories, and ask lots of questions. You'll want to give your child lots of opportunity to do so during your yoga sessions.

- **Plan to keep sessions between 15 and 30 minutes.** In this age group, children's attention spans are improving, so a yoga session of 15–30 minutes is reasonable. As with the 2- to 4-year-olds, be sure to utilize the additional ideas provided with each activity to keep your child in this age group interested, engaged, and having fun.
- **Incorporate themes and stories.** Four- to 6-year-olds become especially engaged when stories and themes are incorporated into their yoga sessions. Themes can be based on any interesting, child-friendly subject. Some theme category ideas include places, animal groups, learning themes such as opposites, things that grow or things that fly, feel-good themes such as happy poses, seasons or occasions, hobbies or interests, and of course, stories and adventures! You can make up your own stories or use a picture book as a guide. Books with animal adventures work best. Inspiring your child's imagination and creativity is easy with yoga!
- **Use props.** Four- to 6-year-olds enjoy props, so you will want to create a stash of props to have on hand that you know your child will enjoy. As with the younger children, refrain from making your yoga session focused on the props and rather bring them out as needed to regain attention or just for fun while expanding upon a pose or activity. A good rule to follow: Only use one major prop per yoga session.
- **Allow your time together to be playful.** Yes, yoga is a contemplative practice, but with children under 7 or 8 years old, it's important to engage all of their senses through the process, eventually coming to a quieter, more reflective place during breathing exercises, centering, and relaxation activities. Remember, yoga for children is fun!
- **Begin to slowly incorporate the Yoga Principles.** Four- to 6-year-olds are beginning to develop a conscience, so very basic, simple discussions of the Yoga Principles are now appropriate. It's best to introduce just one at a time—even focusing on one over many sessions—so that your child is not overwhelmed.

7- to 10-Year-Olds

Your 7- to 10-year-old is . . .

Developing opinions

Looking to "lead"

Seeking approval from adults and friends

With this age group, things begin to look a little bit more like adult yoga. You can sustain your child's attention for a longer period of time, and he is ready for deeper introduction to the Yoga Principles and visualization and relaxation techniques. With your 7- to 10-year-old, you can begin to explore and set up the basic building blocks of a typical formal yoga class. But don't let them fool you—7- to 10-year-olds are still interested in being playful and having fun, so you will want to make sure to incorporate lots of yoga games and songs to encourage playfulness and keep them engaged in the learning process.

- **Sessions can now range between 20 and 40 minutes long.** Your child's attention span is growing, so you can plan for longer activities, or more activities in a session, and spend more time on each activity, delving deeper with the learning process.
- **Begin to focus on proper alignment.** With your 7- to 10-year-old, you can begin focusing a bit more on proper alignment in yoga postures, while also attempting more challenging postures. Begin to introduce flowing sequences, and incorporate more partner work. You can also more deeply explore breathing exercises and relaxation techniques—all of the features of a typical yoga class in a studio.
- **Fully explore the Yoga Principles.** As you probably know, your 7- to 10-year-old loves a good discussion and he is developing a sense of morality and opinions of his own ("That's not fair!"). This is the perfect age to delve into deep discussions on the Yoga Principles. You may choose to emphasize those Yoga Principles that focus on feelings of acceptance, empathy, and civic concerns. As most children this age are working to improve their reading and writing skills, you might use a whiteboard, chalkboard, or shared journal onto which the two of you can write your thoughts as you discuss a given principle.
- **Allow your child more opportunities to lead.** Kids in this age group are also beginning to seek more independence. They may not be as open to being

"instructed" as they were when they were younger. However, they still seek adult guidance and assurance. Allow your child opportunities to take the lead on choosing what to focus on in a yoga session. Ask him, "How are you feeling today? In your body? In your mind? What do you want to focus on?" Suddenly, the yoga session is "his." Before you know it, he'll be teaching *you* a thing or two. Honor him and watch the respect and connection between you grow.

- **Explore the visualization techniques during relaxation.** Seven- to 10-year-olds especially enjoy the use of visual imagery and stories. Now that they have a longer attention span, you can really explore the relaxation and visualization techniques in Chapter 9. The use of creative imagery and stories helps relax children, while also improving their creativity. Try to tie in the theme or Yoga Principle discussed into the story or visualization to help bring it to life.

Preteens (10–12 years)

Your preteen may . . .

Have a strong need to fit in and be respected

Express pessimism

Be modest, embarrassed about physical changes

Be experiencing hormonal changes, mood swings, and interest in the opposite sex

Be experiencing increasing pressures and stress

By this age, children are ready for a full yoga session. You have your child's attention, and can incorporate all of the foundations of yoga found in this book. With your preteen you will find that the Yoga Principles will become a key part of your yoga sessions, offering a chance to open discussion and connect deeper with your preteen as he faces the challenges unique to this age.

- **Plan to spend 20 minutes to up to an hour practicing yoga with your older preteen or teen.** At this age, you can easily fill an hour with poses and plenty of discussion. Keep a steady pace and add variety to your sessions—lots of poses, discussion, partner work, and relaxation activities.
- **Encourage proper alignment.** Children at this age are just starting to grow in their bodies and therefore can exhibit clumsiness. If you are a yoga teacher

or avid yoga practitioner, don't be afraid to model proper alignment and encouragingly suggest adjustments to help your child gain more confidence in the postures. Otherwise, learn and experiment together, following the photos and descriptions as your guide, and then move on to the Internet for extra assistance.

- **Take into account developmental changes.** Hormonal changes in preteens can cause unpredictable moods, weepiness, increased sensitivity, negative thinking, as well as an interest in the opposite sex. In addition, your preteen may be starting to challenge your authority and rules, testing boundaries as she experiments with her growing independence. Preteens can also be self-centered. This is all normal and is mostly due to the many changes occurring in the brain during puberty and beyond. Be patient and note that these changes are, to a large extent, out of her control.

- **Strive for positive discussions based on the Yoga Principles.** The Yoga Principles can provide a framework for thinking about and processing the many pressures your child faces at this age. Start to observe your child and listen carefully to what she says about her day or experiences as you seek opportunities to open discussion and learn together.

- **Create a safe, judgment-free space.** As with all ages, it is essential to create a safe, judgment-free zone for your preteen. Offer general words of encouragement throughout your yoga session and/or during relaxation. As your child rests with her eyes closed while listening to soft, soothing music, encourage her to be with her feelings, letting them well up from her heart and dissipate out into the safe, compassionate space that surrounds her. This means tears are okay. It's healthy to feel our feelings! Providing an opportunity for children to release their emotions without judgment or the need to "fix" or "control" is a tremendous gift from a parent to a child.

- **Remember that preteens like to have fun!** After all, yoga is a time to connect and bond, and preteens can sometimes be overly serious and moody. Partner poses are a great way to lighten the mood and be playful!

- **Invite your preteen to set up an "altar."** Invite your child to set up an altar of items that are important to her or for which she is grateful either in or near the yoga space, or perhaps in her room. She might also like to put up pictures of positive role models such as celebrities or athletes doing yoga—this will help gain her "buy-in" to the practice and may appeal to her need to fit in.

- **Invite friends.** Is your child most interested in hanging out with her friends? Invite them to join you! Get a group of preteens doing yoga together at your house and you just might become the coolest parent around.

The Preteen Brain on Yoga

Beginning in the preadolescent years, the development of the frontal lobes of the brain responsible for language lags behind the amygdala, the part of the brain responsible for emotions. It's no wonder that preteens and teens have a reputation for being emotional and unreasonable at times! Interestingly, researchers are now showing that when children in this age group are able to hone skills that foster self-awareness, self-regulation, empathy, and interpersonal relationships, they are happier and healthier emotionally and academically. The practice of yoga and mindfulness helps preteens and teens develop these essential skills.

CREATING THE YOGA SPACE

Establishing a special place in your home where you and your child can share yoga time will only enhance the experience. The best yoga space in your home will be one that is relatively quiet and distraction free, has nice light, a safe, solid floor, an open wall, and room for a couple of yoga mats, a storage bin or organizer for props, and a music player. Optionally, you can add a place for an altar or other designated area where you and your child can place meaningful photos and objects. But remember—you can practice yoga anywhere with your child, so don't feel restricted when thinking of where to practice. You can even go outside, in your backyard, or if you don't have a backyard, to a nearby park. Here are a few things to keep in mind when thinking about where you practice:

- **Choose a space with safe, comfortable flooring.** The best flooring for yoga is flooring that has clean, smooth wood with no nails, splinters, or wide grooves, or one that has very low-pile, industrial-type carpet. The floor should be comfortable under bare feet and bodies.

- **Choose an area with natural light.** Whenever possible, the best lighting for yoga is natural light. If it's an option, choose a space with windows.
- **Choose a room that is neither too warm nor too cold.** Ideally, your yoga space should be set at a comfortable temperature, warm enough to keep everyone comfortable—warm and limber—but not so hot that your child (or you!) become cranky and lethargic. A temperature between 65–78 degrees Fahrenheit is usually sufficient.
- **Fresh air is important.** The smell and feel of fresh air cleanses the senses and is especially grounding, so you might try opening windows when the weather allows. Having living plants in the space will give it a healthy, living energy and an ongoing fresh supply of oxygen. Be sure to clean the space regularly with natural cleaning solution to prevent the accumulation of debris, bugs, and germs that can all contribute to stale air and the spread of viruses.
- **Have a clock handy.** It is helpful to have a watch or a clock with a second hand nearby. A clock can be helpful for timing various activities, such as Silent Seconds, or when you are challenging your child to hold a pose for a certain length of time.
- **Ensure a clear space.** The less distraction in the room, the more focused your child will be on the yoga practice. A general rule of thumb: the younger the child, the less stuff should be in eyesight.
- **Finally, make sure the space is quiet.** It is important, particularly for children with special needs such as ADD, ADHD, autism, Asperger's syndrome, or Sensory Integration Disorder, that you choose a quiet room/space in the house for regular yoga sessions. This will limit input and distraction and set the tone for a peaceful session.

THE MATERIALS

What will you need to practice yoga at home with your child? You don't need much—simply a mat (in some cases, not even that) and maybe a few items found around the home. Since they have special significance to your child, your child's toys can be used as props, an easy way to add comfort and familiarity to your child's practice. To save money, you can even make your own props. Get creative!

- **Yoga Mats.** In my group classes with children under 4, I prefer not to use yoga mats as they have proven to be a tripping hazard. As well, they turn into playthings, a potential distraction. Having said that, with a one-on-one yoga session where there will not be too much movement on and off a mat, and certainly with older children, I find yoga mats to provide a helpful "home base."

Yoga mats can be an actual sticky mat (preferred on a wood floor), a beach towel, or even a blanket. As children get older and yoga postures become more challenging, the ability of a sticky yoga mat to prevent slipping becomes increasingly important.

Keeping an all-natural spray cleaner and paper towels on hand makes it easy to keep mats clean. Involve your child in the process of keeping the mats clean by making a ritual of cleaning them before putting them away after each yoga session. This is a wonderful example of the practice of discipline or *tapas* (see The Yoga Principles in this chapter).

Yoga mats are available at all major retail stores and can be found for less than $10 at discount chain stores such as Five Below and Big Lots.

- **Heavy Cotton Blankets.** The warmth and weight of a classic Indian blanket (or other heavy cotton blanket) is quite comforting and grounding during the relaxation portion of a session. Have one blanket for each family member neatly stacked up and ready for use during relaxation.

- **Eye Pillows.** Lavender-scented eye pillows are wonderfully relaxing and they can also help weight the eyes and block out the light during the relaxation portion of your yoga sessions. Try making your own (see sidebar).

No-Sew Eye Pillows

You will need a bag of white rice, a few drops of lavender essential oil, and a recycled pair of cotton tights or a sock (think hole-toed or mismatched tights and socks), some rubber bands, and some pretty ribbon. Make tubes of approximately 10 inches by cutting off both ends of the socks or tights. Seal off one end of the tube using one of the rubber bands, leaving about 1½ inches of fabric off the end of the elastic. Mix 1½ cups of the rice with several drops of lavender essential oil. Pour the lavender rice mixture into the tube. Seal off the other end with another rubber band. Now, tie on pretty ribbons to hide the rubber bands.

- **Yoga Blocks or Similar.** Traditional yoga blocks have many creative uses, such as "stepping stones" in yoga games or balancing rocks. Of course, they can also be used to help with support of yoga postures. Find them anywhere that sells mats, blankets, and eye pillows. If you have some hardcover books of varying widths, these can be used in place of blocks.

THE BASIC PROPS

In addition to the basic materials for yoga, here are some basic props that are well suited to a child's yoga practice.

- **Yoga Wand, Chime, or Other Attention Gatherer.** To gain your child's attention or to begin and/or end a yoga session or specific activity, try using a chime or yoga wand. They have many uses referred to throughout this book. Any object with a peaceful bell or chime sound will do. You can even make your own (see sidebar).

Make Your Own Yoga Wand

Purchase a wand-length wooden dowel and a handful of small bells from an art supply store. Find a girl's hair elastic with ribbons and sparkles at any department or drugstore. Elasticize it around the end of the dowel. Use additional pieces of ribbon to string a few bells, and add the bell ribbons to the end of the dowel by tying them into the elastic. Use the yoga wand as a talking stick, to gather attention, or to sprinkle magic yoga dust on your resting child during relaxation.

- **Scarves.** Pretend to be wind or ocean waves. Support a yoga pose. Provide a visual for a breathing exercise. Enhance focus skills through juggling. There are endless ways to use scarves in a yoga session. Raid your closet or attic (and your mother's), yard sales, and recycled clothing stores such as Goodwill to find flowy silk scarves of varying sizes.
- Digital Camera. Taking photos to instantly show your child what he is accomplishing is empowering and fun! Photos allow children to see themselves

succeed in a pose, enhance awareness of their bodies and posture, and effectively engage visual learners. Seeing a photo of himself doing a posture can be inspiring and help build his confidence: "Oh, I can do that!"

- **Pose Cards.** There are many varieties of card decks that can prove very useful when sharing yoga with children. A kid-friendly yoga deck such as *Yoga Pretzels* or the *Yoga 4 Classrooms*® cards can be used as inspiring visuals. Affirmation card decks such as *Power Thoughts for Teens* or *Manifest Your Magnificence* (for younger children) can serve to create a theme, the basis for discussion or journaling, or can be used just for fun. For younger children, a deck of animal cards can be used to help make the connection between a specific animal and a yoga pose being taught. Don't be afraid to try making your own (see sidebar).

How to Make Your Own Pose Cards

Purchase 8.5" × 11" pieces of colored cardstock. Turn the paper horizontally and clearly print the name (child-friendly version) of a pose at the bottom. On the left side, draw or paste an image of the relevant object or animal. On the right side, draw or paste an image of a person in that pose.

- **Beanie Buddies.** Small bean bag–type stuffed animals are popular toys that can be effectively used as engaging props for yoga sessions. The weight and size of the buddies, along with the fact that they shape to whatever surface they are on, make them ideal for use in a variety of yoga games, balance challenges, and breathing activities, as well as during relaxation. Search your attic and yard sales.
- **Die-Cut Letters.** Die-cuts can be used in many different ways with various age groups, from helping children learn letters and sounds to using them in games such as Alphabet Soup (Chapter 7).
- **Balls.** An all-time favorite prop is the classic, plastic beach ball. Use beach-type balls to play Gratitude Ball (Chapter 7). Use Pilates or larger yoga balls

creatively as needed for balancing postures, core-strengthening exercises, and the Ball Smoosh (Chapter 9, Relaxation and Visualization).

- **Magic Mist.** Magic Mist is created by simply mixing water and a few drops of lavender essential oil in a small misting/spray bottle. Spraying the Magic Mist around the room, or high over the head of your child as he rests with eyes closed, produces an almost immediate calming effect. The use of Magic Mist can be incorporated into stories as jungle mist, ocean spray, or a rain shower. It can also be integrated into centering and relaxation activities.
- **Gratitude Rocks.** Gratitude Rocks are small stones, rocks, or smooth glass stones that can be used to store gratitude to refer back to later on. These can be purchased inexpensively by the bag at craft stores or discount stores. See Gratitude Relaxation in Chapter 9 for suggested use.
- **Other Props.** There are many other props you can use in your yoga sessions with your child. Be creative! Think about what your child enjoys. For inspiration, here are just a few items you could use:
  - ··· Musical instruments
  - ··· Animal figurines
  - ··· Yoga straps (old neckties work great, too!)
  - ··· Wooden dowels
  - ··· Yoga pose figurines
  - ··· Glow sticks (for glow-in-the-dark yoga!)
  - ··· Hula hoops
  - ··· Hoberman Sphere®
  - ··· Journals

WHEN TO SHARE YOGA WITH YOUR CHILD

Though having a special yoga space and time each day to share yoga with your child is a wonderful goal, the reality is that yoga can be shared anywhere at any time. You can practice yoga:

- In the morning before breakfast
- When your child is tired or drained
- While in the car
- Any time your child needs to calm excess energy
- As a fun activity to share when your child has friends over

- When your child needs a confidence boost
- When you child needs to dispel negativity
- While waiting in line
- Any time when focus and attention begin to diminish
- When your child is feeling anxious or stressed
- To stretch the body before athletics or as a break from long car rides
- To celebrate/just for fun
- As a family time activity
- Before doing homework or as a homework break
- As a transition to nap or bedtime

As you and your child become more familiar with the activities in this book, you'll learn to notice your needs, and those of your child, at different times and places during the day, and you'll begin to apply the relevant activities at those times. For example, you might notice your child becomes quite anxious in new situations. You've noticed in your yoga sessions that she enjoys and has noted that she feels calm after practicing Balloon Breath. What might you do together in the car before you drop her off at a birthday party? You got it! See Chapter 10 for more ideas on sharing short or long sequences during particular situations or times of day.

TEN TIPS FOR SUCCESS

Here are ten suggestions to help ensure sharing yoga with your child is a success.

- **Center yourself.** It is crucial to have your own practice, whether it be a walking meditation, consistent yoga class, or other contemplative practice. Be sure to take a moment (or a few minutes) to center yourself before practicing yoga with your child. From a pure and centered place, you'll be better able to enter all situations with a clear mind, firm hand, and loving heart. Not surprisingly, when you are in a pure and centered state, your child will reflect the same back to you. Perhaps you have noticed this and also the opposite effect. Being present, content, and grounded will create a warm and safe space for your shared practice.
- **Have realistic expectations.** Avoid disappointment and frustration, and instead create opportunity for success by having realistic expectations. For example, though your 2-year-old may sometimes seem disinterested, he is most likely still learning. He may seemingly take nothing in, only to practice

what he learned later in the grocery store. In general, don't expect your sessions to look like your classes at the studio. Sessions with your child may be louder, more active, and much more playful. Let them be!

- **Respond to your child's current needs.** Notice your child's state of being. Does he need a pick-me-up? Is he bouncing off the walls with a need to dispel some energy? No matter what you have set up for your session, try to be flexible, and change your routine to suit your child's current needs and energy level. Choose yoga sequences and activities accordingly to maximize the benefits of having this special one-on-one practice opportunity! Listening to your child's needs in this way will also enhance your connection over time.

- **Gain buy-in.** Help your child make a commitment to practicing yoga by gaining his buy-in. As a parent, you know your child best. What is important to him? What does he enjoy doing? What are his interests? Use what you know about your child to help him understand how yoga can be beneficial to him, personally. For example, if your child is an athlete, explain how yoga can help build his muscle strength and coordination, and increase energy—all ways to improve performance on game day. Do an Internet search together to find out which athletes are doing yoga regularly (there are many!). If your child is shy, note how yoga can build his confidence and reveal all of his amazing qualities. Or discuss how the discipline gained from developing a yoga practice can support the discipline needed to study and get good grades. Use the Yoga Principles in this chapter to start a discussion on yoga as a lifestyle and engage his interest by showing how yoga connects to his personal daily life. Soon, he'll start to make these connections on his own.

- **Be consistent.** Provide consistency in when, where, and how you share yoga with your child. Using a quiet, soothing space with limited distractions where you commit to practicing together each day will lead to long-term success. Maintain some consistency in the flow of your yoga sessions (Chapter 10). Use an attention-getting instrument ritually, such as a yoga wand or chime, establishing early what the expectation is when you sound the object ("We come into Mountain Pose," etc.). Finally, you might consider having a set of "Yoga Time Rules" posted in your yoga space (see sidebar).

- **Model.** Practice yoga alongside your child. For younger children, demonstrate poses for him first so he can observe the pose, then practice by his side, making sure to be on hand for any adjustments.

- **Engage.** Engage your child in this new practice. Allow your child to decorate your yoga space, set up an altar, choose the music, and with practice, even organize the session sequence. Ask open-ended questions while you practice, and include "fun facts" about the animals you are imitating by doing a little research before your session. Allow your child to be the leader, and offer him jobs to do before, during, and after your sessions. Ask about his experiences with the poses as you go along, and finally, be flexible and follow his lead to help him stay happy and engaged as you practice together.

- **Be safe.** Be extremely attentive to your child while he is attempting poses. Make sure to spot all inversions and offer the proper adjustment as needed to prevent any accidents or injuries. If practicing on a wood floor, make sure to use a mat to prevent slipping.

- **Have *fun*!** Adopt an attitude of openness and playfulness as you practice with your child. When wagging your tail in Down Dog (Chapter 6), go ahead and bark! Yoga time can be noisy and active as well as calm and soothing. Be warm, patient, loving, and nonjudgmental. Notice what your child has to teach *you*. What you emanate will be reflected back to you tenfold!

- **Integrate.** Once your child becomes familiar with the various activities in this book, begin to incorporate them any time. When your child is feeling frustrated, you might practice Geyser Pose (Chapter 6) or Count Down to Calm breath (Chapter 5) together. Your child will begin to become more self-aware and spontaneously use his yoga tools throughout the day, as needed.

Yoga Time Rules

Having a set of rules or guidelines can influence children's behavior, cooperation, creativity, independence, and passion for learning. Positive rules can also reflect a family's values. Work cooperatively with your child or family to come up with your own Yoga Time Rules. Here are a few ideas to get you started: "We are respectful and kind in our words and actions." "When we hear the chime, we come to (Easy Pose, Mountain Pose . . .)." "We always try our best." "We listen to our bodies."

THE YOGA PRINCIPLES

Yoga is so much more than poses. It is a discipline focused on improving health of the whole person. As with any discipline, yoga includes a set of principles, or guidelines, upon which its philosophy is based. Centuries ago, a great sage named Patanjali wrote the *Yoga Sutras,* a sort of "how-to guide" to yoga, which is more or less still followed today. Outlined in the *Yoga Sutras* is the eight-limbed path of yoga, the first two of which describe the *yamas* (attitudes or values) and *niyamas* (personal healthy habits) that Patanjali considered to be an essential part of the yoga practice. These pieces of wisdom are considered the major foundational principles of the yogic lifestyle. As it ends up, they are also universal concepts supporting character development, respect of self and others, and healthy living.

To truly build a complete yoga practice with and for your child, include these Yoga Principles in your practice together. The Yoga Principles included here are the most meaningful and comprehensible to a child. They've been rewritten and combined in some cases to be child-friendly and easy to understand. There are many ways to incorporate them into your practice. You can use these principles as discussion starters at any time during your practice, or use them as themes upon which to build a session. As you grow more competent, you may even begin to match activities to principles. Feel free to use these principles any time the opportunity arises—don't restrict them to your practice together. They can be incredibly helpful tools to bridge discussions over difficult issues and bring you and your child closer.

Each of the following principles includes a description and instructions for practicing it. Ideas about what to avoid, practice, and cultivate, are offered as discussion starters, as it is sometimes helpful for children to understand the opposite in order to fully grasp a new concept. Where appropriate, real-life examples of the principles in action are provided. As part of the learning experience, you might encourage your child to come up with her own examples as well. Related book suggestions are also offered for further discussion. For your older child, asking her to journal and/or draw about a given principle at the end of a session is a wonderful way to help deepen understanding.

Yoga Principle #1: Practice Peace

Surround yourself with love and kindness. Be gentle and peaceful in your thoughts and actions. Be respectful. Show kindness. Do not harm anyone or anything. Practice tolerance.

Avoid: mean or malicious thoughts or actions, ignorance, restlessness, swearing/ cussing, selfishness, closed-mindedness (fear resulting from misunderstanding or intolerance breeds anger and hatred), violence

Practice: openness, compassion, love, understanding, patience, self-love

Example #1: Instead of wishing the school bully would be hurt, send him compassion in your thoughts and actions and watch what happens!

Example #2: You listen to your body as you practice yoga poses. If something hurts, you treat yourself with kindness and respect by backing off and going only so far as is comfortable and healthy for your own body, regardless of what everyone else is doing.

Suggested Reading

- *The Peace Book*, by Todd Parr
- *Hey, Little Ant*, by Phillip M. Hoose, Hannah Hoose, and Debbie Tilley
- *The Colors of Us*, by Karen Katz
- *Unstoppable Me!*, by Dr. Wayne W. Dyer, Kristina Tracy, and Stacy Heller Budnick
- *Zen Shorts*, by John J. Muth
- *Each Kindness*, by Jacqueline Woodson and E.B. Lewis

Yoga Principle #2: Be Honest

Be truthful in your actions, thoughts, and speech. Tell the truth. Be yourself. Be true to you.

Avoid: dishonesty/lying, deception, manipulation, holding grudges, pretending to be someone else, not being honest with yourself

Practice: giving constructive feedback, forgiveness, nonjudgment, assertiveness, owning your own feelings and behavior, honesty, being true to yourself

Example #1: You are at your friend's house after school and he offers you his homework to copy. Though it would certainly be easier, it would also be dishonest and so you choose to do the assignment yourself.

Example #2: Some "friends" want you to try smoking with them, but you and your parents have agreed that smoking is unhealthy and that you will not try it. You say "no" as you don't want to deceive your mom, nor do you want to be a follower just to fit in. Be honest and true to you!

- *"Slowly, Slowly, Slowly," Said the Sloth*, by Eric Carle
- *The Wolf Who Cried Boy*, by Bob Hartman and Tim Raglin
- *Unstoppable Me!*, by Dr. Wayne W. Dyer, Kristina Tracy, and Stacy Heller Budnick
- *The Empty Pot*, by Demi

Yoga Principle #3: Be Generous

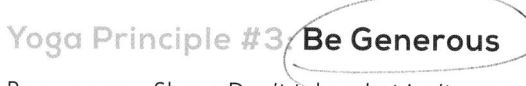

Be generous. Share. Don't take what isn't yours.

Avoid: jealousy, hoarding, plagiarizing, stealing anything—including property, ideas, or attention

Practice: sharing, using objects correctly/the right way, utilizing time responsibly, giving back, generosity

Example #1: You vow not to interrupt your brother when he is telling a story—choosing to allow him the spotlight, rather than steal attention.

Example #2: You love animals and decide to volunteer a few hours per week at the local animal shelter.

Suggested Reading

- *The Selfish Crocodile*, by Faustin Charles and Michael Terry
- *How Leo Learned to Be King*, by Marcus Pfister and J. Alison James
- *Unstoppable Me!*, by Dr. Wayne W. Dyer, Kristina Tracy, and Stacy Heller Budnick

Yoga Principle #4: Practice Moderation

Remember to do all things in moderation. Practice self-control.

Avoid: doing/indulging in too much of anything, whether it be thoughts, speech, or use of your body

Practice: self-control and moderation in all areas of life

Example #1: When you see all your friends coming to school in the latest brand design of sneakers, you immediately think you must get a new pair, too. But then you remember that your sneakers are fine, still fit, and have a lot of wear left. Having yet another pair would be somewhat wasteful as they are not really needed. You decide to be content with, and grateful for, what you've already got.

Example #2: (for preteens and teens) Sensual urges are part of the hormonal changes going on in your bodies. Work to control them such that you won't diminish or disrespect anyone, including yourself. Discuss your feelings with a parent or other trusted adult and find healthy outlets for these emotions, such as exercise, yoga, reading, and meditation/relaxation.

Suggested Reading

- *It's Not What You've Got*, by Dr. Wayne W. Dyer, Kristina Tracy, and Stacy Heller Budnick
- *The Greedy Python*, by Richard Buckley and Eric Carle
- *Howard B. Wigglebottom Learns Too Much of a Good Thing Is Bad*, by Howard Binkow and Susan F. Cornelison

Yoga Principle #5: Be Clean

Take care of yourself, body and mind. Take care of your surroundings, community, and earth.

Avoid: littering, "dumping" on others, filthiness, substance abuse, junk food, swearing/cussing

Practice: keeping oneself and one's surroundings physically clean, eating healthy foods, exercising, cleaning up the earth, being responsible in action and words, being respectful of yourself and others, using good manners

Examples: Brush your teeth at least twice a day. "Just say no" to drugs and alcohol. Eat nutritious, whole foods and get lots of exercise. Choose to recycle. Avoid using foul language.

Suggested Reading

- *The Earth and I*, by Frank Asch
- *Why Should I Recycle?* by Jen Green and Mike Gordon
- *Unstoppable Me!*, by Dr. Wayne W. Dyer, Kristina Tracy, and Stacy Heller Budnick
- *The Care and Keeping of YOU: The Body Book for Girls*, by Valorie Schaefer and Norm Bendell
- *The Boy's Body Book: Everything You Need to Know for Growing Up YOU*, by Kelli Dunham and Steven Bjorkman

Yoga Principle #6: Be Content

Be content with yourself. Celebrate your uniqueness. Maintain a positive outlook. Have an internal sense of peacefulness. Practice gratefulness.

Avoid: being negative and down, being pessimistic, being ungrateful

Practice: making the best of any situation, being grateful, being calm and joyful, not depending on "things" that are outside yourself to make you happy, enjoying daily tasks, focusing on the positive, being happy for others

Example: After losing the soccer game, you're disappointed. Rather than acting angry or grumpy about it, you remember that your team showed great sportsmanship throughout the game and you feel proud.

Suggested Reading

- *The Little Rabbit Who Wanted Red Wings*, by Carolyn Sherwin Bailey
- *I Like Myself!*, by Karen Beaumont and David Catrow
- *Cinderella* (various authors)
- *Unstoppable Me!*, by Dr. Wayne W. Dyer, Kristina Tracy, and Stacy Heller Budnick
- *Zen Shorts*, by John J. Muth
- *I Think, I Am!*, by Louise L. Hay, Kristina Tracy, and Manuela Schwarz
- *The Mixed-Up Chameleon*, by Eric Carle
- *A Bad Case of Stripes*, by David Shannon

Yoga Principle #7: Work Hard

Be disciplined. Always try your best. Establish good habits. Finish what you start. Persevere: Don't give up!

Avoid: being lazy, unmotivated, giving up easily

Practice: perseverance, developing good habits, having determination and enthusiasm for daily and long-term goals

Example #1: You find Sun Salutation difficult and decide to practice five Half Sun Salutes each day upon waking, until you reach your goal of touching your toes.

Example #2: You decide to establish the habit of completing your homework right after school, before heading out to play. You know that doing so will ensure that your homework gets done on time and does not get forgotten. Plus, it's a good habit that will serve you well in the short and long term.

Suggested Reading
- *How Leo Learned to Be King*, by Marcus Pfister and J. Alison James
- *Unstoppable Me!*, by Dr. Wayne W. Dyer, Kristina Tracy, and Stacy Heller Budnick
- *Sally Jean, the Bicycle Queen*, by Cari Best and Christine Davenier
- *The Boy Who Invented TV*, by Kathleen Krull and Greg Couch

Yoga Principle #8: Have Alone Time

Be reflective. Spend time with yourself. Know yourself. Take the time for quiet. Be still.

Avoid: being too busy, being superficial/looking outward or to others for answers to who you are

Practice: enjoying peaceful moments in solitude, being reflective, looking inward for answers and ideas, pondering the question "Who am I?", meditating

Example: Rather than hopping online to check your e-mail when you get home from school, you choose to head up to your favorite corner of your room. You turn off your phone and play your favorite calming music for 10 minutes while sitting in Easy Pose with your eyes closed. You feel refreshed and calm and confident about your ability to do a great job on your writing assignment.

Other Ideas: Sun Salutations in silence, pre-rise breathing, journaling

Suggested Reading
- *I Believe in Me: A Book of Affirmations*, by Connie Bowen
- *The Way I Feel*, by Janan Cain
- *I Take a DEEEP Breath!*, by Sharon R. Penchina
- *Chicken Soup for the Preteen Soul 2*, by Jack Canfield, Mark Victor Hansen, Patty Hansen, and Irene Dunlap
- *The Affirmation Web: A Believe in Yourself Adventure*, by Lori Lite and Helder Botelho
- *Is There Really a Human RACE?*, by Jamie Lee Curtis and Laura Cornell

Yoga Principle #9: Believe in Something Bigger

Think about or even commit to something larger than yourself based on your beliefs. Or, simply connect with all things. Aspire to and appreciate that ideal. Provide a purpose, focus, or "backbone" for your values, principles, and actions.

Discussion Starter Ideas: Talk about connections to nature, the meaning of *Namaste*, Earth Day, and the adage "Do Unto Others."

Suggested Reading

- *All I See Is Part of Me*, by Chara M. Curtis and Cynthia Aldrich
- *The Story of Jumping Mouse* (Native American folktale: various authors)
- *Good People Everywhere*, by Lynea Gillen and Kristina Swarner
- The Bible, Torah, Koran, and other religious texts
- *The Bhagavad Gita*, or other classic yoga texts

PART II

Building Blocks of Yoga for Children

Now that you have learned about the special considerations for each age group, discovered what you need to set up your practice, and explored the basic principles of yoga, you are ready to learn the typical components of a children's yoga practice. Here you'll find information on mindful meditations, breath work, poses, games and creative movement, songs and chants, relaxation, and visualization. Mindful meditations and breath work are the exercises that "yoke" the mind to the body to center your child. Poses provide the physical postures of the practice, including variations for you and your child to do together. Family yoga games are fun, connecting activities that can extend your practice to include the whole family (as well as friends and neighbors). Songs and chants can be used in your practice to add life and reinforce learning. Here, you'll learn how to include songs that link lyrics to poses, which children love! Finally, you'll discover relaxation and visualization exercises to bring your child to a calm, relaxed state, usually at the end of a session. All of the poses, activities, and exercises presented in this part of the book are designed for you to form your own routines, but know that you can call upon them *any time*!

CHAPTER 4

Mindfulness Meditations for Children

DISCOVER MINDFULNESS

Mindfulness—the practice of cultivating awareness and acceptance, free of judgment—has always been inherent in the teaching and practice of yoga. In fact, you cannot truly practice yoga without practicing mindfulness. While yoga and meditation practices are usually the first to come to mind when thinking about mindfulness and the idea of being "aware" or "present," there are, in fact, many ways of cultivating mindfulness. Practicing an instrument, reading a book, painting—these are all activities that promote mindfulness. Being present in the moment is important, but so is how we consider our past experiences and actions. Ultimately, mindfulness allows us to see things as they are, as they are happening, without an emotional response. Cultivating this ability allows us to be the best we can be in any given moment. Being mindful allows us to be more patient and compassionate toward others and releases us from the impulse to "react," which leads us to better, more rational decisions. In addition, the practice of mindfulness raises our threshold for discomfort and stress, helps us regulate our own moods, and makes us more empathetic people overall. Through the practice of yoga, you can develop and enhance these important skills in yourself and your child.

To practice mindfulness, an adult might find a place on his mat, close his eyes, focus on his breath, and bring his awareness to the present moment in a matter of seconds. Not surprisingly, a child can find it quite challenging to bring his mind and body to stillness in this way; in fact, it is an unrealistic expectation.

The approach to teaching mindfulness to children, therefore, is unique. Activities that focus on using the five senses or movement are more developmentally appropriate ways of teaching children this practice. Moments of silence, structured relaxation times, visualization exercises, and activities that foster intentional movement are relevant and engaging for children. Once children have discovered that place of stillness within themselves and become more connected and present through mindful meditation exercises, they often wish to return to that place again and again. Children really do crave opportunities to be quiet and connect within! Over time and with practice, don't be surprised to find that your child begins to initiate these activities on his own, without your guidance. And, beyond that, you will both be increasing your ability to "see clearly" in every moment, without judgment or the impulse to "react" emotionally. What a gift!

Talking Trees

This is a great activity to help your child understand yoga and mindfulness. Begin by having your child stand in Tree Pose. Ask him to tell you about what he had for lunch yesterday, where he was, and who he was with, etc., and while he does, play loud music and try to "bother" him by clapping near his ears. Then have him stop and take his pulse, notice what his mind is doing, where his breath is, and what is going on in his body. Then have your child come into Mountain Pose (Chapter 6), establish a focus point, and take several deep, focused breaths. Encourage him to mindfully come through the sequence of steps to come into Tree Pose on one side and then the other. When finished, discuss with your child the two experiences. Where was his mind the first time? What was going on with his breath? What was happening to him physically? And the second time? Of course, the second experience will be different, and your child will most likely share that he felt more balanced, focused, and calm. Talk with your child about the power of mindful breathing and taking a moment to center and focus and how that related to his ability to practice Tree Pose (yoga is the integration of mind, body, and breath!). How can this lesson be applied to everyday life—at home, at school, on the playground? Assist your child to come up with examples using your own stories as examples.

MINDFULNESS MEDITATION: EXERCISES

The following mindfulness exercises are specially designed for children. They focus on the use of the five main senses of vision, hearing, touch, taste, and smell on movement (Mindful Movement Meditations) and on reflection. Many examples of the other types of activities previously described are presented throughout this book. These mindful meditation activities serve well as ways to open a yoga session, transition to relaxation, or assist any time your child needs calming, centering, or help in gaining new perspective.

Touch Meditations

BACK WRITING

Benefits

| Builds focus and concentration |
| Engages positive touch |
| Promotes literacy and spelling skills |

WHAT TO DO

Back Writing requires your child's full attention; it is engaging for children, and feels good, too. It can serve as a wonderful transition to a yoga session that promotes calm, positive touch, and a bit of fun. Pair it with Partner Massage (see sidebar) for a calming, pre-bedtime activity. Sit down behind your child and use your index finger to firmly write letters or simple shapes on his back, and have him guess what you have written. For older children, try writing full words or even sentences! No matter the age of your child, try adding more challenge over time as you gauge his ability to successfully guess what you write or draw. And don't forget to take turns by having your child write or draw on your back!

WHAT TO SAY

Sit down in front of me and get comfortable. I'm going to write/draw something on your back, and then you tell me what you think it is. Ready? . . . What did I write/draw? That's right! Let's try another one. Careful, this one is a little trickier . . . now, my turn!

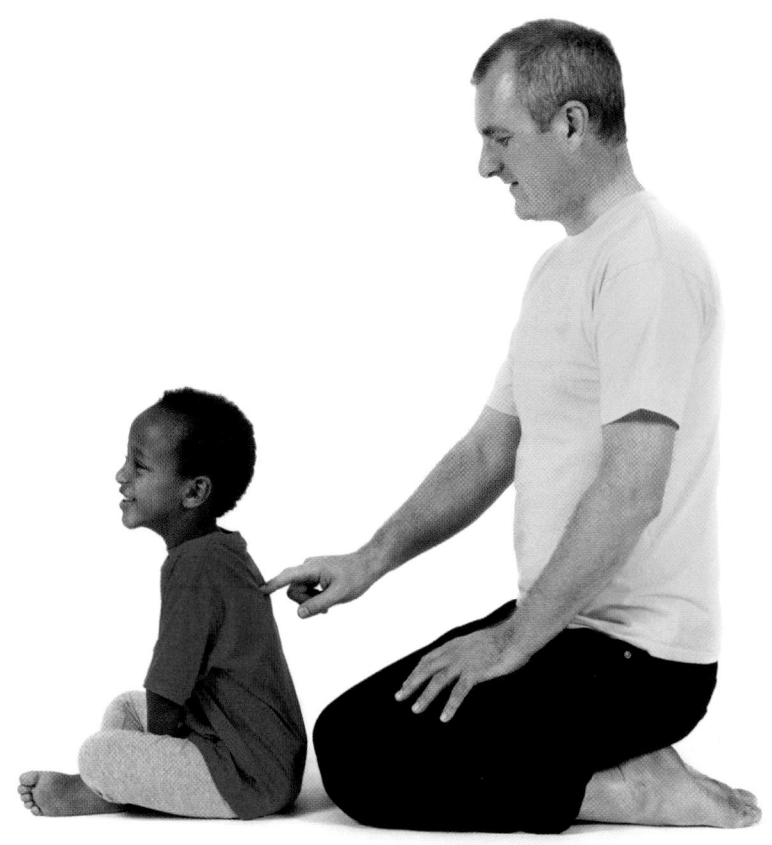

★ Back Writing

Partner Massage

Take turns giving each other a nice back and neck massage. Model for your child compassionate communication by asking him if he would like a softer or firmer touch and asking him where he is holding tension so that you can focus your attention in that area. Of course, be sure he returns the favor! With a group or whole family, sit one behind the other to make a "massage train." When finished, turn around to thank your partner and return the favor.

Benefits

Calms and centers

Dispels excess energy or negativity

WHAT TO DO

Do this exercise any time your child's energy level is high, or is experiencing the grumpies. You might set the stage with soft instrumental music or music with ocean waves in the background. A spritz of Magic Mist will also help soothe the senses (see Magic Mist in this chapter).

At the base of the spine, just above the sacrum, there is a place where many nerve endings come together (think of the location of your back belt loop on a low-slung pair of pants). In her yoga program and book focused on yoga for babies and toddlers, Itsy Bitsy Yoga® founder Helen Garabedian suggests tapping on this area to help comfort and calm a colicky baby. She says, "It's like a burp for the nervous system." Rest and Press is a variation of this idea, but is designed to benefit children and adults.

With your child in Child's Pose (Chapter 6), stand or sit behind him and firmly draw your hands down his back from top to bottom. This will stretch his spine a bit, opening up the space between his vertebrae. Come to rest your hands at the base of his back, where his belt loop would be. Your hands should be stacked palm over palm with your fingers facing forward (think CPR). Breathe in with your child. As he exhales, press into the area with your palms using your own weight for added pressure. As you press down, also pull back energetically. His hips should lower slightly. Be sure to ask your child about the pressure. Is it too little, too much? Try visualizing love, peace, and positive energy coming out through your hands as you touch your child. Breathe with him in and out three times or more before gently jiggling your child side to side, dissipating any stagnant energy.

Still your hands and then draw them, one over the other, firmly down your child's back one last time before gently releasing them from your child's back.

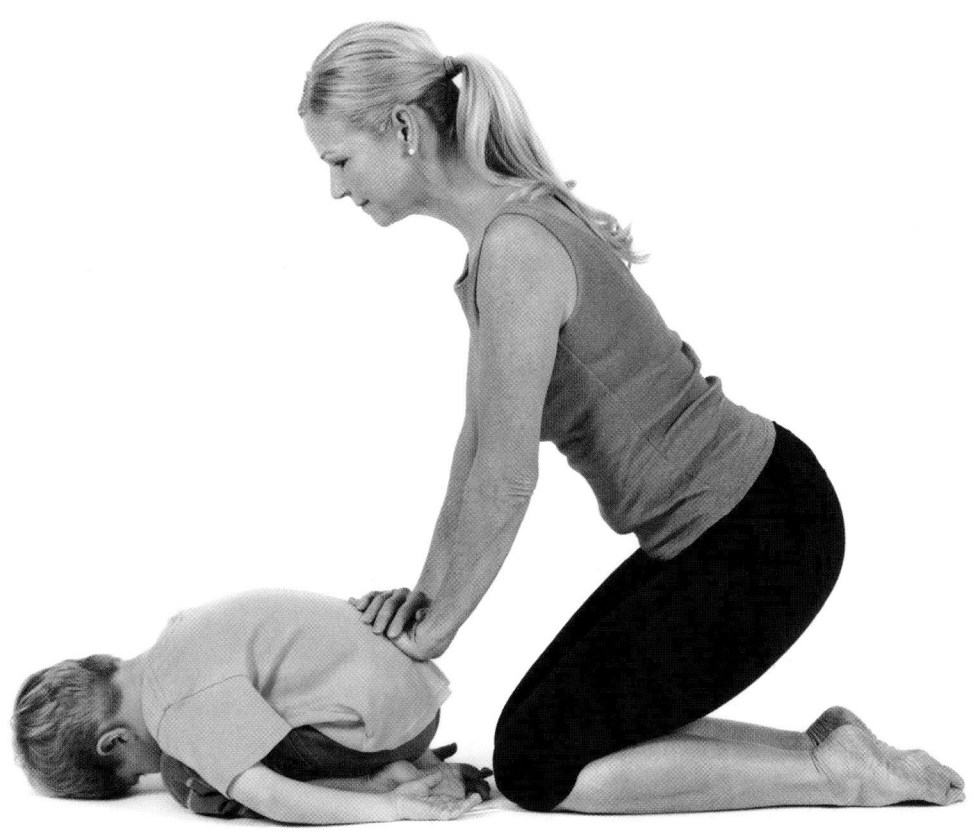

★ Rest and Press

WHAT TO SAY

Come into Child's Pose. Is it okay if I press a bit on your back? Good. I'll give you a turn and then maybe you can give me one. Go ahead and take a nice deep breath as I rub your back. Just breathe in and out, in and out. (Continue on with instructions, checking in with your child along the way.) All done now. Let's take a nice deep breath in and out together. Very, very slowly come to sit up. How do you feel?

MAGIC MASSAGE

Benefits

Relieves stress and tension

"Clears the slate," improves concentration

Encourages self-care

WHAT TO DO

This is a simple self-massage activity that your child can master and use any time. It can be practiced in a seated pose like Easy Pose (Chapter 6), standing, or even lying down. The verbal instructions will walk your child through the steps.

WHAT TO SAY

When you're comfortable, close your eyes and focus on your breath. Using your fingertips and small, firm circular movements, massage the top of your head . . . your temples . . . now your forehead and over and around your eyebrows, spending a little extra time on any areas that need it. Good. Now, move your fingers to your ears. Press and massage your earlobes between your fingers and then gently tug open your ears. Now, move your fingers to the back of your neck and shoulders, massaging into any areas that are holding tension. Now, find your collarbone. Bring your fingers down about one inch or so to find the soft spots on either side. Massage gently for 10 seconds or more. Cross your arms over your chest and give yourself a squeeze. Squeeze into your shoulders and then down your arms; squeeze, squeeze, squeeze. Clasp your hands and rock them from side to side, making a figure eight. Did you hear your wrist crack and pop a bit? That's because you've released some air pockets built up between the joints. Now, take your left hand into your right. Press your thumb into the soft spot between the thumb and the palm, and then down along each finger. Switch hands. Go ahead and rest your hands on your lap and continue to keep your eyes closed. Breathe evenly and deeply for a few moments. What sensations do you notice? How do you feel?

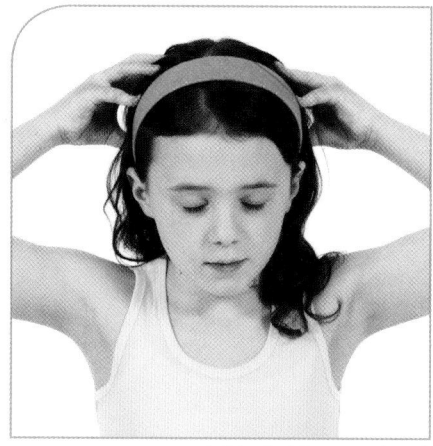

★ Magic Massage, head

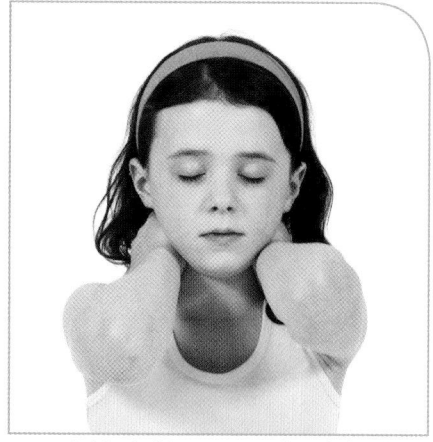

★ Magic Massage, neck and shoulders

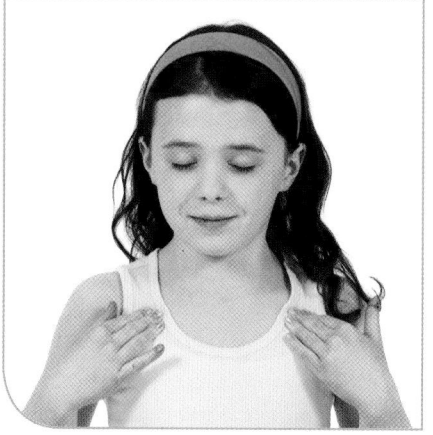

★ Magic Massage, below the collarbone

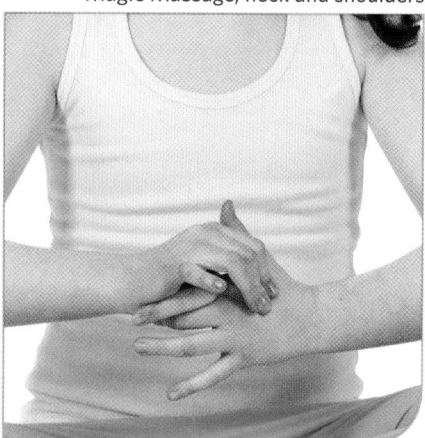

★ Magic Massage, hands

Refresh and Wake Up the Brain!

Magic Massage is restorative, especially after a long period of concentrating or writing. This self-massage sequence stimulates blood flow to the brain and other areas where we typically hold tension, such as the neck and shoulders. The increased blood flow helps improve concentration skills required for reading and writing, while the muscle massage soothes and releases tension.

Benefits

Enhances focus and concentration

Promotes sensory processing

WHAT TO DO

You will need a bag or basket and some animal figurines, items from the doll-house, matchbox cars, or any other similar-sized, yet different small objects that are familiar to your child. Put the objects into the bag. After covering your child's eyes with a blindfold or by pulling down a knit hat, have him reach in with one hand to try to find a particular object (the cat figurine, for example) using only his sense of touch to determine one object from another. The older your child, the more similar the objects should be. For example, if your child is into matchbox cars, put a few different types of cars in the bag and have him try to find a specific model. You can also challenge your older child by having him use his nondominant hand to reach in to find the object. When playing this game with a younger child, have him reach into the bag with both hands. Or, just simplify it by handing him a single, recognizable object, and having him guess what it is.

WHAT TO SAY

I have a bunch of interesting objects here in this bag. Your job is to reach in with one hand and try to pull out the object that I call out. To make sure you can't peek, we're going to cover your eyes with this blindfold (or hat, etc.). Okay, can you see anything? No peeking! Now, reach your hand into the bag and feel around to see if you can pick out the _____. Take your time. Think of the shape of the _____ and see if your fingers can "see" it in the bag. I'm going to be silent now so that you can concentrate. Aha, what do you have? Did you find the _____? (If not, have him set the object aside and try again.)

Sight Meditations

CANDLE GAZING

Benefits

Calms and centers

Focuses attention

WHAT TO DO

Light a candle and place it between you and your child. Use your best judgment as to whether your child should be around a real flame or not. Certainly, if your child is younger than 7 years old, use a flameless tea light candle. In fact, a color-changing LED tea light or pillar candle is especially engaging for all ages. Challenge your child to hold his gaze for longer periods of time with each session. You might begin with 20 seconds and work up to 2 minutes or more over the course of your sessions together.

WHAT TO SAY

Find a comfortable position such as Easy Pose, Hero Pose, or lying on your belly in Sphinx Pose (Chapter 6). Focus your eyes on the candle flame as you practice your Balloon Breathing (Chapter 5). Breathe in . . . breathe out . . . good. Keep your body still as I time you. I will tell you when the time is up. You did it! I wonder if we can do candle gazing even longer next time. What do you think?

MANDALA COLORING

Benefits

Soothes the nervous system

Calms and centers

Inspires creativity

WHAT TO DO

Mandala, in Sanskrit (the language of yoga), means "circle." A mandala is any circular, geometric design, and represents unity, connectedness, and wholeness. Looking at, creating, or coloring a mandala is a long-practiced exercise for promoting focus, concentration, and an overall meditative state. Before you begin this exercise, or the Mandala Movement Meditation found later in this chapter, share with your child some examples of mandalas on the Internet or from a book.

Coloring in a predesigned mandala is a wonderfully meditative activity for any age. Get out markers, crayons, or colored pencils and let your child use his creativity to color his mandala in whatever way he wishes. You are encouraged to color your own alongside your child. Compare and celebrate your unique creations when you are done! There are many mandala coloring books on the market. There are also free mandala coloring pages of all kinds available on the

Internet. Empower your child by letting him choose from a selection you have printed out. A good rule is: the younger the child, the simpler the designs should be, and the less options he should be given. To set a meditative tone, playing soft music is an option. Perhaps your child can choose the music as well!

WHAT TO SAY

It's mandala time! Here are some options—you choose which one you'd like to color today. You can choose from crayons, markers, or colored pencils, and use any colors you wish. I will play the soft music you have selected and we will sit and color together until we finish our designs. Let's sit up tall in Easy Pose and breathe for a minute to prepare our minds and bodies for coloring. Good, now we are ready . . .

Smell Meditation

MAGIC MIST

Benefits

Calming

Encourages deep breathing

WHAT TO DO

Magic Mist contains lavender essential oil, which is known to have a calming effect. (See Chapter 3 to create your own.) Spray a bit of Magic Mist around an area or room to encourage a peaceful, calm atmosphere. This is especially suited to enhance your yoga sessions with your child or to set the tone for relaxation, nap, or bedtime. Encourage your child to inhale and smell the mist, enhancing the breathing component of the exercise. For another smell meditation, see Stop and Smell the Flowers in Chapter 5.

WHAT TO SAY

I've made some Magic Mist to help us become calm and peaceful. I'll spritz some now and then we can breathe together. Do you smell the lavender fragrance? Breathe in the fragrance through your nose, and fill up your belly. Exhale and say, "Ahhhh," because it smells so good! Let's do that two more times.

Taste Meditation

Benefits

Focuses attention

Promotes mindful awareness

Encourages mindful eating

WHAT TO DO

This exercise introduces your child to mindful eating. Mindful eating is practiced in a relaxed, seated position such as in a chair, or in Easy Pose or Hero Pose (see Chapter 6). For this exercise, you will need a small food item such as a blueberry, an M&M, a raisin, or a goldfish cracker. Don't let your child know what you are giving him. If your child is a "peeker," use a blindfold. Have your younger child answer your questions out loud as you ask them. Encourage your older child to answer the questions silently to himself, waiting until the end of the exercise to share his experience. Once you've practiced this exercise with your child a few times using familiar foods, move on to foods that may be less familiar.

WHAT TO SAY

Sit and close your eyes and hold out your palm. I'm going to put a small object in your hand. Go ahead and touch it gently and carefully using your fingers. Is it smooth, rough? What is the shape? Can you guess what it is without peeking? Now bring the item up to your nose. Does it have a smell? What kind? Now, bring it up to your mouth. Place it on your tongue and gently close your mouth. Do not chew yet! Think of words to describe the flavor of the object. What about its texture? Now, begin to slowly, mindfully chew the object. What is the taste like? Sweet, salty? Go ahead and swallow now. Have you guessed what it is? What did you notice about it now that you have eaten it so mindfully?

Sound Meditations

CHIME LISTENING

Benefits

Builds listening skills, focus

Encourages mindful awareness

WHAT TO DO

For this exercise, you will need a chime. When rung, your child will focus on the reverberating sound of the chime until it stops. Before you do this exercise, try centering first by practicing Ocean Breath or Balloon Breath (Chapter 5) together.

WHAT TO SAY

Sit in Easy Pose or Hero Pose (Chapter 6) with your hands in your lap. I'm going to ring the chime, and then you listen closely as the sound of the chime sings. Try closing your eyes. You may notice that your sense of hearing is enhanced when your eyes are closed. Silently raise your hand when you can no longer hear it. Ready . . .

Pass the Chime

For a variation, ring the chime, then pass it back and forth between you (or around the circle if you are working with a group or your family) with the goal of returning it to the starting person before the sound of the chime stops. Be careful! If you touch the metal part of the chime, it will stop the sound, so pass it around *mindfully*.

FOLLOW THE SOUND

Benefits

Builds listening skills, focus

Promotes mindful awareness

WHAT TO DO

For this exercise, choose a simple piece of instrumental music that uses just two or three recognizable instruments, no more than two instruments for children under 8 years and up to three for children 8 years and up. Begin by doing Ocean Breath or Balloon Breath (Chapter 5) together. This exercise can be practiced sitting up as a centering exercise or lying down in *Savasana* (Chapter 6).

WHAT TO SAY

Sit in Easy Pose or Hero Pose (Chapter 6) or lie down. I'm going to play a piece of music that involves two (or three) instruments. When the song begins, choose one instrument sound and try to follow just that instrument as it plays through the song. When you lose track and find yourself starting to follow another instrument, say to yourself, "Oh, I lost track. Where is my instrument? There it is," and then gently bring your focus back to follow the sound of your instrument once again. Closing your eyes will be helpful. Otherwise, you can also focus on a spot on the floor in front of you. When I see that you are ready, I will start the music . . .

Discuss to Learn

As with all of the mindfulness and centering activities, discuss the experience with your child. For this exercise you might ask her, "Which instrument did you try to follow? Was it difficult or easy to stay focused on one instrument? Tell me about that. Do you ever find it challenging to focus on one thing at a time when there is a lot going on around you? What tools can we use to assist us in finding our focus again?"

OUTSIDE IN

Benefits

Builds listening skills, focus

Promotes mindful awareness

WHAT TO DO

This activity can be practiced anywhere, from your child's bedroom to the car, or even as a break from a busy family function as a way to encourage your child's awareness to come inside. Your child can sit in Easy Pose or Hero Pose (Chapter 6), lie down, or sit in a chair. Start by practicing some calming breaths together and encourage your child to close his eyes. When practicing this activity with your younger child, keep it simple by having him focus only on sounds around him (including those outside) and those within him.

WHAT TO SAY

Find a comfortable position. Close your eyes and open your listening ears. Let's practice Balloon Breath together . . . in and out . . . continue to breathe and bring your awareness to the outside of this room. Note to yourself any sounds that you hear. If you hear a car, say "Car," to yourself. Then move on to listen for and note other sounds. (After a minute:) Bring your awareness into this room. Notice what sounds you hear around and within this space and note them to yourself. (After a minute:) Now, bring your awareness into the space near you. (After a minute:) Now listen for sounds and notice sensations within your own body. Again, note them to yourself. (After a minute:) How do you feel? Where is your awareness now? Tell me about what you noticed and heard as you brought your attention from the outside to the inside.

PRACTICING PEACE

Benefits

Encourages reflection
Promotes sense of connectedness
Calms

WHAT TO DO

Life isn't always peaceful for a preteen. Sports practices, hours of homework, and their changing bodies can make for a very hectic life. While peace signs may be hip and appear on everything from their backpacks to T-shirts, preteens may be far from understanding what peace really feels like. Abby Wills of Shanti Generation offers a wonderful meditation exercise that can help your preteen lock into the idea of peace. This meditation is best practiced outside or by an open window, but you can also play nature sounds from a noise machine, iPod, or CD. Following this exercise, encourage your preteen to write or draw about his experience in his journal (see Reflection Journaling later in this chapter). See also "Chants" in Chapter 8 for other sound meditations.

WHAT TO SAY

Sit comfortably with your hands resting on your thighs. Draw your attention to your quiet and gentle breath. Begin to notice the sounds and sensations around you: Maybe birds are singing, perhaps a gentle breeze is blowing . . . what else do you hear? They may not be peace-evoking sounds. Life isn't always peaceful, so it's helpful to learn to integrate and accept abrasive sounds along with those that inspire tranquility. Begin to collect and mentally overlap sounds you hear until they begin to blend into one, long sound. On your next inhale, begin to draw this universal, peaceful sound into your inner self. Notice the sensations these sounds create inside your body and mind. Can you sense the peace of all things being connected? Can you connect to the world around you and feel this peace inside of yourself? What does this feel like inside? Can you describe it?

Movement Meditations

SCARF MEDITATION

Benefits

Calms, centers
Promotes mindful movement
Encourages body awareness

WHAT TO DO

Structured activity with colorful, flowy scarves is a always a child favorite. Give your child one small scarf for each hand or one large scarf to hold with two hands. Become seaweed, ocean waves, wind, water, etc., and move rhythmically to the music. Experiment with changing up the music from slow and flowing to wild and jagged, etc., but always ending with peaceful and slow. Encourage your child to use his scarf to become the music. Be sure to discuss the experience with your child. What did the fast-paced, loud music feel like in your body? And the peaceful music? What happened with your breathing? Your movements? For older children, challenge them to stay focused on moving peacefully and slowly while breathing deeply and easily even when the music is rapid and frenetic. This exercise can lead to some wonderful discussions about our power to regulate our own state of being with focus and breath, regardless of what may be transpiring around us.

WHAT TO SAY

Hold this scarf. I'm going to play some different types of music, starting with slow and peaceful, and let's see if you can match your movements and rhythm to the music. After a while, I might change the music. See then if you find you want to change your movements as well, moving your scarf along with you in whatever directions feel right. Ready?

SCARF JUGGLING

Benefits

Encourages focus and concentration

Builds confidence

WHAT TO DO

Juggling is engaging, is great for building concentration skills, and is incredibly empowering for children 7 and up! First learn to juggle three different color scarves using a simple juggling kit or online instructions. Then, teach your child. It's not as tough as you might think! The key is to start by holding two scarves in one hand and one in the other. Then toss the first one up from the hand holding two, then alternate tossing and catching with each hand. Call out the colors as you catch them up in the air to help you stay focused, "red, yellow, green, red, yellow, green," etc.

WHAT TO SAY

Let's juggle! Watch me juggle first and then I will show you how. Notice that I'm holding two scarves in my right hand and only one in the other. Once I get going, I only want to be holding one scarf in each hand. Here I go. "Red, yellow, green, red, yellow, green!" I did it. Did you see how I focused my eyes up on the scarves? Now you try! That's right. Hold the red and green with your right hand and the yellow with your left. Adjust the red scarf in your grasp so that you can toss it up first. Ready? . . .

METAMORPHOSIS

Benefits

Encourages mindful movement and grace

Calms

Enhances focus and concentration

WHAT TO DO

The following description utilizes the metamorphosis of an acorn growing into a tree. However, this exercise can be adapted for anything that changes or grows from one thing into another such as a caterpillar to a butterfly, a bird hatching from an egg and learning to fly, or a deflating balloon or melting ice cream cone as described in Chapter 9. Set the tone and pace by playing very soft, slow music.

Encourage your child to move slowly and mindfully. Ask "How *slow* can you go?" in a soft tone and relaxed pace as you guide her. Remind her to breathe as she goes through her metamorphosis. When she has morphed into a tree, have her practice her balance by holding Tree Pose while you pretend to be a big gust of wind to "blow her leaves" to and fro. To keep the mindful moment going or to transition to relaxation, your child can "fall" softly like leaves blowing in the wind before coming to settle on the mat or blanket.

WHAT TO SAY
Come into Child's Pose (Chapter 6) to make your body teensy tiny. Imagine you are a tiny acorn tucked snugly down into the earth where it is warm and cozy. If you are very still, you might feel some rain fall on your back (patter your fingers lightly on your child's back). When you feel the rain, inhale and start to slowly, slowly begin to grow up and out of your seed. Trees grow very slowly. How slow can you go? First, put up one shoot . . . then another . . . and slowly start to stand up. Keep breathing . . . now come onto one foot to grow your trunk strong and tall. Start to grow your branches and leaves up to the sky. Now, sprout some new baby acorns by spreading your fingers out wide, "Pop, pop, pop." You did it!

MANDALA MOVEMENT MEDITATION

Benefits

Encourages mindful attention

Boosts creativity

Encourages self-expression and appreciation of diversity

Builds community

WHAT TO DO
Look around your home for small, colorful items that can be organized in groups. Such typical household items could include things like ribbons, buttons, scraps of colorful paper or fabric, scarves, dried beans of varying colors, items from a dollhouse, matchbox cars, figurines, your sea glass collection, rocks, coins, etc. Set up bowls of each type of item around the room, leaving open space in the middle in which to create the mandala. Before starting the exercise, encourage your child to be mindful by staying silent and moving slowly throughout the activity. Try playing quiet music to set the pace and tone. When you've run out of materials or you both decide your mandala is complete, be sure to celebrate your

collaborative creation by taking a picture (over time, you may find you have a beautiful collection of mandala creation photos!). Then, when you're ready, take the mandala apart item by item in the same mindful fashion.

WHAT TO SAY

We are going to create our own mandala by taking turns placing items in this circular space on the floor. I will start by placing this _____ at the center. Now, it's your turn. You can choose any one item from any of the bowls. Choose just one and place it into the circle. You can place it next to mine or somewhere else— wherever you wish to place it is perfectly fine. Now, let's keep going. We are both going to continue to choose one item at a time and silently and mindfully walk in and out of the circle to place it down wherever we feel it would look best. When we've used up all the items in the bowls, we'll come to sit quietly in Easy Pose or Hero Pose (Chapter 6) to gaze at our creation in silence as we breathe together for one minute. Let's do three calming, Flying Bird Breaths (Chapter 5) together now to get our bodies and minds ready to be quiet and mindful before we begin . . . good. Let's begin.

Take It Outdoors

Incorporate this activity with a nature hike (see Nature Walk Meditation later in this chapter). As you walk, gather nature's decorations such as sticks, rocks, flowers, or leaves, and use those items to create a mandala outdoors in an open area. On a snowy day, you might go outside to a freshly snowed lawn or field and create a mandala design by simply walking one foot in front of the other, allowing your footprints to provide the form and design.

WASHING MACHINE

Benefits

Dissipates anxiety, worry, anger

Integrates and organizes

Energizes

WHAT TO DO

This movement series is based on a Qigong ("Chi Gong") exercise and is wonderful to use after a long day. It's a great way to release tension and stress, integrate both sides of the brain, organize the body, and energize. End with Power Breath to energize, or Flying Bird Breath to calm (Chapter 5).

WHAT TO SAY

Stand with your feet about 12 inches apart. Relax your knees and begin to turn your upper body from side to side so that your arms swing out and around your body, back and forth. Think of what you would like to "wash out"—anger, hurt feelings, or worries— and "wash" them right out of your body. Imagine that heaviness is being washed down the drain away from your body and into the ground. When the wash cycle is over, shake yourself dry! Stand in Mountain Pose (Chapter 6), and take a deep breath. Using both sets of fingertips, begin to gently tap yourself. You might like to tap in positive, peaceful thoughts. Begin at your head and tap, tap, tap all the way down the front of your body . . . now, tap all the way back up the back of your body. Tap down each arm, beginning at the shoulders. Wrap your arms around yourself and tap your sides. Switch your arms and do it again. Lower your arms and close your eyes. Notice how you feel.

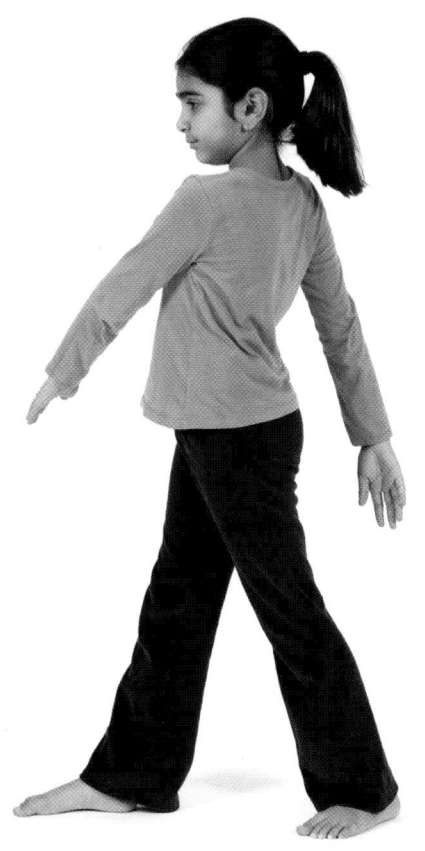

★ Washing Machine

NATURE WALK MEDITATION

Benefits

Promotes body awareness

Encourages mindful attention

WHAT TO DO

The simple act of walking is a repetitive movement that can be quite meditative. Walking outdoors, your child will have a wide range of things to see, hear, touch, and smell—all awakening his senses and bringing him to a deeper awareness of his surroundings and his own body. Take a nature walk with your child at a nearby park or nature preserve. As you walk, have your child focus on every step he takes. Exaggerate and demonstrate the movements involved in taking a single step, and have your child follow after you. Practice mindful walking, and then experiment with pacing. As you walk, ask your child what he sees and hears, and invite him to touch and smell anything (safe!) that interests him.

Reflection Meditations

SILENT SECONDS

Benefits

Enhances focus and attention

Quiets the mind

Calms and centers

WHAT TO DO

Silent Seconds gives your child a chance to bring her attention to the present moment through the practice of focusing on her breath. Use Silent Seconds with children 4 years and older who are familiar with using the breath upon which she will focus, typically Balloon Breath or Ocean Breath (Chapter 5). Time your child as she practices focusing on her breath, starting with 15 seconds and working up to 2 minutes or more over the course of your sessions together. The older your child, the longer you can expect her to be successful practicing Silent Seconds. If your child has a tough time keeping her eyes closed, have her watch the second hand on the clock or give her another small visual upon which she can focus her eyes, such as in Candle Gazing (see Sight Meditations).

WHAT TO SAY

Sit in Easy Pose or Hero Pose (Chapter 6), whichever is more comfortable for you. Press your hands together in front of your heart or rest your hands on your thighs or belly. Begin to practice Balloon Breathing (Chapter 5), breathing in to fill up your lungs and belly, then breathing out slowly to release all the stale air. Continue to breathe while your body remains silent and still . . . when you feel your mind begin to wander, you can say to yourself, "Oh, my mind is wandering. Where is my breath?" and then bring your mind back to your breathing again. Notice how the air feels going in and out of your nose. Can you focus on the feeling of your belly rising and falling with your breath? In . . . out . . . good. I'm going to time you as you focus on your breath in Silent Seconds. I will tell you when . . .

REFLECTION JOURNALING

Benefits

- Encourages self-reflection and self-awareness
- Promotes creativity
- Strengthens bonds and builds community

WHAT TO DO

Having a yoga journal is a wonderful way to help your child process information learned during his practice and discussion. Journals can also be used between sessions as a log for your child to write down thoughts and questions he has that can be brought up at the next session (or any time!). There are a few ways to incorporate journals into your child's yoga practice—you can either give your child prompts to write about between sessions or let him write or draw freely at the end of a session about his experience. If your younger child cannot yet write, you can have him paste photos or magazine clippings, or draw on paper. These are all ways to promote creativity, develop writing skills, facilitate communication between you and your child, and promote a sense of connectedness! Keep in mind your child can choose to keep his journal private or share it with you. Honor his choice.

WHAT TO SAY

(If you want to let your child freely write or draw, simply say:) What did you learn today? What do you still have questions about? Write or draw in your journal to explore your thoughts. (If you want to give them prompts, here are some starter ideas:) How does Tree Pose help you feel strong? What images come to mind while you do Warrior Pose? What does Wheel Pose teach you about the importance of being flexible—in your body and your mind?

THOUGHTS OF GRATITUDE

Benefits

Balances energy
Promotes connectedness
Encourages optimism
Lifts mood
Encourages mindful reflection

WHAT TO DO

A dose of gratitude is always good medicine. In fact, there is nothing more powerful than the experience of gratitude to shift negative energy to positive. Use this meditation to promote appreciation whenever moods are down or your child or family is feeling pessimistic or overwhelmed. (See also Gratitude Relaxation in Chapter 9.)

WHAT TO SAY

Close your eyes and relax your face and neck muscles. Listen to the sound of your breath as it moves in and out of your nose. Begin to think about all in your life that is good. One by one, begin to list them out in your mind. I will do the same as I sit here next to you. After a minute, we can share.

FEELINGS SHARE

Benefits

Encourages connectedness
Promotes self-awareness
Encourages mindful reflection

WHAT TO DO

Enhance your connection with your child by sharing the truth (within reason) about your feelings and encouraging your child to express her honest thoughts and feelings, too. When she does share, be sure to give her your undivided attention by truly listening. Remember, there is no need to "fix" feelings. Model for your child how feelings need not be judged, e.g., "I'm noticing I feel sad today. Sadness is a feeling. It's okay to feel sad sometimes." Simply create a safe space for your child to have her feelings and you yours as you sit side by side sharing and just being together. After you've both shared your feelings now and other feelings you may have had previously, discuss how our feelings are fleeting, changing from moment to moment and certainly over the course of the day. As negative feelings can sometimes be overwhelming to a child in the moment, this introduction to the concept of impermanence can be quite reassuring.

WHAT TO SAY

Let's sit side by side together. What are we feeling? Let's take a couple of nice Balloon Breaths (Chapter 5) together. Ahhh. I think I'm feeling tired and a bit frustrated still by something that happened earlier today. But I'm also feeling peaceful sitting here next to you. How are you feeling right now? Tell me about your day. Did you have different feelings earlier today than you do now? Let's just sit and breathe together, noticing our feelings, knowing that no matter what we are feeling, it's okay. When we are done, you can share with me if you'd like. (With an older child, you might encourage her to follow up this exercise with a journal entry—see Reflection Journaling in this chapter.)

Thank Bank

This simple craft and activity for children (and adults!) encourages gratitude. Make a slit into the top of a child-sized shoe box with a removable top. Have your child decorate the outside of the box. Each evening before bed, or at the start of each yoga session, have your child remember something that took place or something that he noticed for which he is grateful. Have him write it down on a colored slip of paper and stick it in the box (if your child is a pre-writer, you can write what he says). The next time he is feeling grumpy, unappreciative, or sad, encourage him to review the contents. Remembering his blessings will go a long way to improving his mood, and may spark some meaningful discussions.

CHAPTER 5

Breath Work

THE IMPORTANCE OF BREATH

Breathing is arguably the single most important aspect of yoga. You might say yoga *is* breathing. Of course, breathing is the mechanism that sustains life. It brings much-needed oxygen to our organs, muscles, and cells. But through *conscious* breathing, we can actually regulate our mind-body system. When we feel stressed, we can soothe our nervous system, literally "short-circuiting" our stress hormones. By the same token, we can use our breath to energize our bodies and clear and refresh our minds. In a nutshell, when we purposely lengthen our exhalations, we activate our parasympathetic nervous system, which calms us. When we purposely lengthen our inhalations, we increase the oxygen level in our bloodstream, which alleviates fatigue throughout our bodies and brains. Focusing on equalizing the length of our inhalations and exhalations brings our mind and body into balance. But, in order to do this, we must breathe correctly and with intention.

Have you ever watched a baby breathing? Babies come into the world breathing with their entire being. Their bellies fill up completely, rising and falling with each inhale and exhale. During childhood we begin to lose that gift. Over the years, our breathing becomes more shallow, tending to engage the ribs and shoulders rather than the entire torso. In fact, as children and adults, we typically only use about 25 percent of our lung capacity. Although this partial breath may be enough to sustain the body, it can lead to a multitude of problems, including sleep issues, poor focus, low energy, reduced endurance and strength, headaches, sluggish bodily functions, diminished fine motor control, and chronic anxiety. Maybe you've experienced this yourself. Certainly, as parents and teachers, we've seen children struggle with the aforementioned issues, but we may not have associated them with improper breathing.

Of all the physiological systems in the body, breathing is the only one we can consciously control. And this remarkable gift of having the ability to regulate our own breathing allows us to manipulate our ability to respond and adapt, and even alter our state of being. All it takes is attention and practice.

INTRODUCING YOUR CHILD TO BREATH WORK

As a parent guiding your child in the practice of yoga, it is essential that you help her become aware of the power of her breath. When children learn to breathe deeply and fully, they immediately notice a change in how they feel. They often note feeling calmer, more focused, less agitated, and less reactive.

Try to incorporate at least one type of conscious breathing activity into each yoga session, and always point out its benefits by asking questions that help your child notice the effects of the exercise on her own state of being. The benefits and information in the "What to Do" and "What to Say" sections of each breathing exercise can serve as a guide to get those discussions going. For example, you might ask your child how she feels after practicing Power Breath. She might say, "energized," "powerful," or "confident." You might then ask, "Can you think of a time of day or a situation where it might be helpful to practice Power Breath?" Through these discussions, you can help your child connect the exercise to times in her life when the breath could be a useful tool for self-regulation. Over time, hopefully she will be inspired to use these simple, conscious breathing exercises as needed.

You may wonder how much children are learning and how much they will retain after a yoga practice. Over and over again, parents and children have shared how they are able to use breathing exercises the most consistently and effectively as a daily tool. Many children express how focused breathing such as Ocean Breath and Balloon Breath help them fall asleep more easily, settle their nerves before a test or performance, or calm down before hitting their sibling when frustrated. If your child can take away deep breathing skills from your yoga sessions together, then you have done your job successfully as a yoga instructor *and* parent. Breathing activities are simple and quick, and anyone (even a child!) can do them anywhere for instant focus, energy, or calm. Truly, it is the simplest tool for self-regulation.

Discussion: Oxygen = Energy

This is a fun experiment that can help your older child understand the importance of the breath. Be sure to remind your child of your family's rules regarding fire safety. This experiment should only be demonstrated by an adult. Place a glass over a lit tea light candle and discuss what happens. Why did the flame get smaller and then go out? Fire requires oxygen to maintain its energy ("life" or *prana*). Do humans need oxygen to sustain energy and life? What happens when we don't get enough? Have your child slouch over and try to take a deep breath . . . what is the result? Now, light the candle again. Allow the flame to diminish but take the glass away just before it goes out completely. Discuss what happens. Make the connection to the importance of taking time to breathe fully to energize and refresh our bodies and minds.

Consider this: One good breath will allow a child to relax mentally and physically. One good breath will teach a child to pause before committing to her words and actions. One good breath will help a child release her anger and approach difficult situations with a clear mind. One good breath will help a child gather the courage to take a calculated risk, whether it's trying something different or making a new friend. One good breath will improve a child's focus, so she can perform better at school, on the ball field, and at home. One good breath will remind a child to smile, to forgive, to play, to love, to live. If one good breath will help a child achieve all of this, imagine what a lifetime of good breaths will do!

There is truly something profound that happens when a family comes together for the simple purpose of conscious breathing. Take time to breathe together as a family. No words needed! Notice stress levels diminish as connectedness improves, all with a few deep breaths.

BREATHING EXERCISES

Unless otherwise noted, the following exercises can be practiced sitting in Easy Pose or Hero Pose, sitting up in a chair with feet flat on the floor, standing in Mountain Pose, or in some cases, even lying down. The most important consideration is that your child maintains a position where the lungs and diaphragm have space to move and open completely.

For easy reference, the breathing exercises presented are categorized as Energizing or Calming. But keep in mind that depending on the intention and situation at hand, many of these exercises can be energizing, empowering, and calming—all at the same time. For example, a child who's had a bad day at school can release his frustrations and be empowered at the same time when practicing Lion's Breath (categorized as an energizing breath). But, through doing so, he can also calm himself and bring his nervous system back to a more grounded and centered state. Use the benefits of the breath provided to help guide you.

Energizing

Is your child tired from a long day of school, or a long soccer practice? Does your child need to relieve some tension or frustration? Is he feeling downtrodden? Does he need a confidence boost? Choose to practice breathing exercises from this category any time your child is feeling tired or needs to be empowered. You can incorporate these breathing exercises into your yoga sessions when you notice your child's energy is waning.

Benefits

Releases tension

Energizes, empowers

Lifts mood

WHAT TO DO

Conductor Breath is a variation of the traditional Breath of Joy, which is fitting, as it's great fun to practice Conductor Breath! It can provide a quick and easy way to loosen up and gain a new perspective, relieve tension or frustration, and can serve as an energy booster. On the last exhale forward, encourage your child to hang down in Rag Doll Pose (Chapter 6) for several breaths before inhaling to slowly rise back up to standing.

WHAT TO SAY

Begin in Mountain Pose (Chapter 6) with your feet slightly wider than hip distance apart. Inhale through your nose slightly while bringing your arms out in front of you. Inhale a little more and swing your arms out to your sides. Now, inhale all the way as you swing your arms way up over your head. Exhale, "Ha!" and let your arms and torso fall forward between your bent legs. Good! Now, pop right back up to inhale your arms forward, then out to the sides, then all the way up . . . "Ha!" Repeat a few times, using the momentum of your forward fall to help propel you back up to the first inhale. When you are done, come to rest in Rag Doll Pose for a few breaths before slowly rising back up to standing.

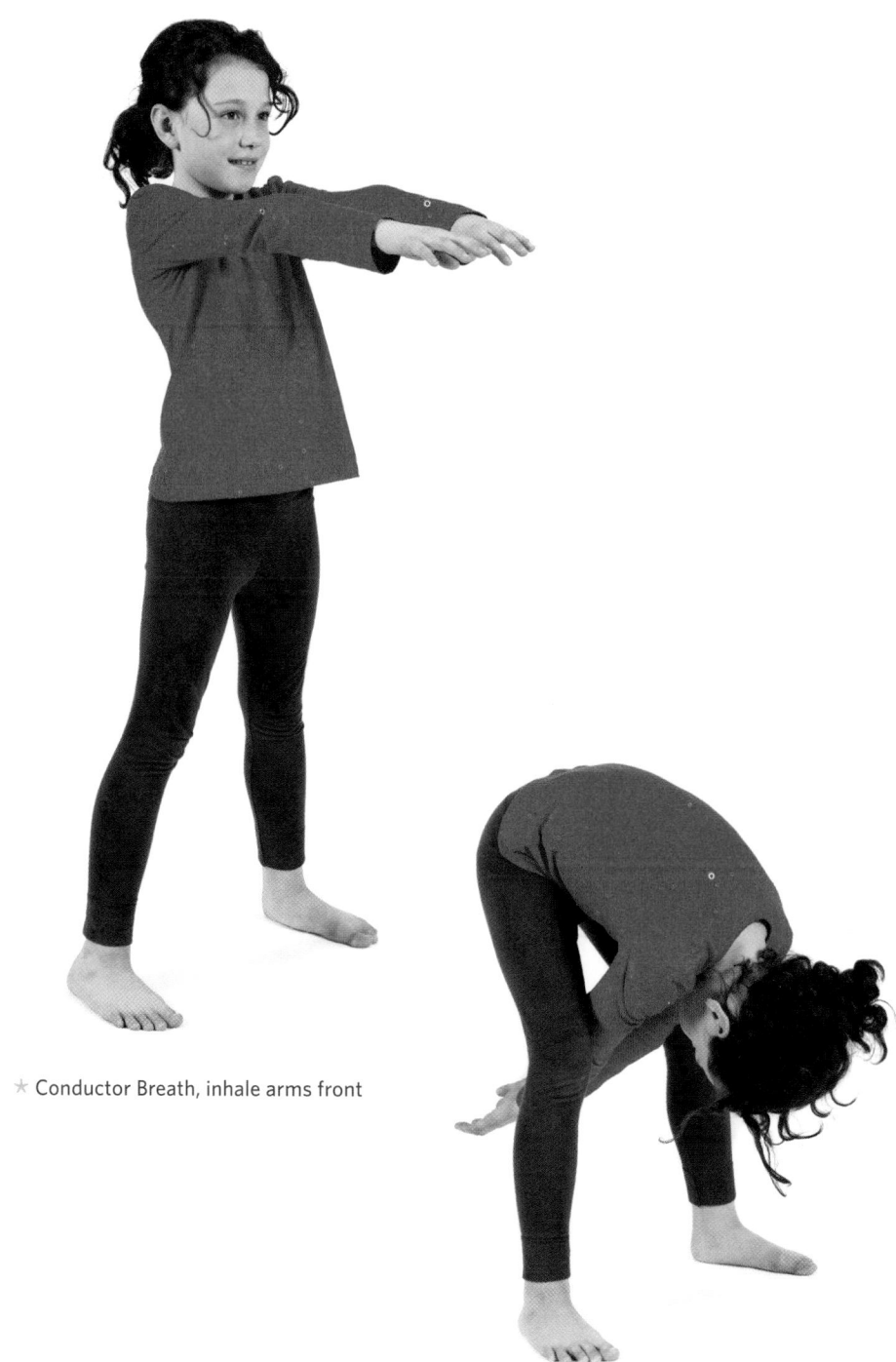

★ Conductor Breath, inhale arms front

★ Conductor Breath, exhale fall forward

Benefits

| Integrates both sides of the brain and body |
| Clears the mind |
| Improves focus |
| Calms and energizes |

WHAT TO DO

This is a kid-friendly version of traditional Alternate Nostril Breathing. Be sure your child does not press down too hard when blocking his nostril so as not to close off the other side as well. To encourage an inward focus, have your child close her eyes. If she has a slightly stuffy nose, this breath may help clear it. However, if her stuffy nose is blocking her air passage completely, skip this exercise until she is feeling better.

WHAT TO SAY

Sit or stand up tall. Gently place your right pointer finger over your right nostril to close it. Breathe in and out slowly and deeply through your left nostril for 3 breaths. Pause and switch to close off your left nostril. Breathe in and out slowly and deeply through your right nostril for 3 breaths. Continue to switch back and forth for 1 to 3 minutes or more. Notice how you feel.

Whole Brain Breathing

Breathing in through the left nostril stimulates the right "feeling" hemisphere of the brain, and breathing in through your right nostril stimulates the left "thinking" hemisphere of the brain. Alternating the breath between both nostrils integrates both sides of the brain for improved brain function. A couple of minutes of Alternate Nostril Breathing before homework time or a test is a great way for your child to access his whole brain for improved performance.

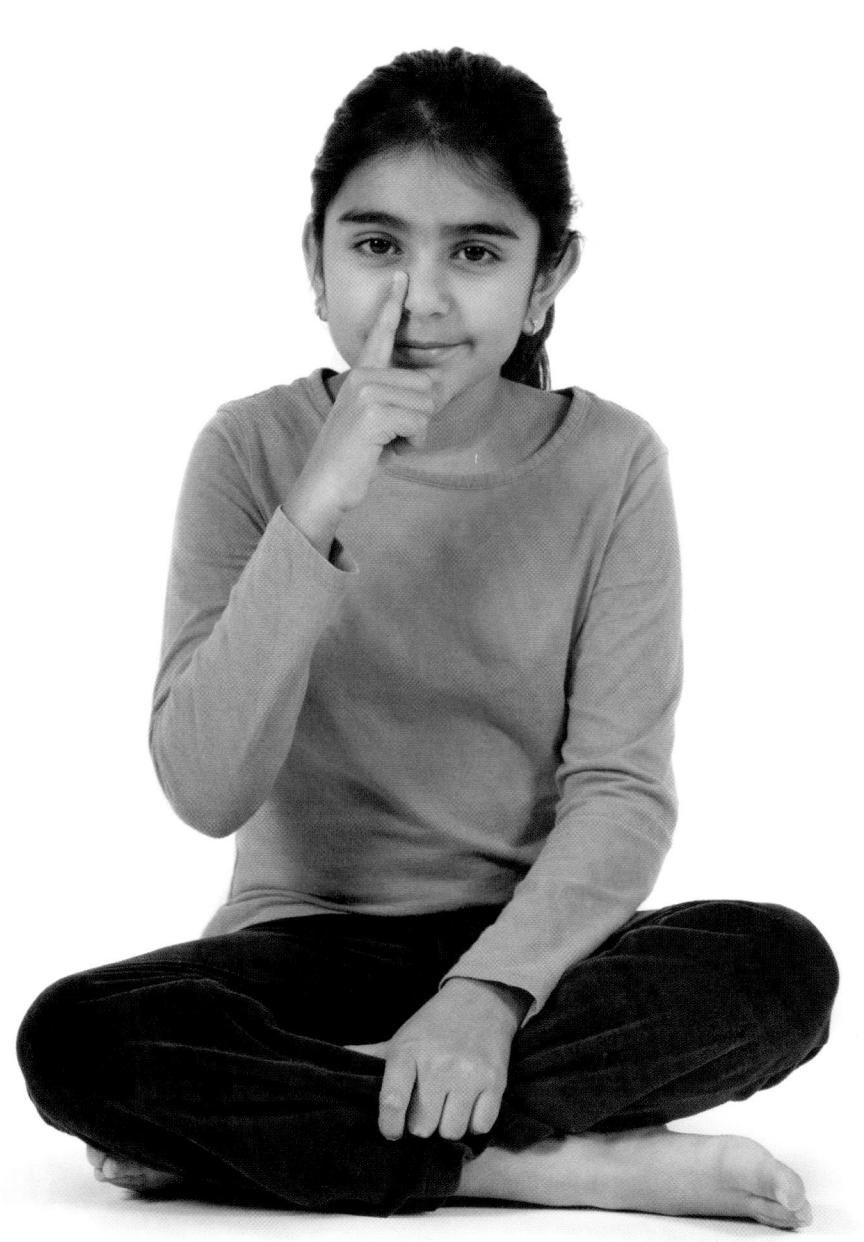

★ Alternate Nostril Breathing

Chapter 5: Breath Work 87

BUMBLE BEE BREATH

Benefits

Encourages an inward focus

Connects to inner self

Promotes speech development

Calms and centers

Promotes new perspective

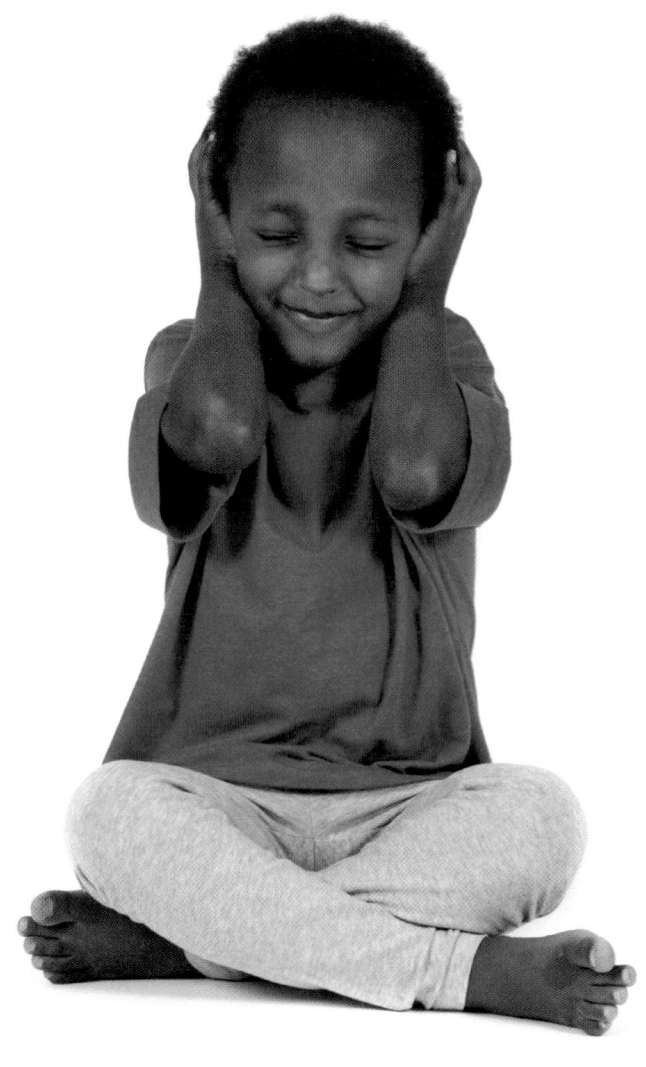

★ Bumble Bee Breath

WHAT TO DO

This breath is presented in three steps, working to bring awareness from the outside, in. After each step, encourage your child to share his experience. Once your child is comfortable with Bumble Bee Breath, have him experiment with breathing out other sounds such as "Zzzzz," "Ohhhh," "Shhhh," "LIII" or "Sssss." Note that some children can be startled or uncomfortable with how loud their hum becomes when their ears are blocked. To avoid this, encourage your child to simply cup his hands over his ears rather than blocking them with his fingers.

WHAT TO SAY

Sit or stand up tall. Take a slow, deep breath in through your nose before exhaling out to "Hummmmmm," as long as possible. Try it again, but this time with your eyes closed. Focus on the humming sound. Notice the vibration created in your lips. Was that a different experience? How so? Now, let's try it again but with your eyes closed and your ears covered with your hands. Where did your focus go? How do you feel? Shall we try that again?

BUNNY BREATH

Benefits

Refreshes and energizes

Clears the mind

WHAT TO DO

It's a fine line between energizing our bodies and minds and over-oxygenating them. When practicing Bunny Breath, only allow your child to do three to five breaths. As well, be sure your child sighs audibly to exhale so that you can ensure she is exhaling completely. Encourage your younger child (or even your older one!) to make bunny ears with her hands, twitch her nose, and hop like a bunny—make it fun!

WHAT TO SAY

Sit or stand up tall. Imagine that you are a bunny sniffing around for some yummy carrots. Take three to five quick sniffs in through your nose. Pause. Exhale out through your mouth with a long, slow, audible sigh. Repeat four or five times.

POWER BREATH

Benefits

Empowers

Boosts confidence

Energizes

WHAT TO DO

Try adding power-boosting affirmations to this breath as you raise your arms up with your child. Try, "I have the sun within me . . . Ha!" or "When I feel anxious, I can breathe in the sun's power . . . Ha!" or "I am filled with energy . . . Ha!" Encourage your child to come up with his own affirmations and take turns saying them as you practice this exercise together.

WHAT TO SAY

Stand in Mountain Pose (Chapter 6) with your feet hip distance apart. Inhale and reach your arms out to your sides and up to the sun. Grab some of the sun's powerful energy and forcefully exhale to say "Ha!" as you pull it down into your own place of power—your solar plexus, located just below your rib cage. Repeat this sequence at least 3 times or until you feel your personal place of power is filled up with power and light. "Ha!" How do you feel?

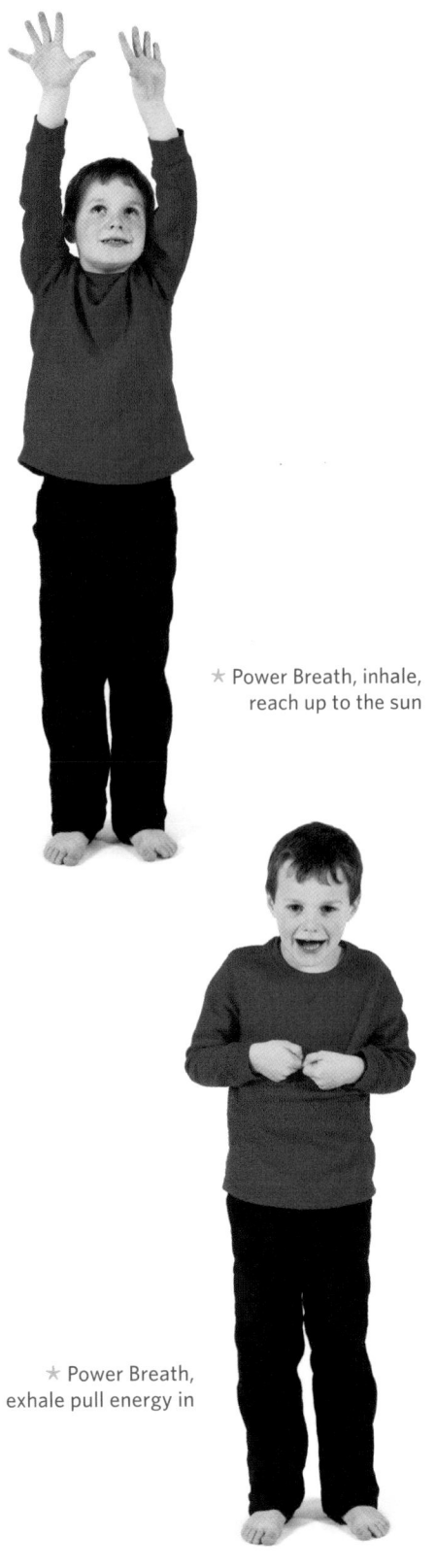

★ Power Breath, inhale, reach up to the sun

★ Power Breath, exhale pull energy in

LION'S BREATH

Benefits

Strengthens the diaphragm

Relieves tension in the face, neck, and body

Connects children to their inner strength

Releases excess energy

WHAT TO DO

This breath can get really loud and it's okay! Encourage your child to connect with his inner strength and courage when practicing Lion's Breath. For extra fun, feign your fear, pretending to cower back from his roar.

WHAT TO SAY

Come into Hero Pose (Chapter 6), close your eyes, and imagine yourself as a strong and fierce lion. Take a deep inhale through your nose. Exhale out through your wide-open mouth, while sticking out your tongue toward your chin. Open your eyes wide and let out a "ROAR!" Yikes, you are fierce!

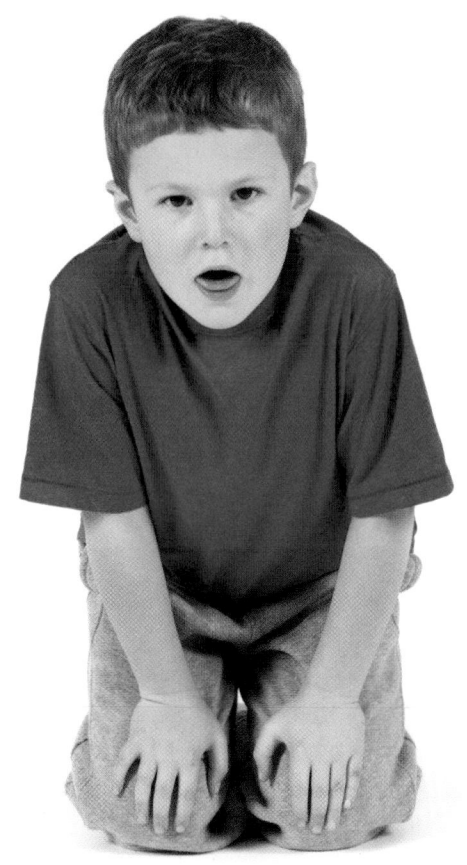

★ Lion's Breath

CALMING

Is your child overstimulated, anxious, or upset? Does your child need to dispel some excess energy? These calming, integrating breath exercises are perfect for opening or closing the yoga sessions with your child, before nap or bedtime, when your child is feeling frustrated, or before starting homework.

COUNT DOWN TO CALM

Benefits

| Relieves frustration |
| Alleviates anxiety |
| Calms |
| Encourages focus |

WHAT TO DO

Slowing and deepening our breath can help us slow down and relax our bodies and minds. Encourage your child to think of times when she could benefit from practicing Count Down to Calm breath. If your younger child has trouble counting with her fingers, have her watch you as you use your own fingers to count. An older child may opt not to use her fingers at all, choosing instead to close her eyes and count silently to herself.

WHAT TO SAY

Sit or stand up tall. Holding up one hand, lift one finger at a time, counting 1, 2, 3, 4, 5, as you inhale. Pause. Exhale and count down backward, 5, 4, 3, 2, 1, as you pull one finger in at a time. Repeat 3 to 5 times or until you feel relaxed and calm.

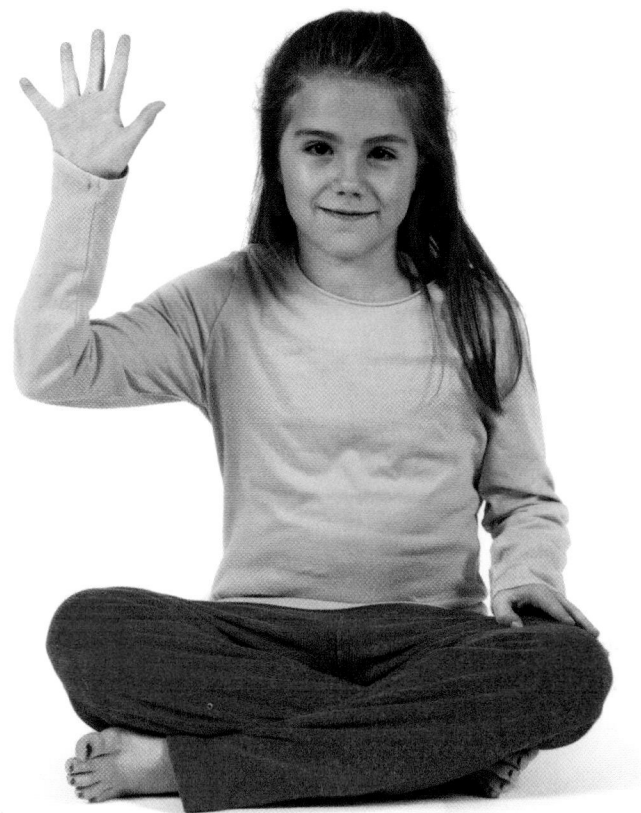

* Count Down to Calm

Start a Breath Log

Count Down to Calm and other breath work can serve as wonderful self-regulation tools that your child can use as needed when she is on her own. Ask your child to think of times it would be good to use this and other types of breathing exercises. Encourage her to start a breath log (maybe you can start one, too!), jotting down when and where she practiced a particular breath and how she felt before and after. Obviously, your prewriting child may need some writing assistance with this exercise. You might even start a sticker chart for the purpose of encouraging the use of these valuable tools.

EXTENDED EXHALE BREATH

Benefits

Calms
Alleviates anxiety
Encourages focus and concentration

WHAT TO DO

With this breath, the exhale is twice as long as the inhale. Count up to 5 as your child inhales slowly, filling up her lungs. Count up to 10 as you encourage her to exhale slowly. It may take a few attempts for your child to judge how slowly to exhale to get to 10 without feeling as if she ends up holding her breath. Part of this exercise is practice! Don't worry if she doesn't understand it the first few times. She will, as long as you continue to guide her over time.

WHAT TO SAY

Sit or stand up tall. Breathe in through your nose, filling up your belly, 1, 2, 3, 4, 5. Pause. Now exhale slowly to 10: 1, 2, 3, 4, 5, 6, 7, 8, 9, 10. Good. Let's try that again. (Repeat 3 to 5 times or more.)

OCEAN BREATH

Benefits

Calms
Promotes focus and concentration
Grounds and centers

WHAT TO DO

This breath is called Ocean Breath because you make the sound of ocean waves by contracting the back of the throat (the glottis) with the inhalation and exhalation. This breath is done through the nose, but it is helpful to introduce it by first practicing breathing through the mouth. If your child is having trouble "hearing" his ocean waves, have him cover his ears while closing his eyes. Is your child a Star Wars fan? He might be interested to know that Ocean Breath is also known as "Darth Vader Breath!"

WHAT TO SAY

Sit or stand up tall. First, take a deep breath in through your nose. Exhale and whisper out the sound "hhhh" through your mouth, as if you were fogging up a mirror. Inhale again through your nose. When you exhale this time, keep your mouth closed as you make the "hhhh" sound. Slowly breathe back in through your nose, keeping the back of your throat slightly constricted. Good! Can you hear the sound of the ocean waves crashing in and flowing out? Continue this breath for 1 minute. In . . . and . . . out.

CRASHING WAVE BREATH

Benefits

Calms
Encourages grace and finesse
Connects and builds community

WHAT TO DO

For extra fun use a scarf for this exercise, but it's not required. Crashing Wave Breath can be practiced alone, together (standing across from one another), or as a family (in a circle) with each person holding a separate scarf. It serves as a wonderful centering exercise to start a yoga session or as a transition to relaxation activities.

WHAT TO SAY

Imagine an ocean wave coming into shore, then crashing and flowing back out to sea. Breathe in slowly and deeply while walking forward like a wave coming into shore. Holding your scarf with both hands, raise your arms up like a growing wave. Now, lower your scarf down as you walk backward. Exhale to make a crashing wave sound, "Psshhhhhhhhh." (Repeat at least five times.)

BALLOON BREATH

Benefits

Improves focus

Promotes clarity

Calms and centers

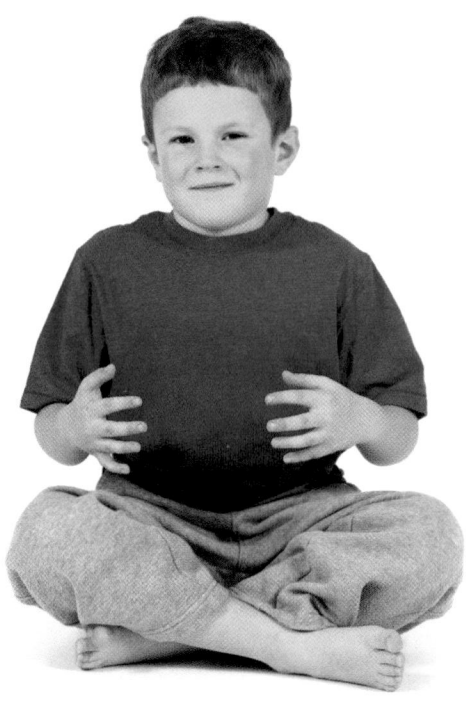

★ Balloon Breath

WHAT TO DO

When leading your child in Balloon Breathing, use your hands to demonstrate the way the belly should rise and fall. Using your hands will also provide a visual guide to the pace at which your child should be inhaling and exhaling. As an alternative, try using a Hoberman Sphere® (Chapter 3), one of the recommended props, as a visual guide to pacing and a wonderfully engaging point of focus for your child. If your child is willing to close his eyes while practicing Balloon Breath, you can provide a visual focus by encouraging him to imagine the color of his "balloon."

WHAT TO SAY

Sit or stand up tall or lie down. Place your hands gently on your lower belly. Close your eyes. Imagine your belly is a balloon. To inflate your balloon belly, breathe in slowly through your nose, filling up your balloon belly. That's right, stick your belly out to fill it up all the way. Now slowly exhale and feel your balloon belly deflate. Let all that stale air out of the balloon to escape out through your nose. (Repeat 4 to 6 times.) What did you notice? How do you feel?

CANDLE BREATH

Benefits

WHAT TO DO

This is a wonderfully simple first breathing exercise for your youngest child. Candle Breath encourages an extended exhale, which stimulates the parasympathetic nervous system and has a calming effect. To avoid over-oxygenation, this breath should be practiced slowly no more than five times with the emphasis on the exhale. For extra fun, have your child hold up the same number of fingers as his age. As with any real or imaginary exercise involving a candle, fire, or flame, be sure to remind your child of your family's fire safety rules.

WHAT TO SAY

Sit or stand up tall. Clasp your hands in front of you. Bring your pointing fingers together and point them up. There's your candle! Imagine there is a flame on top. Breathe in deeply through your nose to fill up your belly. Now slowly blow out your candle . . . let's do that two more times.

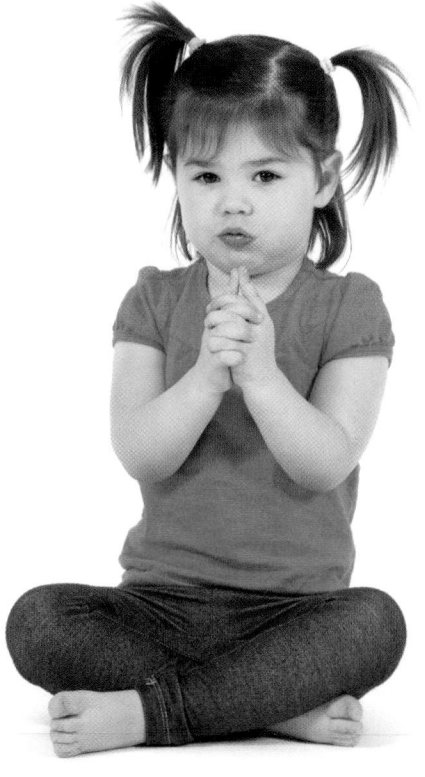

★ Candle Breath

FLYING BIRD BREATH

Benefits

Calms and centers

Promotes body awareness

Encourages poise and grace

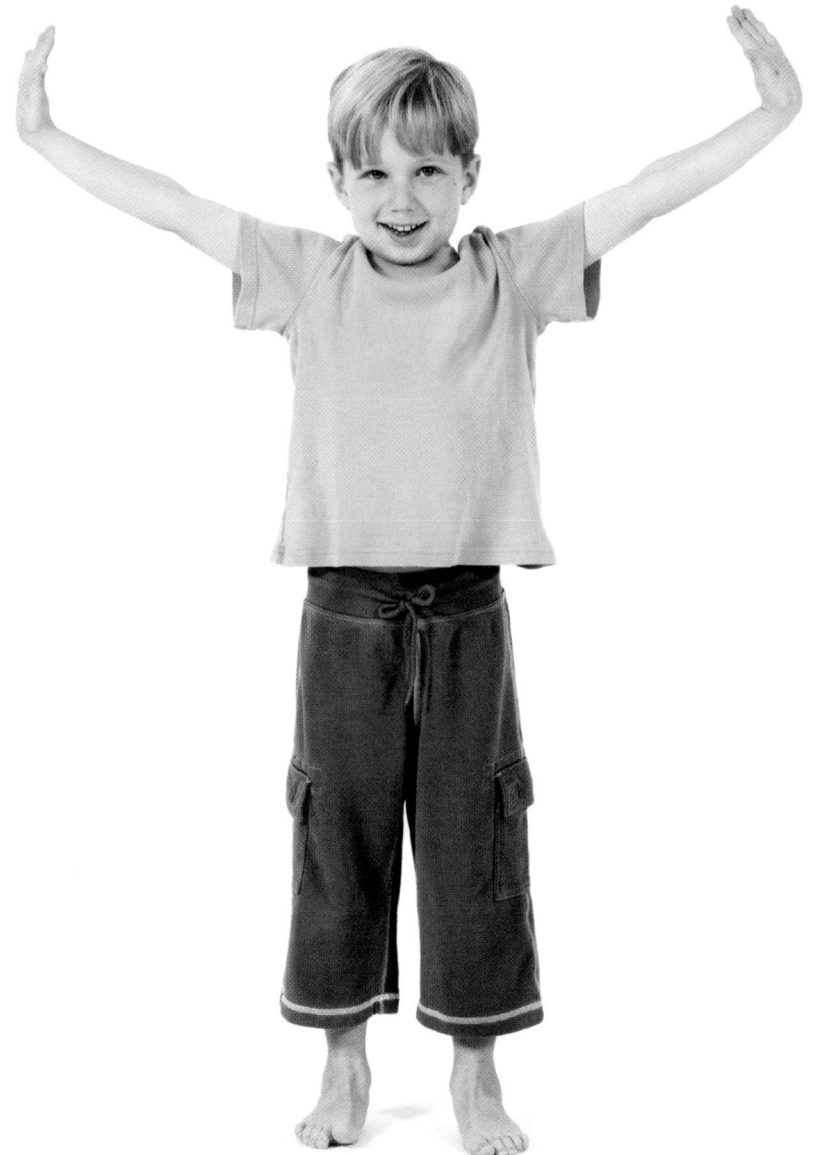

★ Flying Bird Breath

WHAT TO DO

Flying Bird Breath is a simple, calming breath appropriate for all ages. It can be practiced sitting, standing, or even while slowly walking. As you lift and lower your arms, you'll be ensuring a slow pace and providing a helpful visual for your child. To encourage an inward focus, have your child close his eyes if that's comfortable for him. Try using Flying Bird Breath as a transition between one activity and another, or whenever your child needs to catch his breath or take a break during a session.

WHAT TO SAY

Sit or stand up tall and close your eyes. Imagine you are a beautiful, strong bird with large, open wings. Breathe in slowly while lifting your arms out to the sides, palms facing up. Continue to inhale as you reach up with straight arms and touch your palms together above your head. Exhale slowly as you turn your palms down and lower your arms. Repeat several times, slowly and fluidly, as you move with your breath. Notice how you feel.

Adventures in Flying

Flying Bird Breath can serve as a wonderful centering activity. While practicing Flying Bird Breath, have your child close his eyes and imagine he is taking flight. If your child is under 6, guide him to visualize a particular journey and what he might see on that journey. For an older child, ask him questions like "What do you see on your journey?" After a minute or two, guide your child to end his journey and share about his adventure.

DOG BREATH

Benefits

Cools the body and refreshes the mind

Helps dissipate anger and frustration

WHAT TO DO

Curling the tongue or making an "O" shape with the mouth slows the airflow. This is a safe breath for all ages.

WHAT TO SAY

Sit or stand up tall. Stick out your tongue and curl it. If you can't curl your tongue, just form an "O" shape with your mouth. Inhale through your mouth to the count of 3. Pause. Then exhale to the count of 5. (Repeat five or six times.)

BLOW IT BREATHING

Benefits

Strengthens the diaphragm

Promotes speech development

★ Blow It Breathing

WHAT TO DO

Using anything from pretend flowers with lavender scent sprayed on them to pinwheels, feathers, tissues, or cotton balls, you can turn many objects into "blow its." It's a simple breathing exercise that is lots of fun! Do use caution when practicing this breath with your young child, ensuring he emphasizes and extends the exhale/blowing, as opposed to the inhale. As well, Blow It Breathing should only be repeated a few times to avoid potential lightheadedness and hyperventilation.

WHAT TO SAY

Take this pinwheel. Take a deep breath in through your nose. Now, slowly blow on the pinwheel. Can you get the pinwheel to spin? Keep your eyes focused on the pinwheel. Can you keep it moving with your breath?

STOP AND SMELL THE FLOWERS

Benefits

Calms
Expands the lungs
Cleanses

WHAT TO DO

Try using real or artificial flowers sprayed with Magic Mist (Chapter 3) with your youngest child for this exercise. Encourage your child to practice smelling the flowers slowly, taking his time to really fill up his lungs. Then be sure your child audibly exhales so that you can ensure he is exhaling completely.

WHAT TO SAY

Imagine you are in a garden or field full of your favorite flowers. Stop and smell the flowers! Close your eyes and picture your favorite flower in your mind, its color, its shape, and its smell. Breathe in very slowly and deeply to smell the beautiful fragrance of your favorite flower. How does it smell? Say, "Ahhhhh!" as you exhale very slowly. (Repeat Smell the Flowers Breath 3 to 6 times, focusing on the slow pace of the breath.)

GOOD IN/BAD OUT BREATH

Benefits

Encourages perspective change

Empowers

Dissipates negativity

WHAT TO DO

Good In/Bad Out Breath is a wonderful practice for your older child. Preteens and teens sometimes experience a period of negative thinking as a protective mechanism to help them deal with the challenges and changes inherent in being an adolescent. Encourage your child to use this breath any time she needs a confidence boost or perspective shift.

WHAT TO SAY

Find a comfortable seated position, sit up tall, and close your eyes. Think of something positive to say about yourself. Using Ocean Breath as your guide, breathe in a positive thought, letting it get big, flowing into your heart, and out to all the parts of your body. Exhale any negative thoughts that come up. For example, my positive thought might be: "I can do my best." I breathe in the positive thought, then breathe out any negative thoughts that counteract it, such as: "It's too hard. I can't do it." Imagine those negative thoughts releasing out from your body and flowing out through the window and up to the sky. On your last few breaths, just focus on the positive thought, allowing any remaining negativity to scatter away naturally.

BACK-TO-BACK BREATHING

Benefits

Calms

Encourages breath awareness

Promotes connectedness

WHAT TO DO

Back-to-Back Breathing is a partner breath exercise that offers an opportunity to connect with your child in a deep and meaningful way. Use it as a transition to bedtime, sharing time, or any time you need calm and connection.

WHAT TO SAY

Let's sit back-to-back in Easy Pose (Chapter 6). Let the weight of your body push back against me. Can you feel the warmth of my back? I can feel yours. It's a warm, peaceful feeling. Let's practice Balloon Breathing. Breathe in slowly through your nose, filling up your balloon belly. Fill it up all the way so that your entire belly and chest expand. Now slowly exhale and feel your balloon belly deflate. Let all that stale air out of the balloon belly to escape out through your nose. Let's do that again, breathing together. What did you notice? How do you feel?

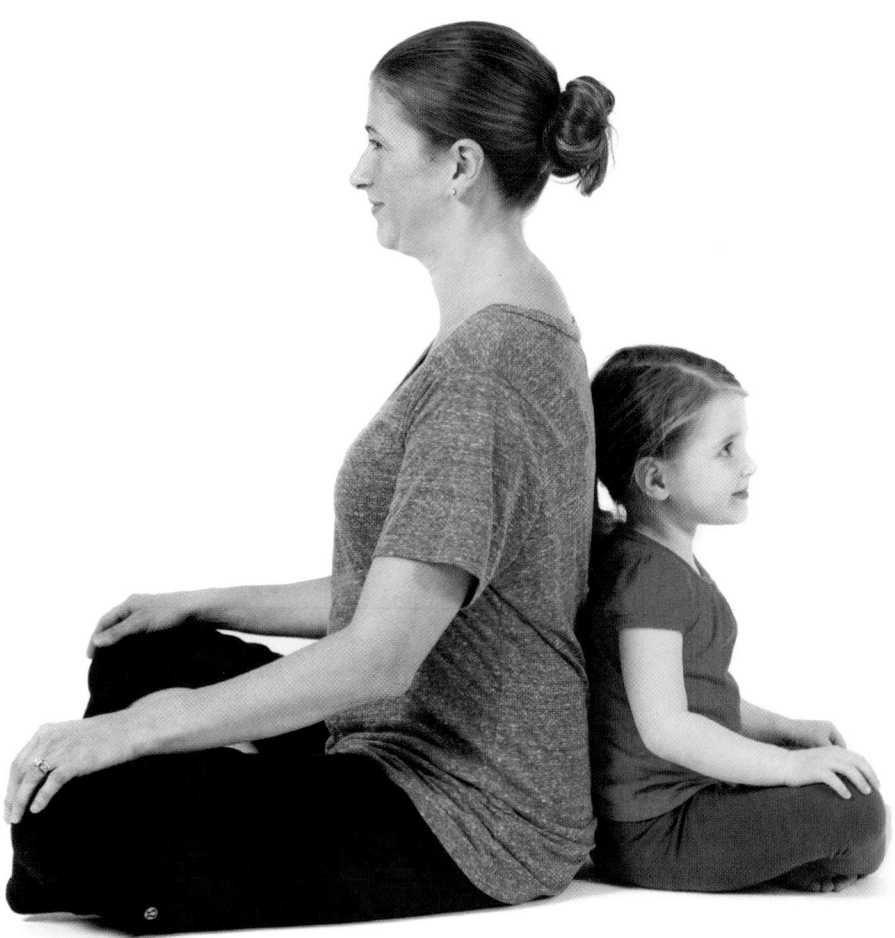

★ Back-to-Back Breathing

CHAPTER 6

Poses and Partner Poses

WORKING WITH POSES

Movement is the basis for physical and cognitive development. Babies begin with body language as their first form of communication. Over time, with experimentation and an open area to move their bodies, babies learn to roll over, crawl and then walk, grasp objects, and later even throw a ball. Today, we often put our babies in carriers, lie them on their backs to sleep (as recommended to avoid SIDS), and are hesitant to put them on the floor. As they grow, they might watch TV rather than play outside, while at school they spend much of the 6-hour day sitting at a desk. Perhaps not surprisingly, children today are being increasingly diagnosed with motor challenges and learning disabilities.

Yoga poses provide the physical component of a yoga practice. Designed to open the joints and stretch and strengthen the muscles, yoga poses and yoga-based movements also move lymph through the body (which plays a critical role in the function of the immune system), help improve coordination, boost circulation, and promote mindfulness through conscious, focused movement. Note that movement is also the foundation for learning. When children fold over in Rag Doll Pose, they're increasing blood flow to the brain; when they balance in Eagle Pose, they're improving concentration skills; when they reach across into Twisty Star, they're performing cross-lateral movements that optimize the communication between the right and left hemispheres of the brain, essential to the development of higher reasoning and motor planning. Structured yoga-based movements provide children an opportunity to become aware of their bodies. When yoga poses are paired with breathing, meditation, and relaxation exercises, children learn to notice how they feel and begin to self-regulate by calling upon and utilizing these simple exercises as needed.

The more traditional poses (though sometimes given kid-friendly names) include basic instructions as it is assumed that you are somewhat familiar with them. There are also many unique, child-friendly poses offered here. Some of the poses include variations, suggestions that really make the pose come to life for children! The ideas include partner versions of the pose to try out with your child, games, creative movement options, or questions—most with the purpose of extending the time the pose is held, making it more educational and/or just making it more fun for kids.

To make them easy to find, all of the poses are listed in alphabetical order. Once you've chosen the intention or theme for your sequence (Chapter 10), you can pick and choose relevant yoga poses from this chapter.

Here are a few general tips to keep in mind as you share yoga poses with your child. Following these tips will help ensure your child is benefiting as much as possible from the practice while also ensuring her safety:

- **Establish foundational poses first.** Teach the three foundational poses first. These transitional poses provide a home base to return to between other poses, encouraging mindful movement. If standing, that is Mountain Pose. If sitting, that is Easy Pose. If lying down, that is lying flat on your back.
- **Encourage breath awareness.** With children ages 5 and up, be sure to encourage the breathing instructions as described in each "What to Say" section.
- **Encourage mindful awareness.** Being mindful means paying close attention to whatever we are doing (see Chapter 4 for more on mindfulness). During your child's yoga practice (and throughout the day), encourage her to get into her "mindful body" and to "be mindful." Bring your child's awareness to the sensations in her body as she practices the poses while teaching her about her body. Ask, "Where do you feel the stretch?" and say, "Notice which muscles are being strengthened. That's the ABC muscle." If your child is struggling, encourage her to notice her challenge without judgment and to modify accordingly. If she complains that something hurts, for example, you might respond, "It's wonderful that you are being mindful of what your body is telling you (focusing on the positive). Could you honor your body by easing off of the pose enough so that it is more comfortable? Here is a modification you can try."

→ beanie babies

- **Establish the "focus point."** When teaching balancing poses such as Airplane, Tree, Eagle, Triangle, or Warrior III, have your child find a "focus point"—something small and unmoving directly across from his line of vision. Remind your child to find his focus point whenever attempting a challenging balance pose.
- **Side bends versus forward bends.** When guiding your child into side-bending poses such as Crescent Moon or Triangle, it can be helpful to have her imagine she is the PB&J between two slices of bread. The sandwich filling squirts out the sides of the sandwich, not the front or back. This visual will help your child maintain a true side bend, as opposed to a forward bend.
- **Challenge counting.** To help engage and challenge your child, try counting out loud as he holds especially difficult poses.
- **Keep instructions and expectations age appropriate.** Use the "What to Say" section as a guideline and age up or down accordingly. A basic rule to follow is: the younger your child, the more simple/less wordy the instructions should be. To learn more about various ages and what to keep in mind for your presentation and expectations, visit Chapter 3.

AIRPLANE

Benefits

Improves balance and coordination

Strengthens and stretches hamstrings, back, and arms

WHAT TO DO
To help ensure success for a younger child, you might suggest she keep her back toe on or close to the floor when attempting Airplane Pose.

WHAT TO SAY
Begin in Mountain Pose, and prepare for liftoff! Find a focus point to help you with your balance. Breathe in . . . breathe out . . . now, extend your arms straight out from your sides like airplane wings and shift your weight to your right foot. Inhale to get tall and stretch your arms out wide. Now, 3, 2, 1, liftoff! Gently lift your left leg behind you. Bend forward at your hips and look ahead at your focus point. Can you keep the plane steady? Try breathing in . . . and out . . . while you fly. Now, get your body ready for a smooth landing: 3, 2, 1 . . . bring your left foot gently back down to earth. Return to Mountain Pose. You did it! Now, switch sides.

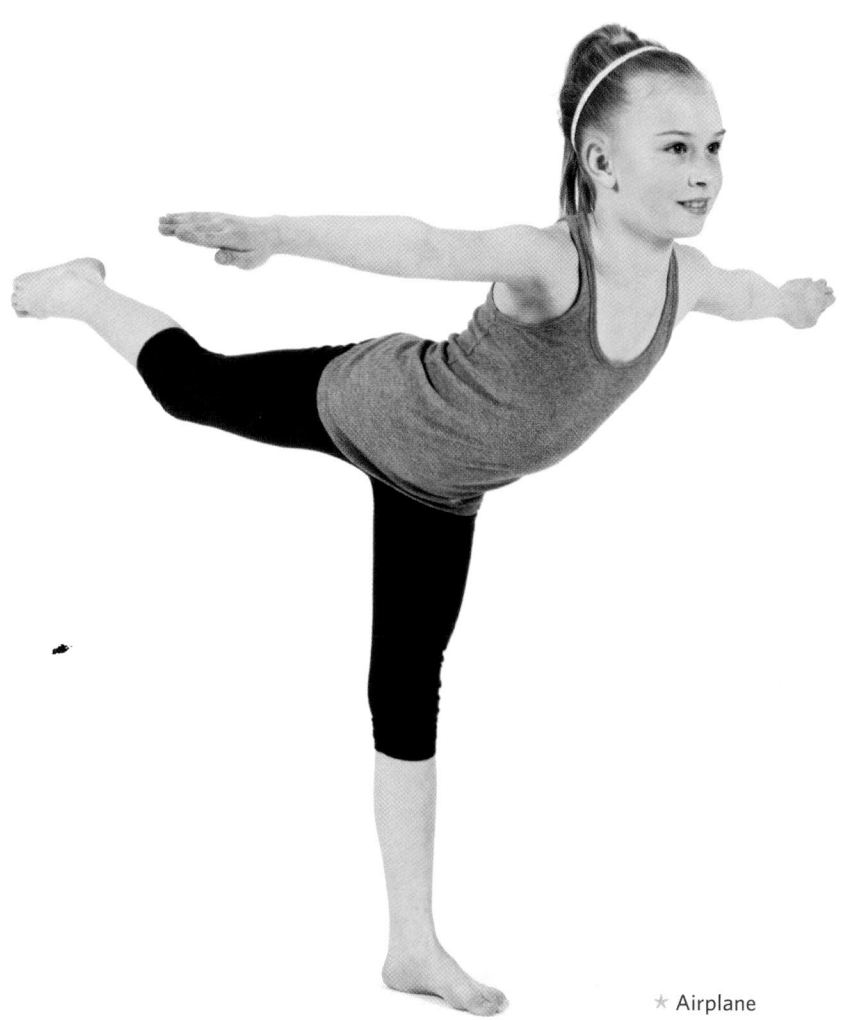

★ Airplane

Fly and Count

Counting out loud while holding a pose is an effective way to engage attention and use the breath, while practicing counting skills. Encourage your child to count to 5 while he holds the pose. Over time and with practice, he might count to 10 or more, providing a sense of accomplishment.

Benefits

| Massages the spine |
| Builds coordination |
| Builds core strength |

WHAT TO DO

To protect the spine, Ball Pose should be practiced on a carpet or thick or double-layered yoga mat. When introducing the pose to a young child or a child with poor core strength, you can support his rolls by kneeling beside him and placing one of your hands behind his upper back and the other under his knees.

WHAT TO SAY

Start in Easy Pose. Place your feet flat on the floor and wrap your arms around your knees. Gently roll back like a ball and inhale. Exhale and use your tummy muscles to pull yourself right back up again to sitting. Nice work! Can you keep the rolling going? Inhale back . . . exhale forward. It's fun to roll like a ball!

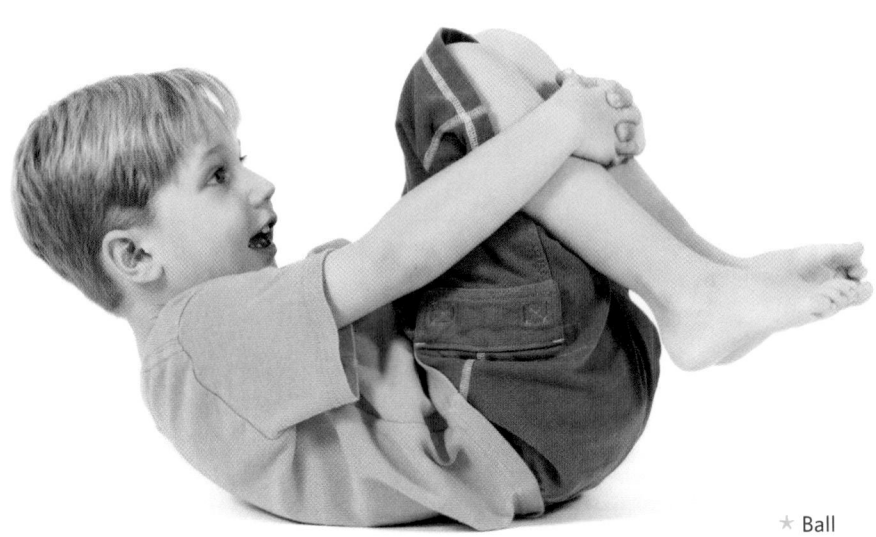

⋆ Ball

BALL VARIATIONS

Ball Pose is a challenging core strengthener. Try these variations of Ball Pose to keep your child engaged and having fun while improving her core strength.

- **Butter-Ball.** A cross between Butterfly Pose and Ball Pose. Roll like a ball while in Butterfly Pose, hands around your feet.
- **Roll and Stop!** Roll back and then come back up to balance on your bottom without touching toes to the floor.

BEE

Benefits

Stretches and strengthens arms and shoulders

Opens chest and lungs

WHAT TO DO

Encourage your child to really pull her shoulder blades back and in toward each other to help stretch her shoulders and open her chest. When she "flies," you can encourage flying around the room or just on her mat, depending on space and energy level.

WHAT TO SAY

Start in Mountain Pose. Make yourself into a bumble bee by putting on a stinger! Roll your shoulders back and reach around to clasp your hands behind you. Good! Now, puff out your chest to fly as you draw your hands up behind you to show off your stinger. Inhale deeply and exhale out, "Bzzzz!" as you fly off to find your beehive.

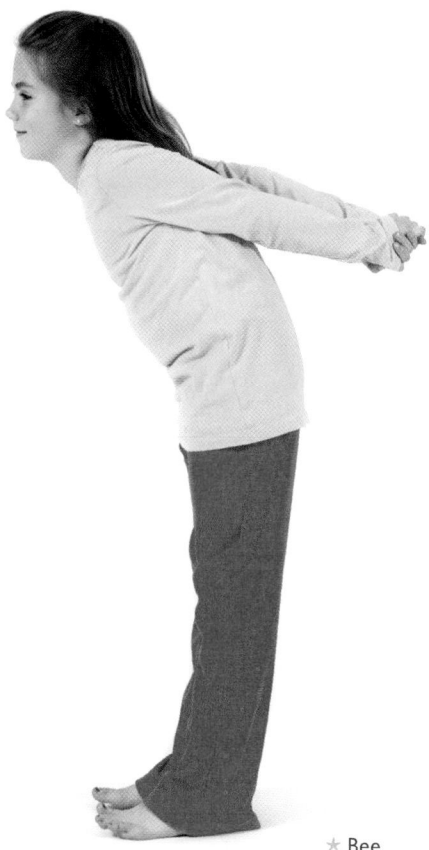

★ Bee

BOAT

Benefits

| Strengthens core muscles |
| Tones kidneys |
| Improves digestion |
| Stretches hamstrings |

WHAT TO DO

To protect delicate tailbones, this pose should be practiced on a carpet or thick yoga mat. Boat Pose is a challenging core strengthener and therefore your child may not wish to practice it or may want to give up easily. Try introducing the pose in stages. First, invite your child to keep her toes on the floor. Once she develops a bit of core strength, try encouraging her to lift her toes off the floor while keeping the knees bent. The final variation, Challenging Boat, stretches the legs and arms out fully. At whatever level your child is practicing, singing the "Row Your Boat" song (Chapter 8) while rowing the arms in Boat Pose is such fun, your child may forget how hard she's working!

WHAT TO SAY

Sit down with your feet on the floor, knees bent. Extend your arms straight out alongside your knees. Engage your tummy muscles to sit up tall. Lift one toe off the floor and then the other, and find your balance on your bottom bones. Be strong and breathe in and out, making sure your boat doesn't "tip over." If you are feeling really strong, try straightening out your legs. Now you're ready to sail! Can you breathe in and out and hold the pose while I count to 5? 1, 2, 3, 4, 5. Relax and rest for a moment and we can try it again!

BOAT VARIATIONS

Older children will be engaged by creative, challenging variations. Try these!

- **Rock the Boat.** Roll back in Ball Pose and then roll forward to come up and balance in Boat Pose. For even more of a challenge, hold the toes or feet in Boat Pose, roll back, and come to sitting in Boat Pose balance.
- **Half Boat.** From Boat Pose, use your tummy muscles to lower yourself down to hover above the water without sinking . . . don't sink! Trying pulling yourself back up to safety. You did it!

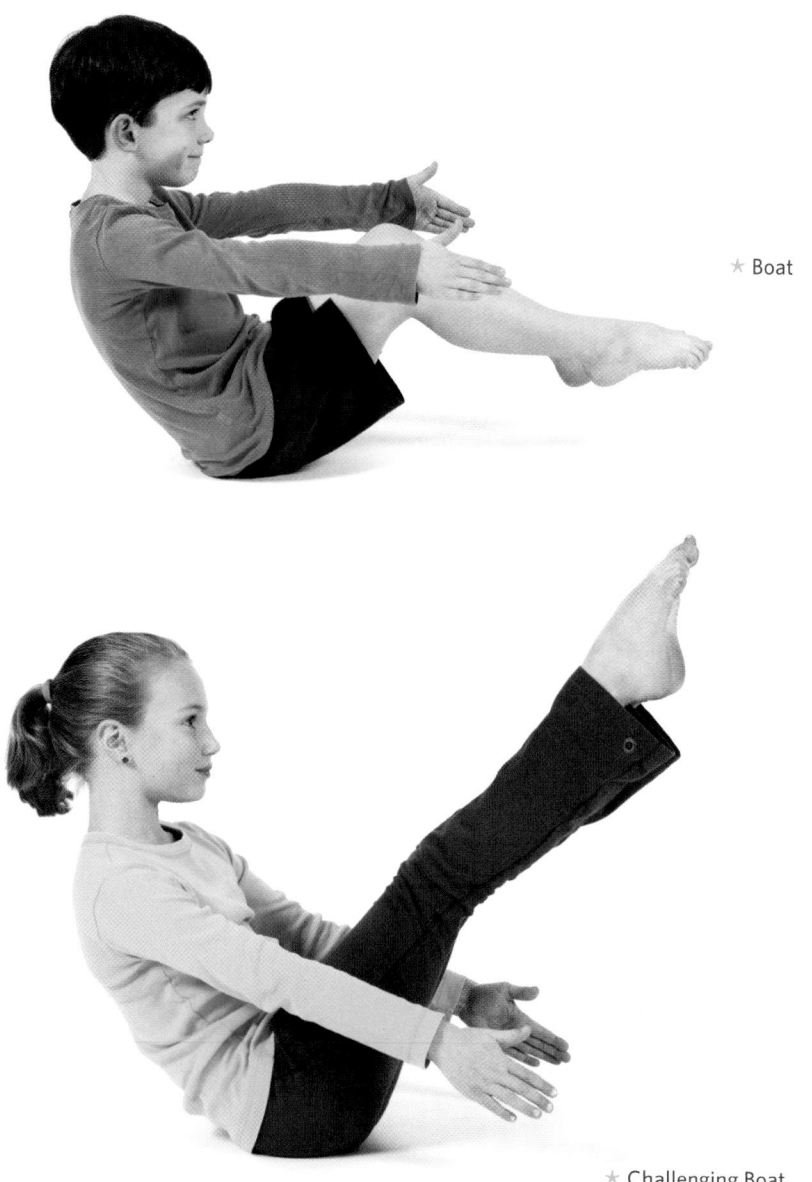

★ Boat

★ Challenging Boat

- **Double Boat.** For a partner version, sit across from your child with your knees bent. Hold hands on the outside of your legs to anchor yourself. Lean back and connect the soles of your feet together. Press into your feet to lift and extend one leg up at a time. It's a Double Boat!

Benefits

Improves posture
Aids digestion
Strengthens and stretches the shoulders, arms, legs, back, and glutes
Opens the lungs

WHAT TO DO

Half Bow and Full Bow Poses are beneficial after a long day of being hunched over a desk at school. These poses help improve posture while opening up the chest and lungs. Encourage your child to breathe with you, deeply and evenly, while practicing the poses. Diaphragmatic breathing is especially helpful for children with asthma or other respiratory challenges, and can be practiced any time energy is low.

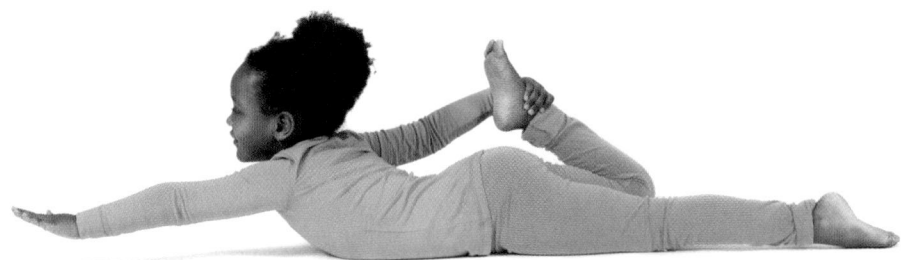

★ Half Bow

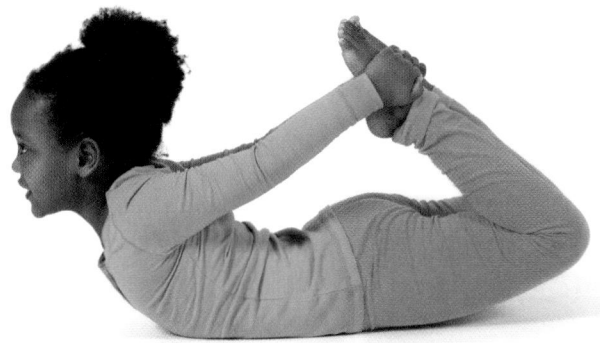

★ Full Bow

WHAT TO SAY

Begin by lying on your belly. Extend your left arm in front of you while keeping your left leg stretched out straight behind you. Reach back with your right hand to grab your right ankle. Press your foot back into your hand and notice your chest expand. You're a half bow! Breathe in . . . breathe out . . . now release to rest your head on your folded arms. Switch sides. Now try Full Bow. Lie on your belly. This time, grab hold of both your ankles. Look ahead and breathe in to lift and open your chest as you push your feet back into your hands. Take a few deep breaths here. Release and rest in Child's Pose.

BOW AND ARROW

Benefits

Opens hips

Lengthens leg muscles

Improves posture and core strength

WHAT TO DO

Encouraging good posture when you introduce this pose to your child will help her improve her core strength, coordination, and balance. If your child is struggling to stay upright, she can keep her opposite hand on the floor behind her, as pictured, or you can support her by holding her back with your hand. Try having your child hold and stretch in the pose for three breaths before switching sides.

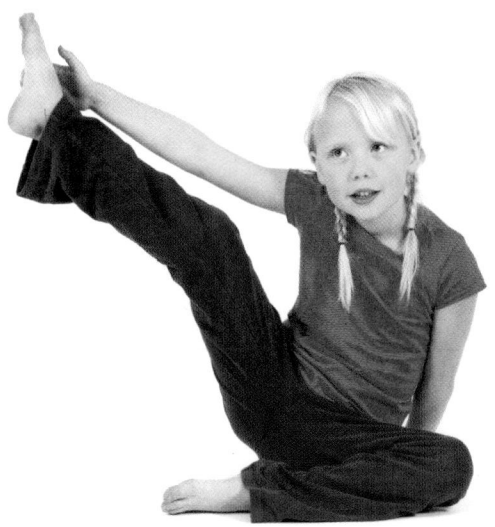

★ Bow and Arrow

WHAT TO SAY

Begin in Easy Pose. Hook your index finger around the same side big toe or the outside of your foot. Extend your leg. You're a Bow and Arrow! Let's hold this pose for three breaths . . . switch sides. (To your older child: Try to balance with both legs extended.)

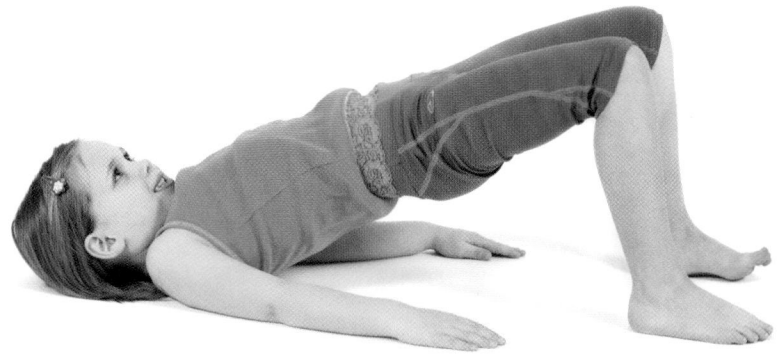

BRIDGE

Benefits

Strengthens legs, back, and glutes

Improves digestion

Opens chest and lungs

WHAT TO DO

For this pose, it helps to visualize a drawbridge and a boat needing to pass underneath. Ask "Can I get by?" as you pretend your hand is the "boat" trying to pass underneath the "bridge." With your younger child, you might even employ a toy boat to "sail" under his bridge when it's up. An older child or teen can try rolling her shoulders back and bringing the elbows closer together to clasp her hands under her body as she lifts her hips up high. Have your child practice breathing in and out 3 to 5 times as she holds the pose before resting for a moment and then trying it again.

WHAT TO SAY

Lie down on your back. Place your feet flat on the floor, hip-distance apart. Here comes the boat! Time to raise the bridge. Keeping your shoulders and feet flat on the floor, lift your hips high into the air. Good! Lift your chest up to arch your spine. (To older children: Shimmy your shoulders back and walk your elbows in to clasp your hands together.) Breathe in and out slowly three times. Now let's lower our bridges. Exhale as you gently bring your hips back down to the floor, rolling slowly down the spine. Rest and repeat this sequence a few times. When you're finished, pull your knees into your chest and rock from side to side to massage and rest your lower back.

BUTTERFLY

Benefits

WHAT TO DO

If your child has tight hips, have her sit on a folded blanket so that her hips are above her legs and feet. For the most benefit, encourage your child to sit up tall while practicing Butterfly Pose.

WHAT TO SAY

Sit up nice and tall and bring the bottoms of your feet together to form your butterfly wings. Breathing in, lift your knees up. Breathing out, lower your knees. You're flying . . . close your eyes and imagine what color your butterfly is and where it might like to fly today. Continue to breathe and flap your wings for a minute.

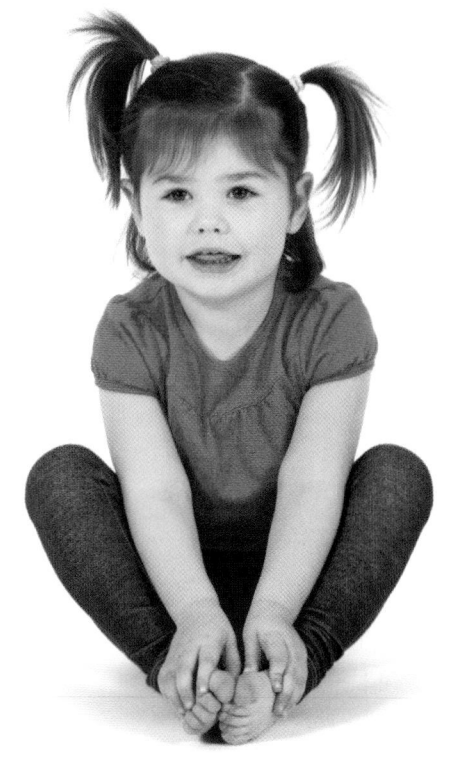

★ Butterfly, flapping wings

BUTTERFLY VARIATIONS

- **Sing the "Butterfly Song."** With your younger child, flap your leg "wings" up and down as you sing the "Butterfly Song" (Chapter 8).

- **Nose to Toes.** Challenge your child to fold forward to draw her nose down to her toes. Alternatively, she can lift one leg and bring her toes up to her nose and then switch sides. "How do your feet smell today?!"

CAMEL

Benefits

Stretches shoulders, thighs, and hips

Strengthens the back

Opens the throat, chest, and lungs

Releases fatigue

WHAT TO DO

For this pose, it's important to move slowly and mindfully to protect the neck and back. The tops of the feet can be flat on the floor, or the toes can be tucked under to bring the heels closer to the hands. The goal is to have your child extend and lift from the lower back, and elongate the neck rather than cranking it back. Your child should use her hands to support her lower back as she arches backward as well as to progress back out of the pose.

WHAT TO SAY

Kneel beside me. You can keep your feet flat on the floor or tuck your toes under to bring your heels closer to your hands. Bring your hands to your lower back, fingers pointing down. Open up your chest wide and breathe in . . . and breathe out. Now, try reaching back with one hand at a time for each of your heels. Press your hips forward, open your chest, and lift and lengthen your chin to the sky. You're a beautiful camel. Breathe in and out slowly three times. Slowly bring one hand then the other back to support your lower back before lifting up out of the pose.

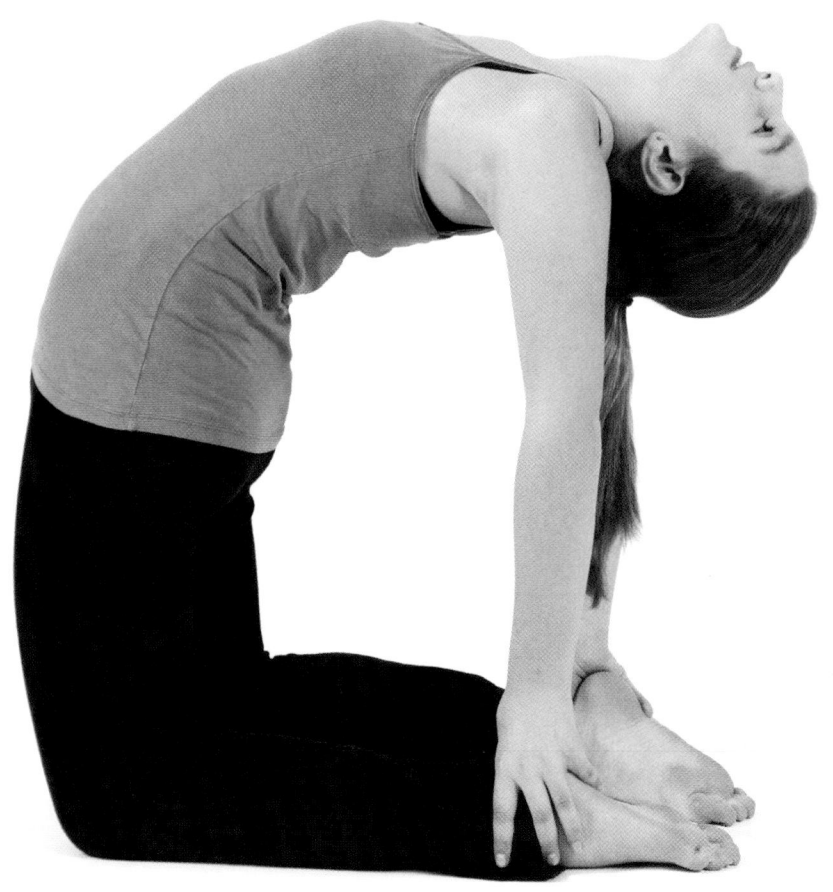

★ Camel

CANDLE

Benefits

Supports endocrine system

Promotes blood flow to the brain

Alleviates sinus issues

Aids digestion

WHAT TO DO

For a simpler version of Candle Pose, your younger child can simply lift her legs in the air, providing the added benefit of strengthening her core muscles (pictured as Candle, modified). If your older child is struggling to come into, but capable of holding, a full shoulder stand version of the pose, try standing in front of her raised legs and gently lifting them up by the ankles, or have her press her feet into a wall. She'll then be able to adjust her shoulders, elbows, and hands to support her weight. Be safe: It's fun to imagine lighting, being, and blowing out candles, but only in our imaginations. Be sure to review with your child your family's rules about fire safety, e.g., playing with matches.

WHAT TO SAY

Lie down on your back. Now swing your legs up into the air and "catch them" with your hands, keeping your arms and elbows on the ground. Can you bring your shoulders closer together? Keep your legs straight and point your toes to the sky! (For younger children: Wiggle your toes to flicker the "flame.")

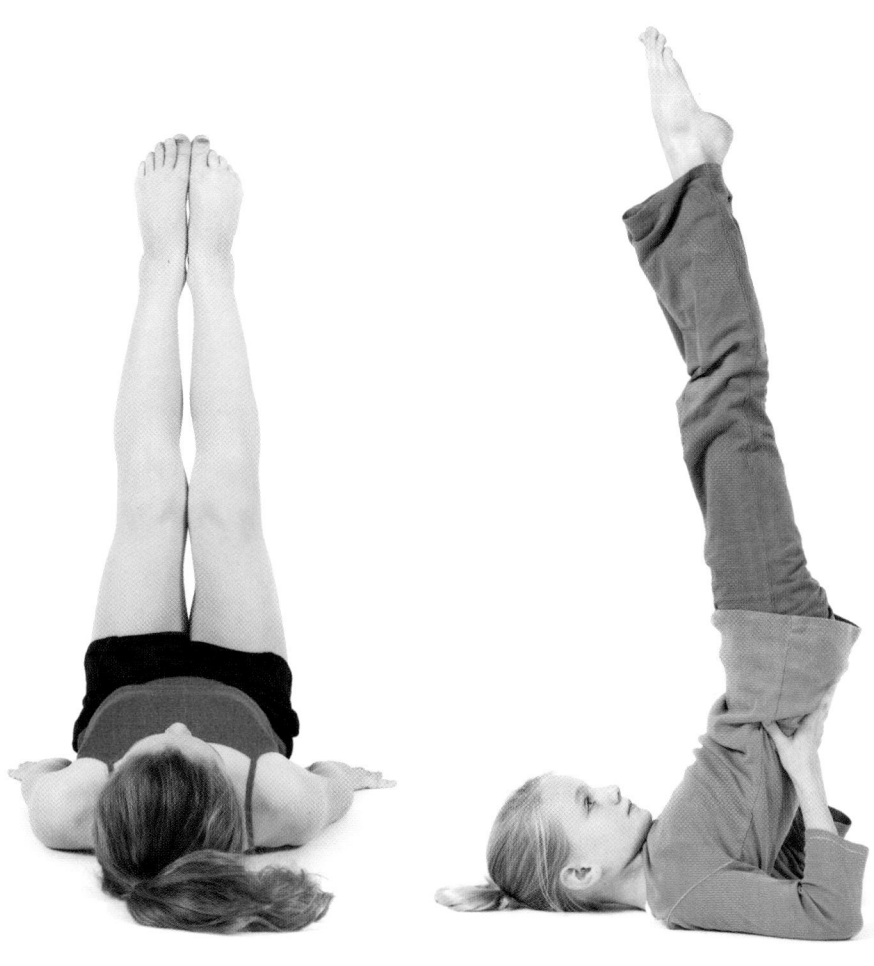

★ Candle, modified

★ Candle

Partner Variation

Twin Flames. Lying down lengthwise, with your heads a few inches apart, come into Candle Pose with your child. Touch your toes with your child's in the air to create twin flames.

CAT (HAPPY CAT/SCARED CAT)

Benefits

Improves coordination

Stretches and strengthens the back and spine

Massages the internal organs such as the kidneys

WHAT TO DO

This moving pose combination requires a level of body awareness and coordination that children of varying ages and abilities may still be developing. Try introducing just one pose at a time and have fun with it, allowing your child to make noise and be silly. When the individual poses are mastered, you can then combine to make a fun and silly flow!

WHAT TO SAY *tell them where to look*

Begin in Table Pose. Breathe in to open up your chest and look up at the sky. Say, "Meow!" You're a happy cat! Now arch your spine up to the sky and look underneath at your belly button. Say, "Hisssss." Inhale, Happy Cat, "Meow!" Exhale, Scared Cat, "Hisssss!" Meow and hiss to move from Happy Cat Pose to Scared Cat Pose several times. What a sweet kitty you are!

CAT VARIATIONS

These add-on poses will help your child develop balance and coordination while strengthening his back, arms, and legs.

- **Cat Stretch.** From Table Pose, lift your right arm straight out in front of you. Now lift your left leg straight out behind you. Balance for one full breath, in and out, before exhaling both limbs back down. Switch sides, inhaling as you lift your left arm and right leg, exhaling as you lower them.
- **Silly Cat.** Starting in Table Pose, stretch your right arm up high into the air. Breathe in deep and look up toward your hand. Exhale, bring your right arm down and underneath your left arm and come down to rest on your right shoulder. Breathe in and out here for several counts. Come back up to Table Pose and switch sides.

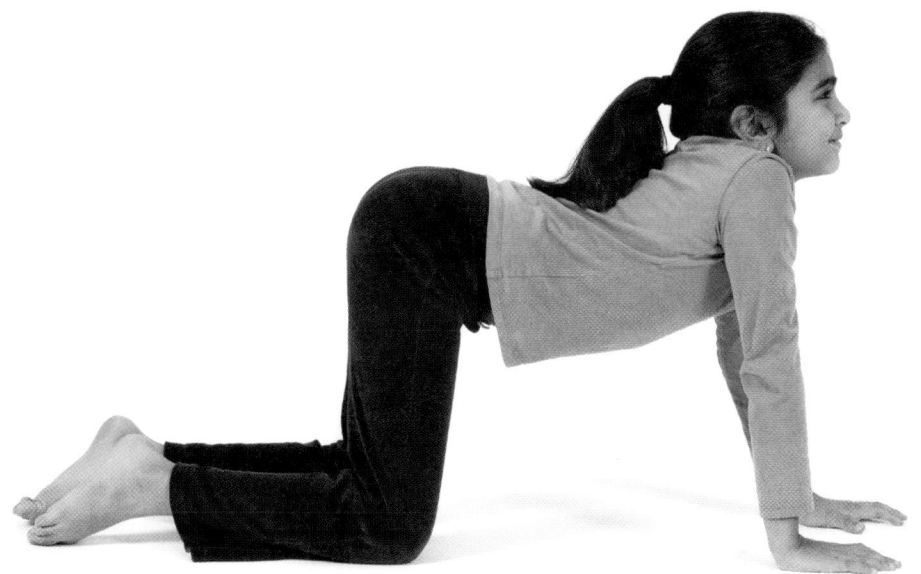

★ Happy Cat

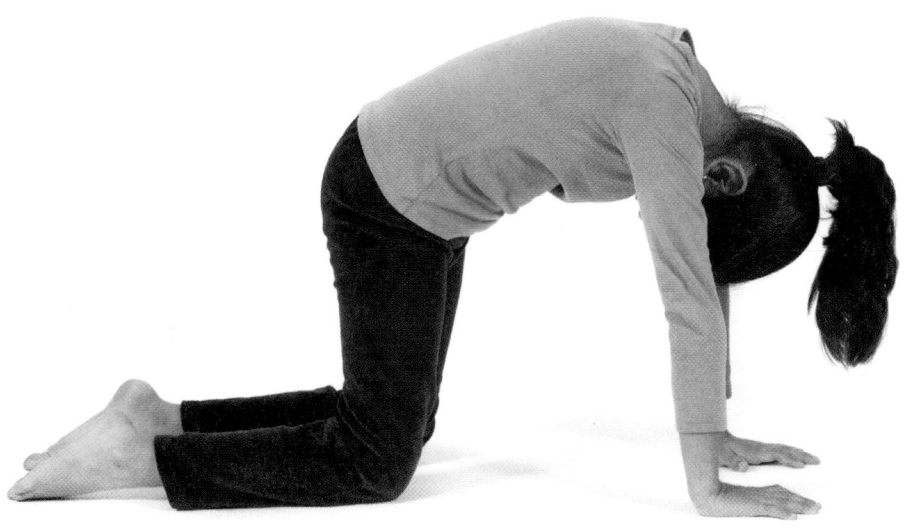

★ Scared Cat

CHAIR

Benefits

Strengthens feet, ankles, calves, and thighs

Strengthens and stretches shoulders, arms, and upper back

WHAT TO DO

One of the best ways to engage your child is to challenge her. When you first introduce Chair Pose to your child, focus only on proper alignment: eyes on a focus point, arms up, shoulders down, knees bent, core strong, tailbone slightly tucked under to protect her lower back. Once mastered, your child will enjoy being challenged to see how long she can hold the pose while breathing mindfully. Use a stopwatch or the minute hand on a wall clock to keep time and start with a 10-second challenge. Increase by 5 seconds each time you practice Chair Pose together.

WHAT TO SAY

Start in Mountain Pose with your feet several inches apart. Find a focus point for your eyes. Inhale and lift your arms up or out in front of you (for balance). Bend your knees and "sit" down as if sitting in a chair. Breathe in and out slowly and evenly for three breaths. How long can you hold Chair Pose? I will time you . . .

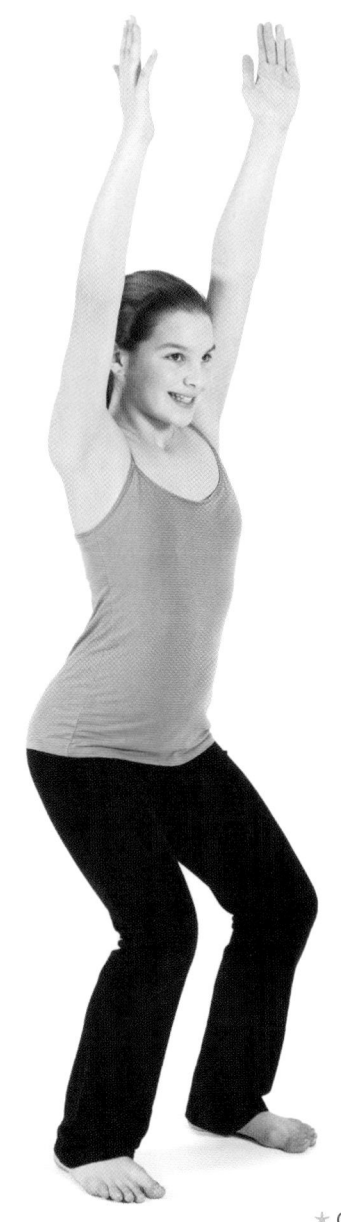

★ Chair

CHILD'S POSE

Benefits

Relieves stress
Serves as a resting pose
Stretches the thighs, hips, ankles, and knees
Relieves back strain

WHAT TO DO

Child's Pose can serve as an opportunity to rest between more challenging poses, or can be practiced any time for calm and focus. For a gentle neck stretch variation, guide your child to turn her head to one side and rest there for a few breaths and then repeat on the other side. For an arm and shoulder stretch variation, suggest your child bring her arms out in front of her for an "Extended Child's Pose."

WHAT TO SAY

Start by sitting on your heels. Separate your knees a little bit. Bend forward to rest your forehead gently on the floor. Let your arms relax down to the floor along the sides of your body, palms facing up. Close your eyes and allow your shoulders, neck, and back muscles to relax. Rest here for several breaths, breathing in and out slowly and deeply.

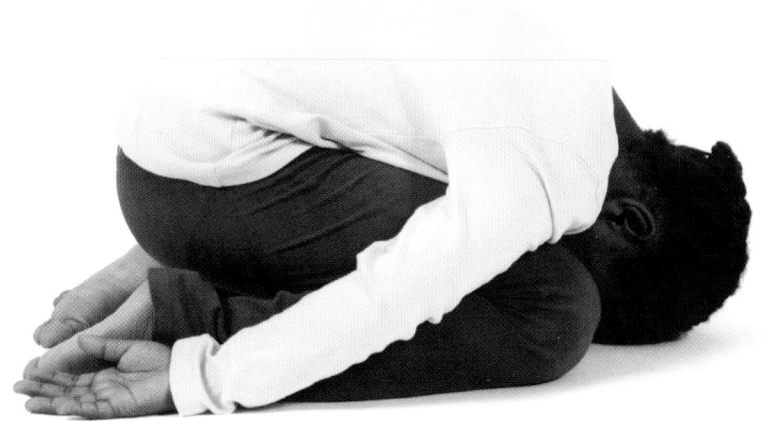

★ Child's Pose

COBRA

Benefits

WHAT TO DO

Encourage your child to keep his neck and spine long, and his shoulders down away from his ears. As opposed to simply pushing into his hands, encourage your child to lift up using his lower back muscles. For extra fun, have him "snake race" by slithering using only his hands and arms to move (this is best practiced on a slippery floor). Slithering like a snake builds upper body strength and coordination.

WHAT TO SAY

Start on your belly with your legs together like a long snake tail behind you. Put your hands on the floor directly under your shoulders. Inhale and lift your chest, using your hands for support. You are now a spitting cobra! Exhale out "hissss" to lower down to rest. Try it again. This time show me a silly, scary snake face when you hiss out. Ready . . .

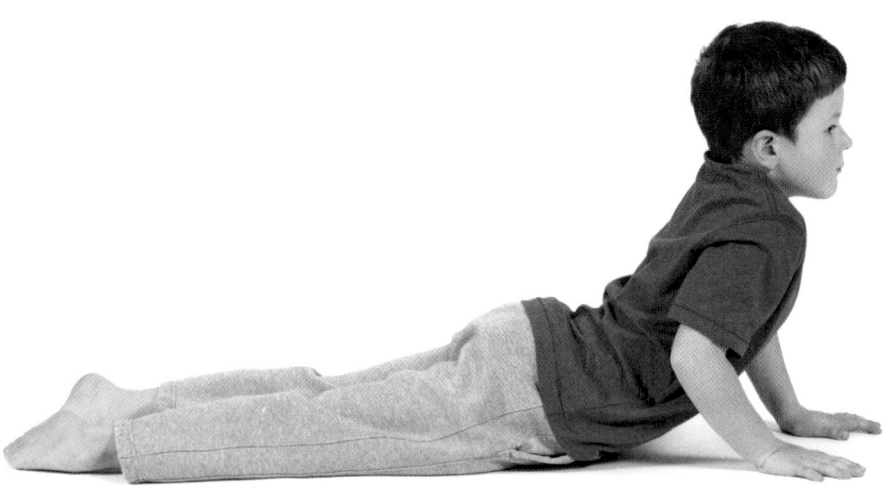

★ Cobra

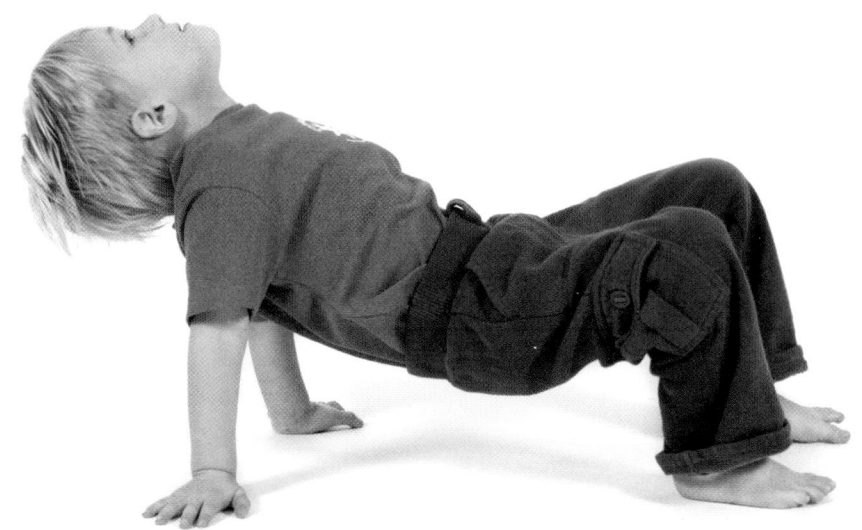

★ Crab

CRAB

Benefits

Builds strength in core, arms, and legs

Improves coordination

WHAT TO DO

Crab Pose engages many muscles of the body at once, making it a strength challenge. Be sure to include the variations to keep your child engaged as he strengthens his muscles and builds his coordination.

WHAT TO SAY

Start by sitting on your bottom with your knees bent, feet flat on the floor. Put your hands on the floor behind you, fingers facing forward. Lift your belly to the sky. Up, up, up! Good! You're a crab! Try crab-walking. Crabs can walk forward . . . backward . . . and side to side . . .

CRAB VARIATIONS

Encourage a playful connection with your child with these Crab variations.

- **Crab Dance.** Lift and lower your right foot and then your left, alternating feet to create the "dance." To rest, lower your bottom to the floor, hug your knees in, and take a deep breath in and out. For extra fun, play some lively music.
- **Crab High-Five.** Touch feet with your child one at a time. "High-Five, Dude!"

- **Crab Race!** From a start to a finish line, race going forward, backward, and sideways.
- **Crab Soccer.** Set up goals with books or cushions and use a soft, inflatable beach ball. This game is especially fun in a larger, open space with at least two people on each team!

CRESCENT MOON

Benefits

Stretches and strengthens waist, core, and spine
Aids digestion
Massages abdominal organs

WHAT TO DO
Crescent Moon is a side-bending pose that can be practiced sitting or standing. A slight variation of this pose is to have your child keep her right arm down at her side (or if sitting, with her right hand on the floor at her right side) as she reaches up and over to the side with her left arm before switching sides.

WHAT TO SAY
Begin sitting in Easy Pose or standing in Mountain Pose. Bring your arms up over your head, and either press your palms together or clasp your hands together with your pointer fingers pointing upward. Inhale and stretch up tall. Now exhale and bend to your right. You're a beautiful crescent moon! Inhale back up and exhale to the left. Use your breath to flow back and forth from side to side a few times.

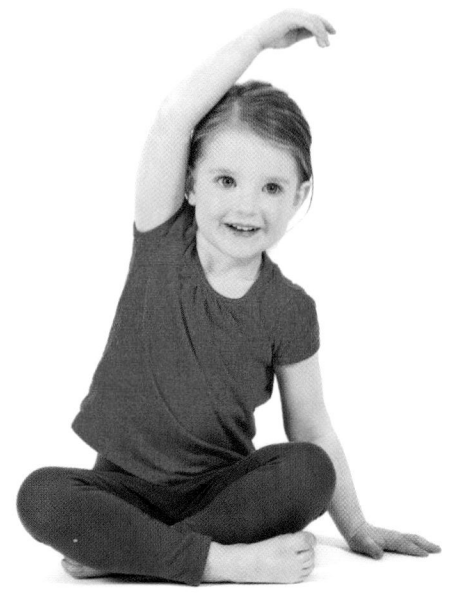

★ Crescent Moon

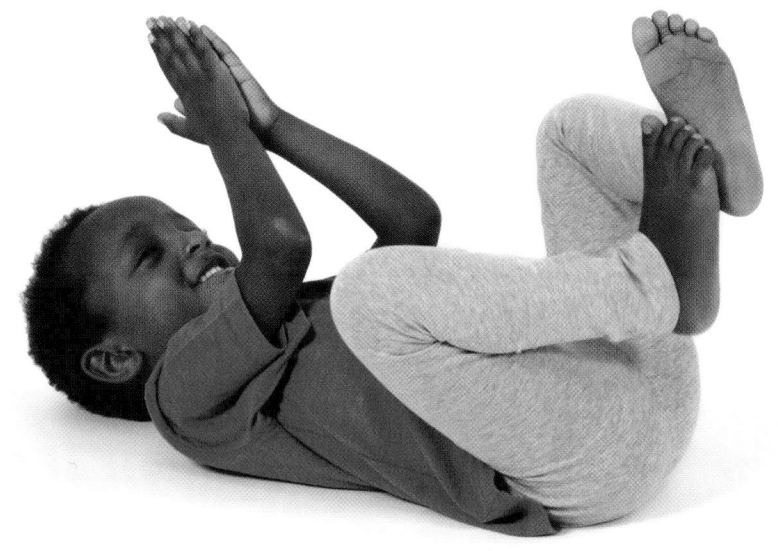

CRICKET

Benefits

Improves coordination

Builds core strength

WHAT TO DO

Crickets are unique in that they live nearly everywhere in the world where there are plants. And their "ears" are located in their front legs. Search the Internet and share with your child some interesting facts about crickets.

WHAT TO SAY

Lie down on your back. Lift your feet and hands into the air. Place your hands together and the bottoms of your feet together and rub hard and fast to create friction. That's it! Can you hear the crickets?

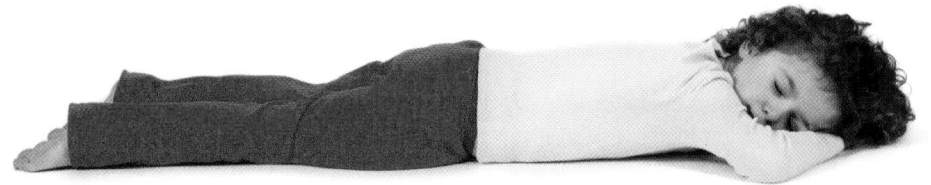
* Crocodile Pose

CROCODILE POSE

Benefits

Relieves tension, headache

Restorative

WHAT TO DO

Crocodile Pose is a restorative pose, similar to *Savasana* or Child's Pose, and can even be used in place of *Savasana* for children who are not comfortable on their backs.

WHAT TO SAY

Lie down on your belly. Separate your legs a little bit and rest your feet flat on the floor (or with your toes angled in toward each other). Bend your arms at the elbows and tuck your hands, palms down, under your forehead. Now, you can turn your head to the side. Ahh. Breathe in and out 3 to 5 times or as long as needed.

DOLPHIN POSE

Benefits

Strengthens the arms, shoulders, and back

Stretches the hamstrings and calves

Brings fresh oxygen to the brain

WHAT TO DO

To protect the neck and head, this challenging, strengthening pose should be reserved for an older child or one with strong enough shoulders and arms to hold the majority of her weight. Her head should not touch the floor. Your younger child can practice and benefit from this pose too, but instruct her to keep her knees on the floor. Encourage your child to rest for a few breaths in Child's Pose between each attempt.

WHAT TO SAY

Begin on your hands and knees in Table Pose. Lower your forearms to the ground, keeping your elbows parallel to each other underneath your shoulders. Now, clasp your hands together, with your thumbs facing up. Keeping your arms and shoulders strong, begin to tuck your toes under and lift your knees off the floor. Good! Straighten your legs and push your heels back, just like you do in Down Dog. Now, relax your head and neck. Can you nod "yes" and "no"? When you're ready to rest, just bring your knees back down to the floor. Rest in Child's Pose and breathe . . .

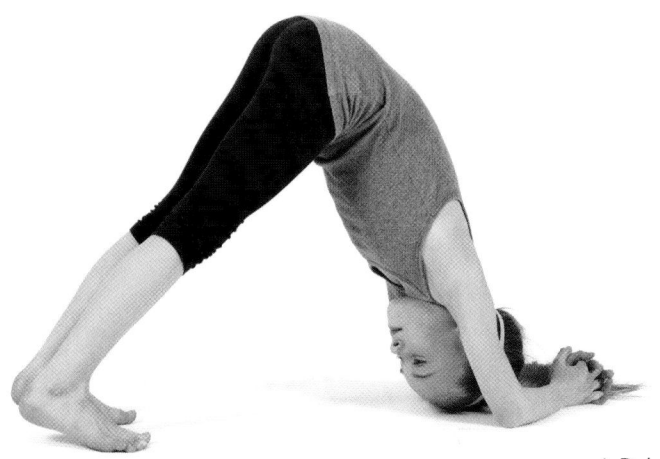

★ Dolphin Pose

DOLPHIN VARIATION FOR OLDER CHILDREN

For older children or those ready to be challenged, try adding this variation of Dolphin.

- **Spouting Dolphin.** With your arms and shoulders strong, roll your body forward into a forearm Plank Pose. Reach your chin past your clasped hands. Breathe out to spout like a dolphin, "Pssssh!" Continue moving back and forth.

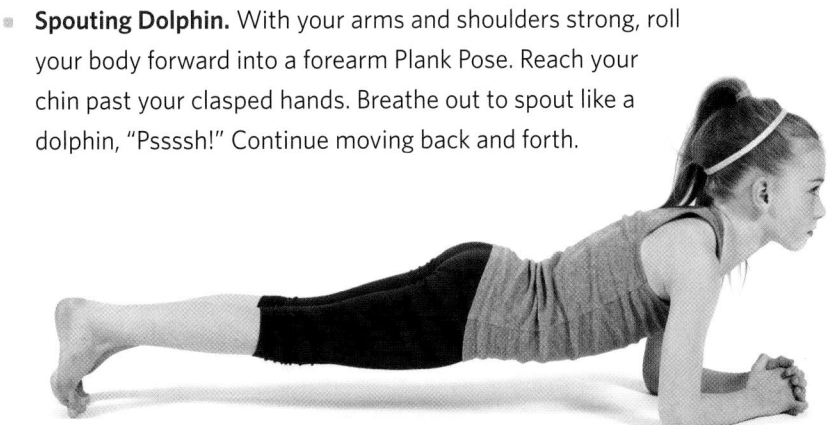

★ Spouting Dolphin

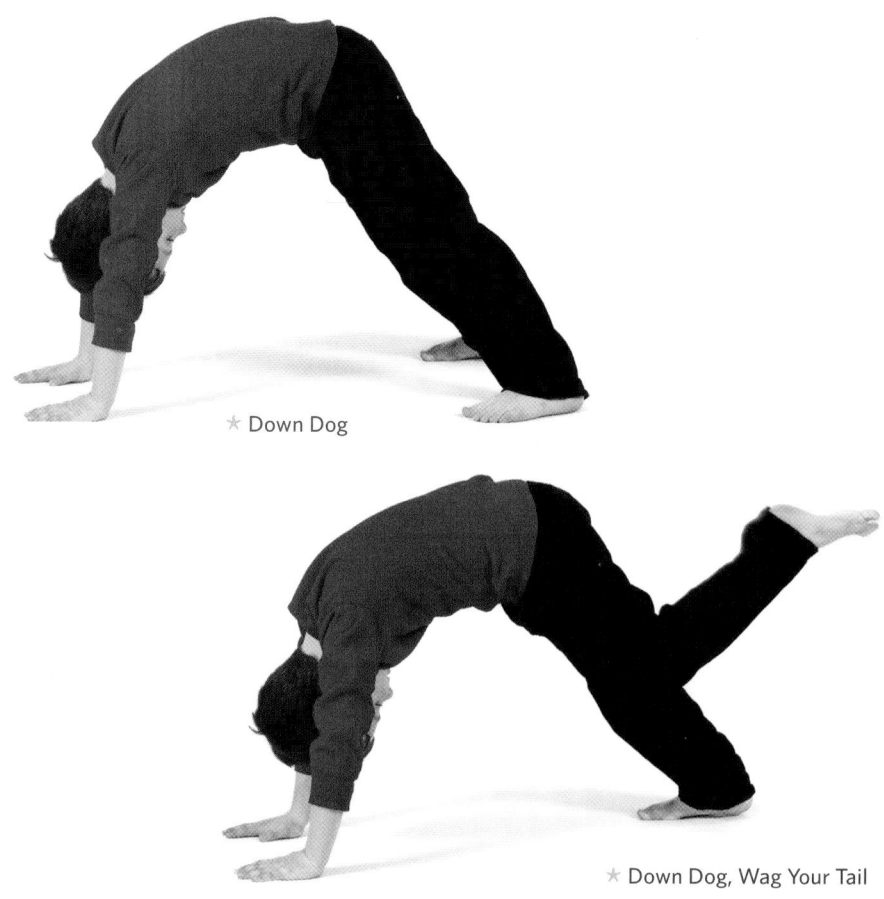

* Down Dog

* Down Dog, Wag Your Tail

DOWN DOG

Benefits

Stretches the shoulders, arms, hamstrings, and calves

Strengthens the arms, shoulders, and back

Encourages flow of oxygen and nutrients to the brain

WHAT TO DO

Remind your child to press his hips up and back while pressing his heels toward the floor. Ideally, his back should be flat, not rounded, fingers spread wide, with shoulders away from the ears. To stretch out the heel cords and hamstrings, have him "wag his tail" by alternately pressing each back to the floor. For a balance challenge, he can "wag his tail" by lifting one leg and shaking it out, and then switching sides. It's okay if his knees bend a bit while he's becoming more flexible!

WHAT TO SAY

Start in Table Pose. Spread your fingers wide. Now, tuck your toes under and push your bottom high up into the air. Check your arms . . . are they straight and strong? Relax your neck and head. Good. Now check your feet. Stretch your heels back as close to the floor as you can. What a beautiful dog stretch! Breathe in . . . breathe out. (For older children: Let's stay here and breathe in Down Dog Pose for three full breaths. For younger children: What sound does a dog make? "Ruff ruff!") Now lower back down to Table Pose and sit back on your heels. Well done!

DOG VARIATIONS

Pretending to be a dog is such fun. Try these add-ons to bring the pose to life!

- **Mark Your Territory.** Raise your right leg up and open your hips to the right. Look up under your right arm. Feel the stretch! Breathe in and out two times before lowering your leg down and switching sides.
- **Double Dog.** For a partner version, one person comes to Down Dog. The second person stands to her left and places her hands 12 inches in front of her partner's, more if her legs are longer than her partner's legs. Next, she slowly raises her right foot and anchors it on her partner's right hip. She will use that leverage to lift up her left foot and anchor it to her partner's left hip.

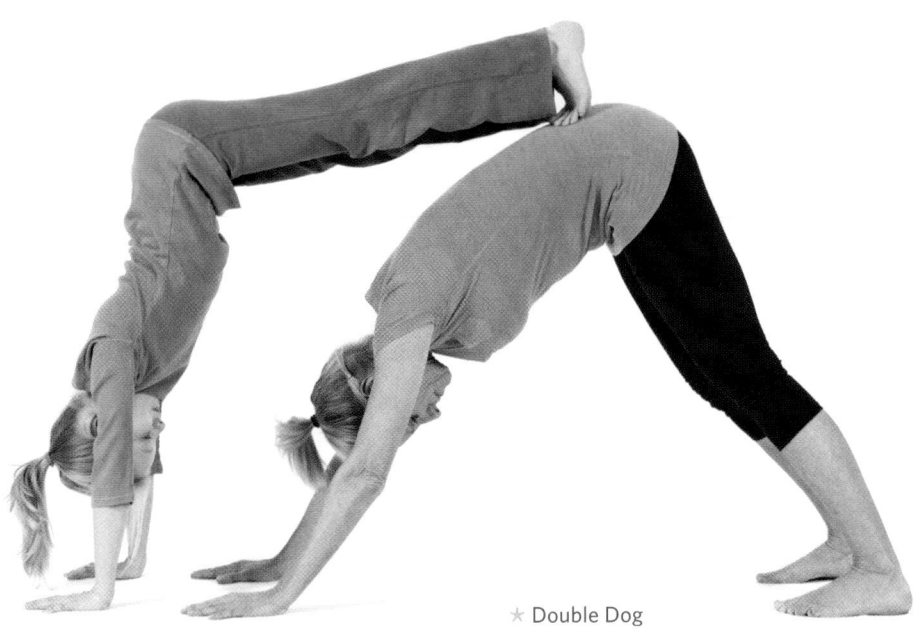

★ Double Dog

Benefits

Helps develop balance and coordination

Encourages focus and concentration

Stretches and strengthens the arms, shoulders, and back

Releases toxins and aids in digestion (twisting dragon)

WHAT TO DO

To protect the knees, practice this pose on a carpet, blanket, or yoga mat. Have your child imagine the qualities of a dragon: fierce, strong, protective. Encourage her to feel those qualities as she practices the pose, perhaps even adding an affirmation such as, "I am fierce!" Adding Dragon Breath provides a constructive, cleansing release for pent-up emotions or excess energy.

WHAT TO SAY

Come down to your knees. Bring your right leg forward and place your foot flat on the floor. Check to be sure your knee is either just above or slightly behind your ankle. Inhale deeply through your nose, bring your arms straight up, and look up to the sky (younger children can face forward). Check your shoulders. They should be down away from your ears. Wow, you are fierce and strong! Now inhale and stretch your arms up to the sky, exhale with a Dragon Breath— "Haaa!"—and bring your arms down in

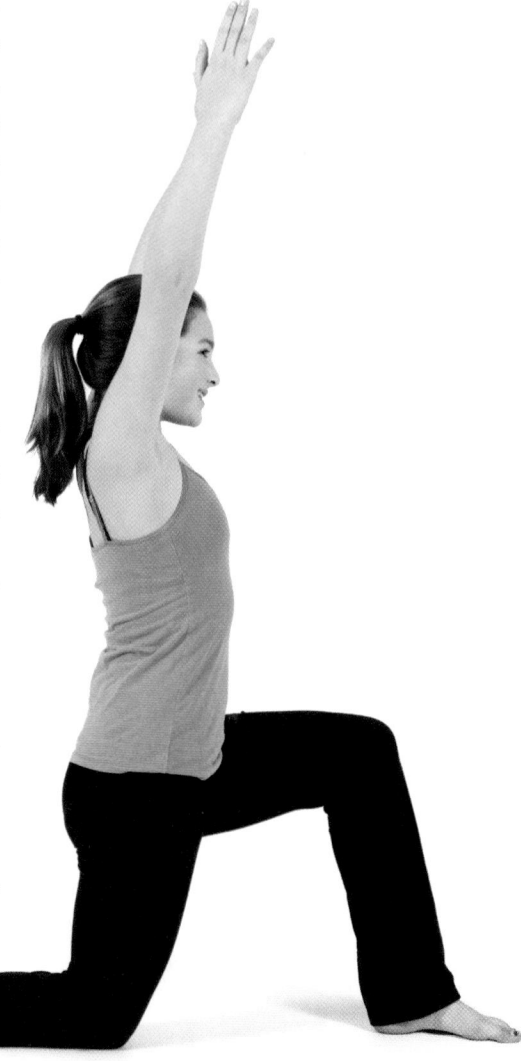

★ Dragon

front of you while you. What fiery breath you have! Try it again. Breathe your arms up . . . and exhale your arms forward. Try it one more time all by yourself. Come down to rest in Hero Pose before switching sides.

DRAGON VARIATIONS

- **Twisting Dragon (or Slayed Dragon).** From Dragon Pose, bring your hands together in front of your heart. Bow forward and cross your elbow over your opposite knee, twisting your torso to the side. Find a focus point on the wall in front of you. Now you're a twisting dragon! Can you balance here and breathe with me? (For an extra challenge: If you are feeling balanced here, try finding a focus point up toward the ceiling.) Hold the pose for a few deep breaths. Release and switch sides.

- **Twin Dragons.** For a partner version, practice Dragon facing each other with your right feet forward. Position yourselves so that the insides of your right knees are facing each other. Reach up to connect hands above and look into each others' eyes. Breathe in and out a few times before switching sides.

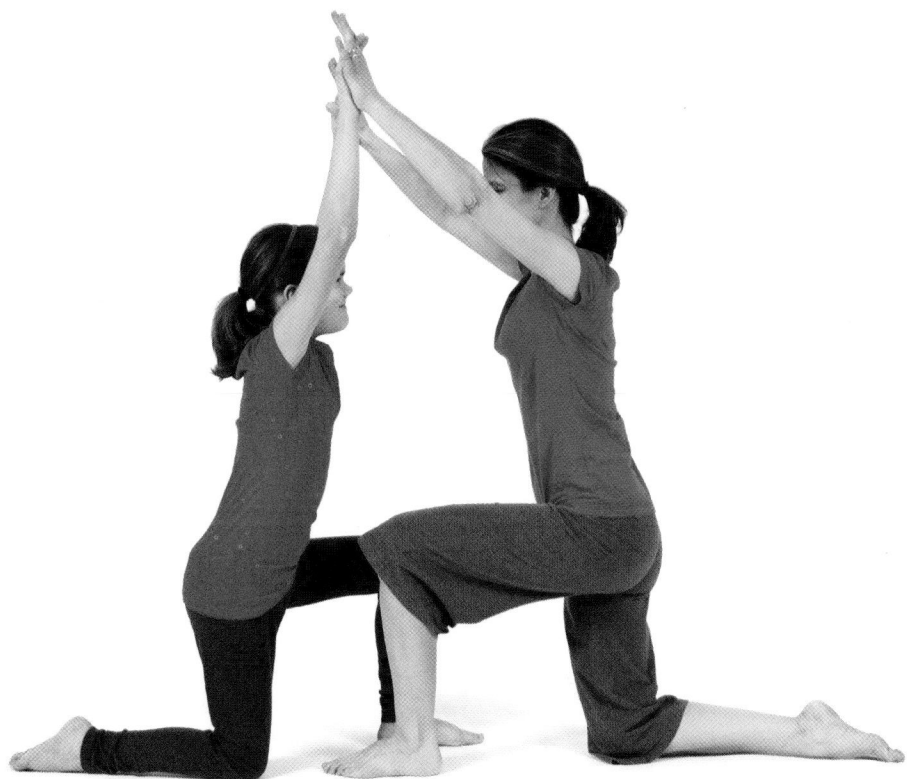

★ Twin Dragons

EAGLE POSE

Benefits

Helps develop balance, coordination, and focus

Stretches shoulders and upper back

Strengthens legs, knees, and ankles

Integrates both sides of the brain

WHAT TO DO

The full expression of Eagle Pose is described below. Similar benefits can be achieved using a simpler version with your younger child. Simply have her cross her arms over her chest and put one leg over the other, keeping both feet on the ground. (See photos for variations.)

WHAT TO SAY

Balance
use animals
to focus

Start in Mountain Pose. Find a focus point. Extend your left arm out and cross it over your right. Bend at your elbows and wrap your forearms together, bringing the palms of your hands together. Now, shift your weight to your left foot and bend your knees slightly. Wrap your right leg over your left. Keep your toe on the floor, or if you are feeling balanced, challenge yourself by drawing your foot around and behind your left leg. You are a wise and regal eagle! Balance in Eagle Pose and breathe in and out several times. When you are ready, inhale and stretch your limbs out wide to soar like an eagle before exhaling back to Mountain Pose. Switch sides.

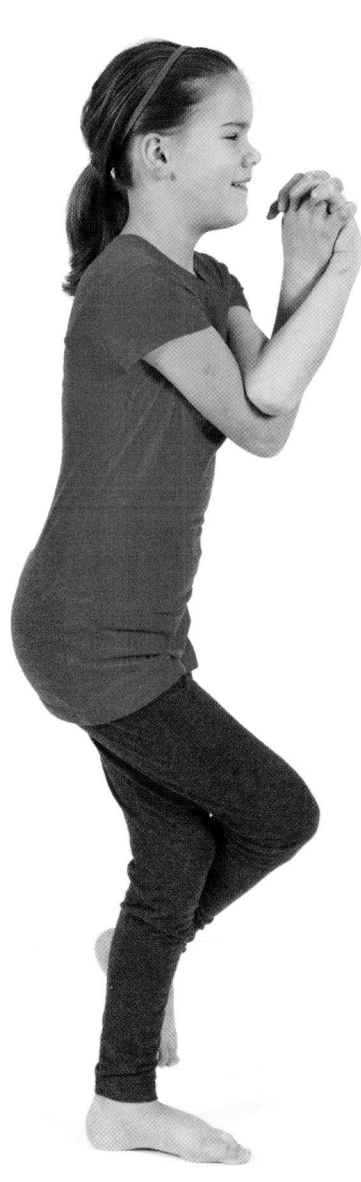

* Eagle Pose

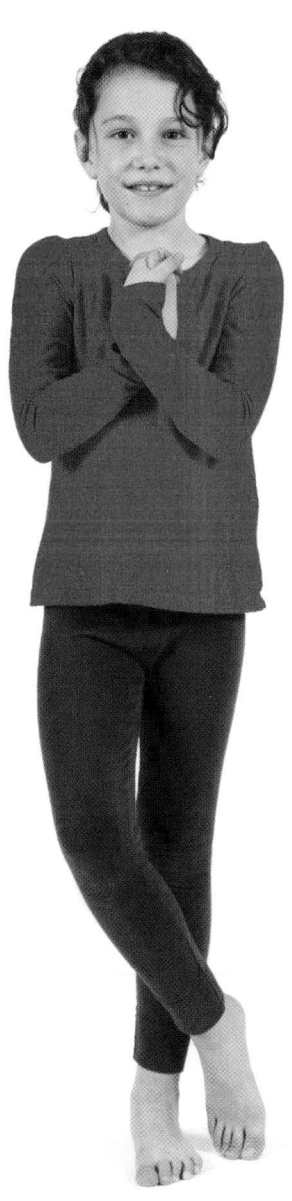

* Eagle Pose, modified

younger kid

Benefits

Calms and balances
Strengthens the back and spine
Encourages good posture
Stretches the legs, ankles, and feet

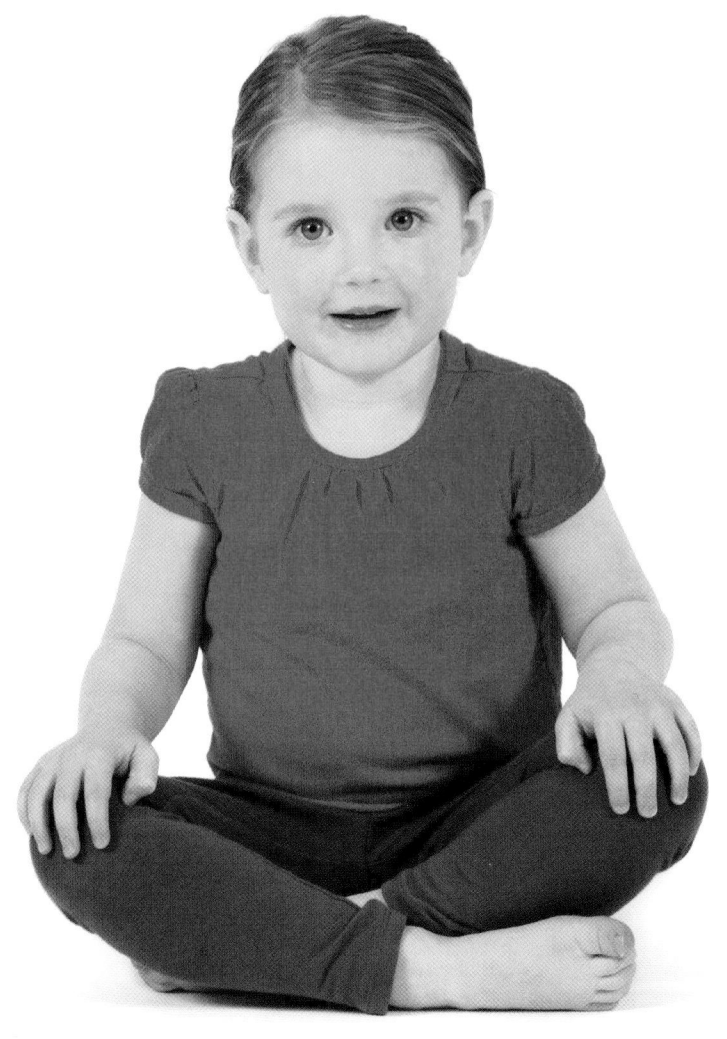

★ Easy Pose

WHAT TO DO

If your child finds it difficult to sit up tall due to tight hips and/or poor core strength, or complains of her lower back hurting, place a folded blanket or yoga mat under her hips so that her sitting bones are on the blanket and her legs are folded in front of her on the floor. In general, placing a blanket under the hips while practicing sitting poses, regardless of core strength, is more comfortable, especially if holding poses for longer than a few breaths.

WHAT TO SAY

Sit with your legs crossed comfortably (like "criss cross applesauce"), hands resting in your lap. Sit up tall, stretching up your neck and spine as if your head is on a puppet string attached to the ceiling. Beautiful! Now, take a deep breath in and lift your shoulders up to your ears. Exhale out, "ahhh," and roll them back and down. Do that again. Now, gently close your eyes. Bring your hands together in front of your heart, thumbs gently pressing into your chest. Breathe slowly and deeply.

Happy or Grumpy?

In any sitting pose, maintaining good posture is essential to reap the full benefits of the pose. Try slouching over, looking grumpy and tired. Ask your child to mimic you and tell how she feels in that position. Tired? Bored? Grumpy? Try breathing in this position together. Is it even possible? Now, encourage her to sit up tall with you. Ask her, "How do you feel, now?" Alert? Happy? Energized? "Can you take a deep breath with me, now?" Note together how your mood and breath change with the better posture. To encourage your child to maintain good posture as you practice together, teasingly ask, "Are you happy or grumpy?" Watch her sit up tall!

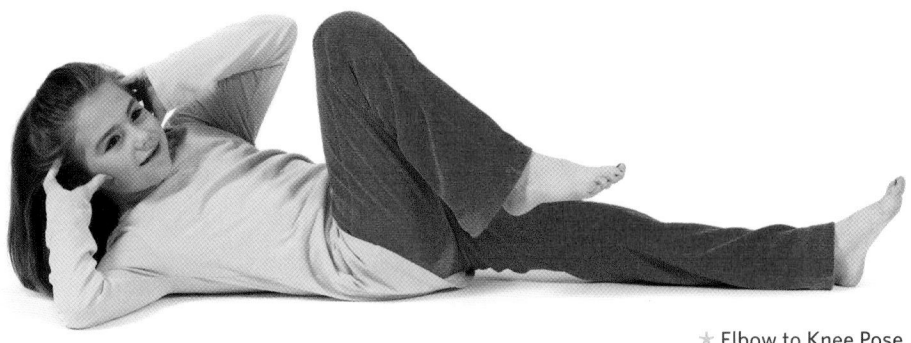

★ Elbow to Knee Pose

ELBOW TO KNEE POSE

Benefits

Aids digestion

Builds core strength

Improves coordination

Brain builder (integrates information flow between both sides of the brain)

WHAT TO DO

If your child skipped crawling as a baby, she may find this challenging, but extremely beneficial as this and other cross-crawl motions help to coordinate the information flow between the two sides of the brain, ultimately helping with physical coordination and learning readiness. For a simpler variation, have your child touch her hand to knee, rather than elbow to knee. Note that crossing the midline, elbow to knee, can also be practiced from a standing position.

WHAT TO SAY

Lie down on your back. Bring your fingers to rest behind your ears, elbows out to the sides. Pull your left knee up and reach your right elbow across to your left knee. Switch sides. Can you go faster, alternating between both sides? That's it! Let's count to 10, counting up one for each movement . . . 1, 2, 3 . . . relax down to the floor to rest, stretching your legs out long and reaching your arms up over your head. Take a deep breath in . . . and out, "Ahhh." Let's try it again. Ready . . .

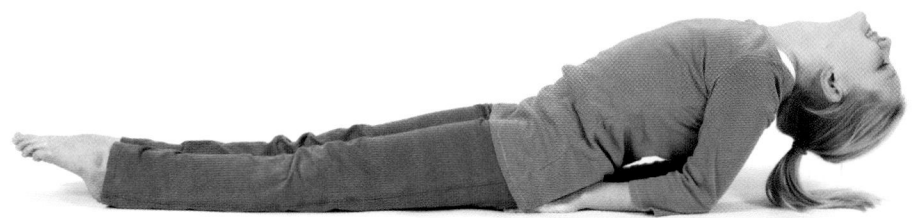

FISH POSE

Benefits

Stretches and stimulates all muscles and organs of the front side of the body

Improves posture

Opens the chest and lungs

Strengthens the muscles of the upper back, shoulders, and neck

make fish face

WHAT TO DO

This is a tricky pose for young children and can be potentially dangerous for the neck if not practiced properly. Only teach this pose if your child has the ability to hold her head off the floor while in the pose, or can safely get in and out of it with your support. Skip this pose completely if your child is under 6 years.

WHAT TO SAY

Lie on your back on the floor with your knees bent, feet flat on the floor. Tuck your hands under your hips, palms facing down. Inhale and open your chest wide as you draw your elbows in under your body. For older children: Extend your legs long. Imagine your legs are your fishtail! Now, press into your forearms to inhale and lift your torso and head up off the floor. Your fish gills are wide open . . . breathe in deeply, in . . . and out . . . very slowly lift your head and lower your upper body back down to rest.

FLAG POSE / Side plank

Benefits

Strengthens the arms, core muscles, and legs

Stretches and strengthens the wrists

Improves balance

WHAT TO DO

Flag, or Side Plank, is a very challenging balance pose that also requires significant arm strength. Try practicing Flag Pose on a wall so that the wall can be used behind the body for support. As well, when first experimenting with the pose, your child will benefit from keeping both of her feet on the floor, one in front of the other, as opposed to stacking the feet on top of each other.

WHAT TO SAY

Begin in Down Dog. Turn onto the outside edge of your right foot. Begin to shift your weight to your right hand as you turn your body to your left. Stack your legs on top of each other and raise your left arm up to the sky. You're a flag! Can you balance and breathe here for three breaths or more? You can do it! When you are ready, come down to take a break and shake out your arms before switching to try Flag Pose on the other side.

★ Flag Pose

Benefits

Promotes focus and concentration

Improves balance

Strengthens the back, thighs, ankles, and feet

WHAT TO DO

Your youngest child may have difficulty with challenging balance poses. You can either assist him by holding his hand, or he can keep his big toe on the floor rather than lifting his knee up. For extra fun, have your child try to balance a beanie buddy on his knee while practicing Flamingo Pose.

WHAT TO SAY

Start in Mountain Pose and find a focus point. Bring your hands up into your armpits to create your wings. Beautiful! Now, shift your weight to your left foot and lift your right knee up as high as you can. You're a flamingo! Can you balance here for a count of 5? 1, 2, 3, 4, 5. You did it! Let's switch sides and try that again.

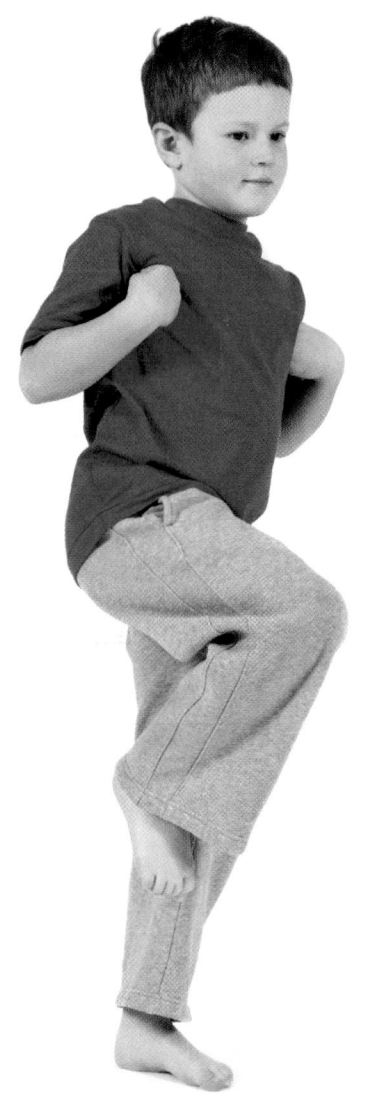

⋆ Flamingo

Benefits

Opens chest and lungs

Stretches neck, shoulders, upper back, thighs, glutes, and hips

Tones internal organs

WHAT TO DO

This moving pose serves as a visual prompt to help younger children learn when to inhale and exhale (inhale to open, exhale to close). As your child inhales, remind her to open her chest and arms wide to gain the full benefit of the pose.

WHAT TO SAY

Begin in Easy Pose. Bend your elbows and place your fingertips just behind your ears. Inhale to "bloom" open your arm petals. Exhale and bring your elbows together in front of your face and down to the floor. Now inhale to "bloom" all the way open while "smelling" the beautiful fragrance of your flower. Exhale back down, closing your petals. Repeat opening and closing your flower petals, using your breath as a guide. Inhale to open . . . exhale to close. Repeat 3 to 5 times or more.

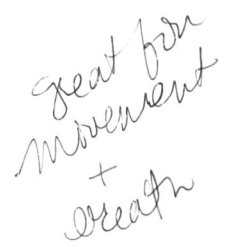

great for movement + breath

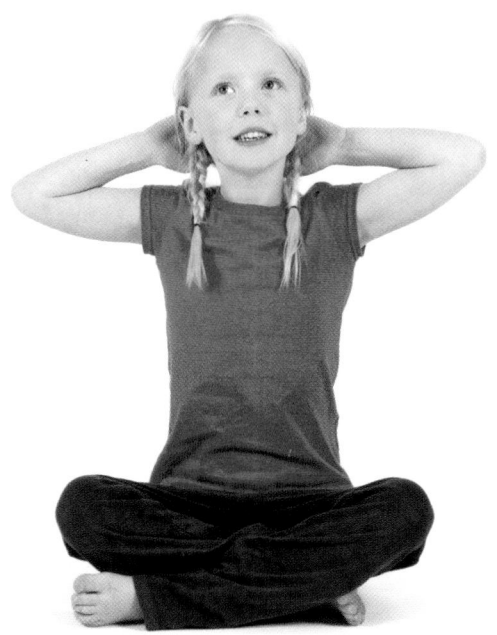

★ Flower, open

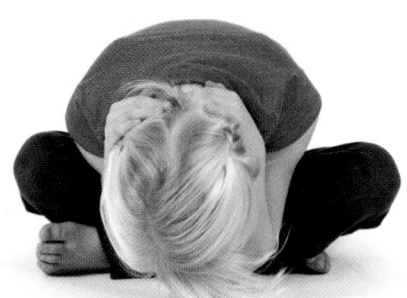

★ Flower, closed

Benefits

Strengthens shoulders and arms

Improves balance and circulation

WHAT TO DO

This pose is a great precursor to Headstand. To protect the neck and head, this challenging pose should be reserved for an older child or one with strong enough shoulders and arms to hold all of her weight with confidence. Her head should not touch the floor. Be sure to spot your child when practicing any inversion pose.

WHAT TO SAY

Begin in Table Pose in front of a stable wall. Bring your forearms down to the floor. Arm check! Are they parallel to one other and stacked just beneath your shoulders? Are your fingers a couple inches from the wall? Good. Now, keep your arms and shoulders strong, tuck your toes, and start to straighten your legs, just like you do in Down Dog. Tiptoe your feet closer to your arms. When your spine is straight over your head and neck, pull in your belly muscles to lift your feet up off the floor, pulling your knees up and in over your torso. Stay here or try straightening your legs to the sky! Breathe here, and when you are ready, come back out of the pose in the same sequence, working backward . . . slowly draw your knees in, lower your feet to the floor, and now your knees. Rest in Child's Pose.

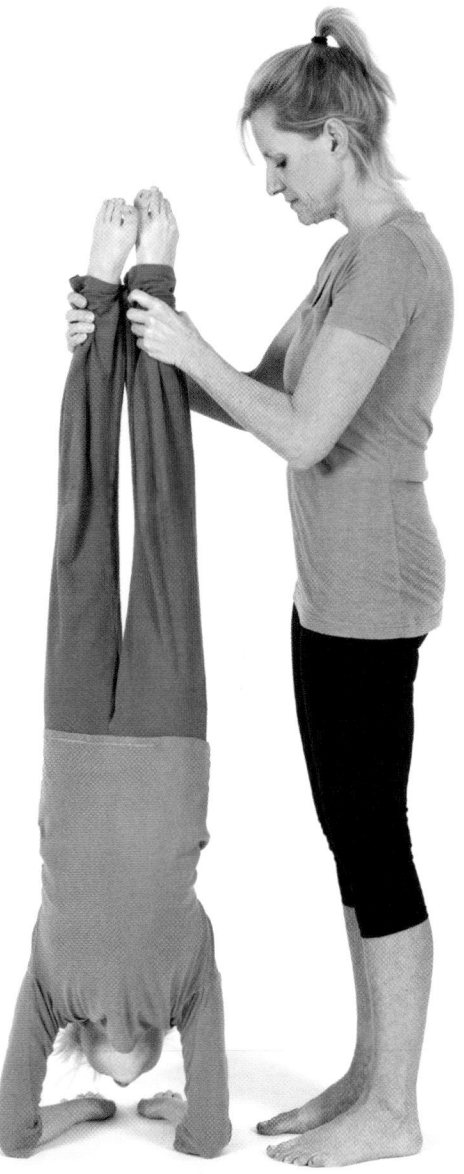

★ Forearm Stand

Do next to a wall only!

Benefits

Keeps legs limber

Stretches the hips and inner thighs

Aids digestion

Improves balance

WHAT TO DO

Note that this version of Frog Pose is more kid friendly than the traditional yoga posture, yet provides similar benefits. Your child may want to balance on her toes, which is fine as it provides a balance challenge. However, to obtain the pose's full benefits, you'll want to encourage her to bring her heels to the floor. This is easier to do the farther apart the feet are placed. As well, using a rolled-up yoga mat or blanket beneath the heels can provide comfort and support.

WHAT TO SAY

Start by standing with your feet a little wider than hip distance apart. Squat down by bending your knees out to the sides until your bottom almost reaches the floor. Can you bring your heels to the floor? Place both hands on the floor between your legs for balance. Now you're a frog! "Ribbit!" Stay here in the pose for several breaths. Stand up to shake out your legs before trying it again!

FROG VARIATIONS

Offer these challenges when your child has mastered the basic pose.

- **_Namaste_ Frog Balance.** Bring your hands to _Namaste_ Pose with your elbows on the inside of the knees, pressing outward. Check your posture and breathe . . . how long can you balance here?
- **Frog Hops.** Hop in place, coming all the way back down into Frog Pose each time. Whoa! How high can you go? Let's count together. 1, 2, 3, HOP! 1, 2, 3, HOP! . . .

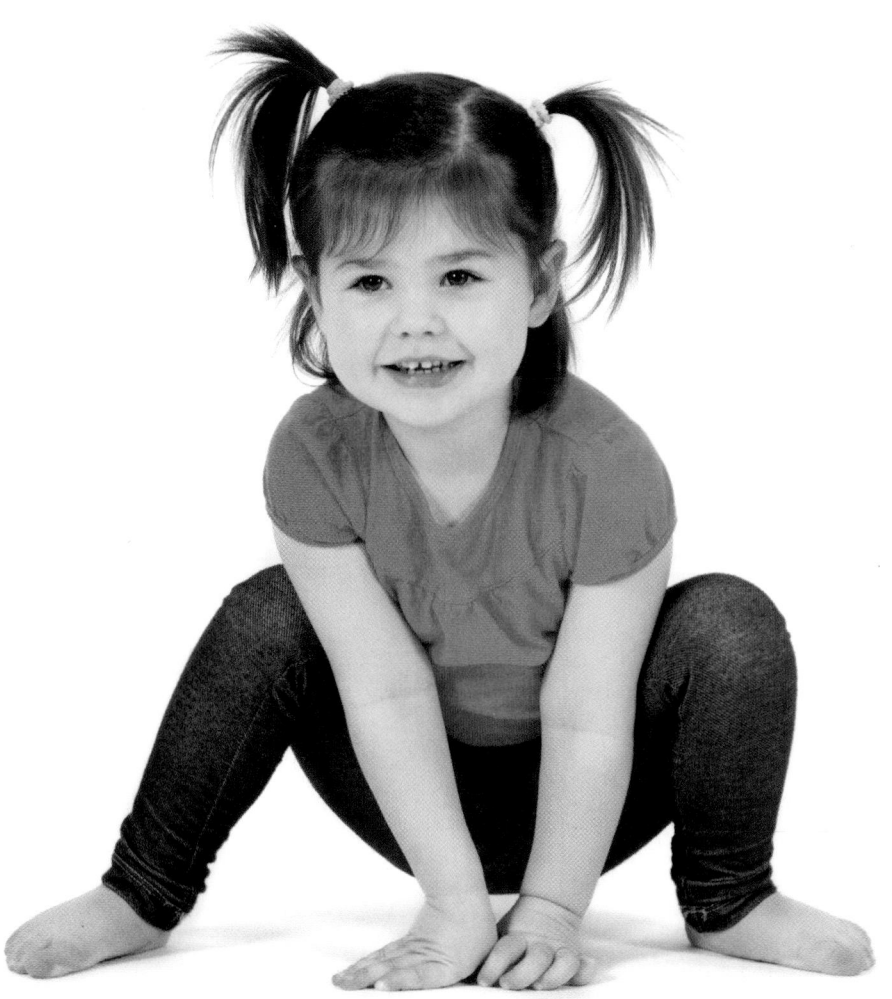

★ Frog

GATE

Benefits

Stretches waist and spine

Improves balance

Cleanses internal organs

Opens the lungs

WHAT TO DO

To protect delicate knees, practice Gate Pose on a carpet, yoga mat, or folded blanket. As well, ensure your child's knee is facing up when extended. To maintain a true side bend, encourage your child to bend sideways from the waist, rather than forward from the hips. His hand will most likely reach to his lower thigh or just below his knee.

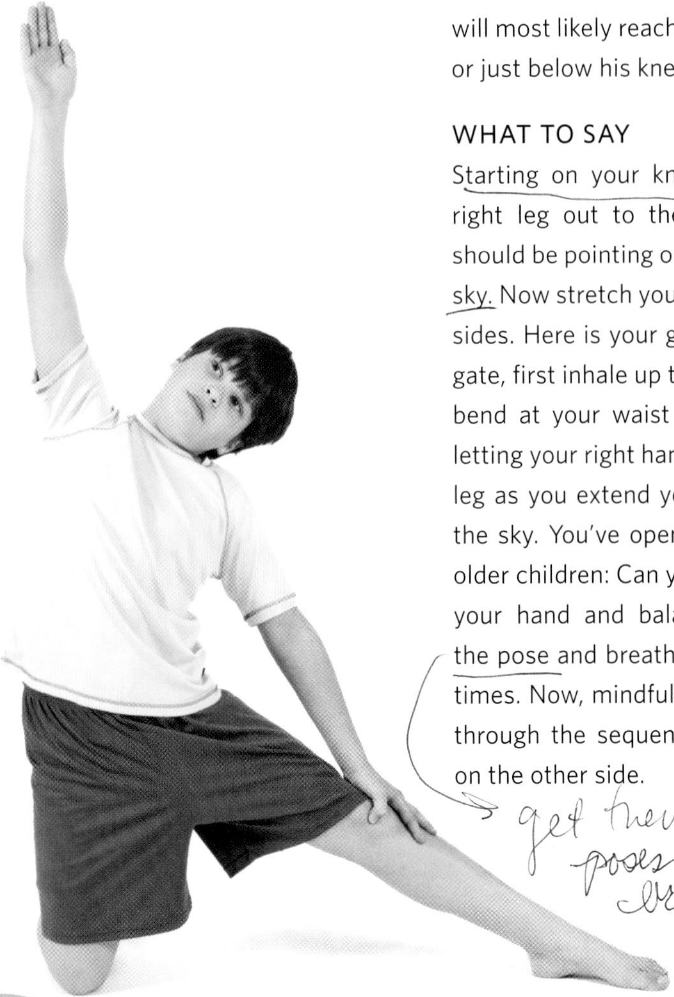

WHAT TO SAY

Starting on your knees, stretch your right leg out to the side. Your toes should be pointing out, knee facing the sky. Now stretch your arms out to your sides. Here is your gate! To open your gate, first inhale up tall. As you exhale, bend at your waist toward the right, letting your right hand slide down your leg as you extend your left arm up to the sky. You've opened the gate! (For older children: Can you look up toward your hand and balance here?) Hold the pose and breathe in and out three times. Now, mindfully come backward through the sequence and let's try it on the other side.

→ get them to hold poses by distraction breathing, noises, counting in Spanish

★ Gate

open & close the gate

Benefits

Relieves tension and stress

Dispels excess energy or negativity

WHAT TO DO

Explain to your child what a geyser is. Try an Internet search and watch the live streaming video of Old Faithful in Yellowstone National Park. After practicing Geyser Pose with your child, discuss these questions: What would happen to the earth without the occasional geyser eruption? What would happen to you if you were not able to release your feelings? Can you think of other peaceful ways to release anger, frustration, and pent-up emotions and energy?

WHAT TO SAY

Start in Mountain Pose with hands together in front of the heart. Close your eyes and look inward to notice if you are carrying around any anger or excess energy inside. Let it bubble up out from your heart and body into your hands. Inhale through your nose deeply and pause. Now, forcefully explode your arms and legs out, making the sound of a geyser releasing hot steam, "Pssssh!" Imagine that

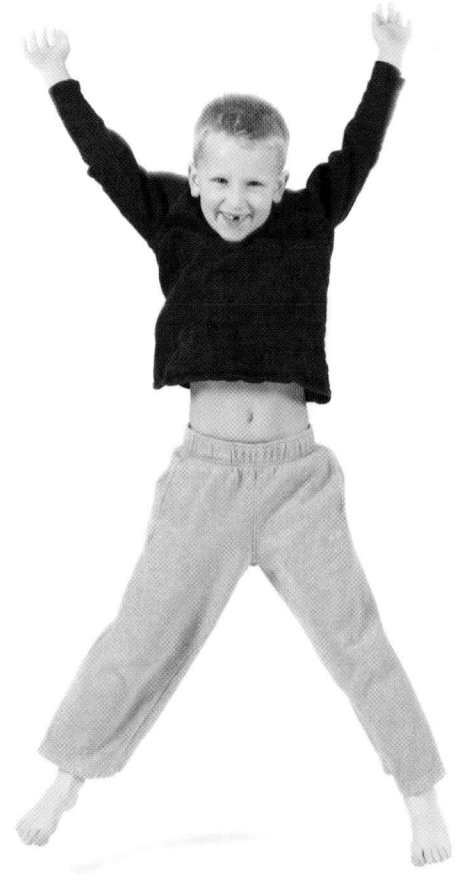

★ Geyser

hot steam leaving your body and mind. Draw your arms and legs down before inhaling your hands back up to your heart, drawing in peace and calm. Repeat 3 to 5 times or until your inner geyser is cooled down and peaceful.

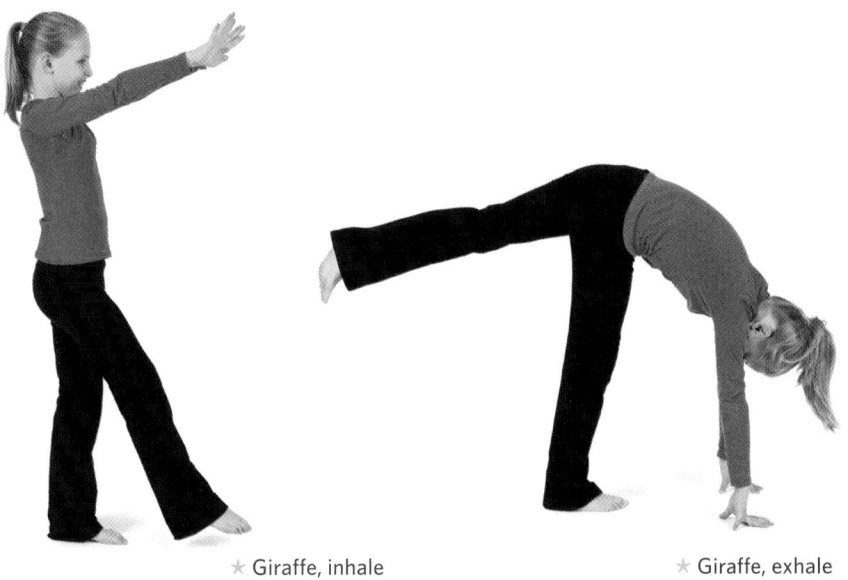

★ Giraffe, inhale   ★ Giraffe, exhale

GIRAFFE

Benefits

Improves balance and focus

Stretches the hamstrings, calves, and hips

Promotes circulation and blood flow to the brain

WHAT TO DO

Giraffe is a moving pose requiring a great deal of balance and coordination. It is recommended for older children who may be confidently seeking a challenge! It can be helpful to have your child imagine she is walking a tightrope when practicing Giraffe Pose. Better yet, roll out an old necktie or a yoga strap to create a real one on which to practice. Have your child try to keep her feet one in front of the other on the tightrope while she's "giraffe walking."

WHAT TO SAY

Begin in Mountain Pose. Keeping both hips and feet facing forward, inhale your arms up to the sky and your right leg straight up in front of you. Keeping both legs straight, exhale and fold forward to bring your arms down over your front leg. Switch sides by standing up and raising your left leg this time to "giraffe walk" forward, legs long and strong. Can you stay balanced? Remember, the slower and more mindfully you move, the more successful you will be. How many giraffe steps can you take while staying balanced?

Benefits

Promotes balance

Strengthens the wrists and legs

Tones spine

WHAT TO DO

Try using a wall when first sharing Half Moon pose with your child. Have her stand against the wall while coming into the pose. The wall will serve to support her balance and help her feel successful. When she is ready, have her move to her mat to try it again.

WHAT TO SAY

Begin in Star Pose. Now come into Triangle Pose, bending to your right. Now, slowly bend your right knee and lean over to bring your right hand to the floor. Bring your left arm up to the sky. Yes, that's it! Now, slowly start to straighten your right leg as you extend your left leg out. Keep your eyes on your focus point in front of you on the wall. (For older children: Now, try turning your gaze up to the sky.) Can you hold the pose and breathe for 5 seconds? I will count . . . great work! Slowly come back out of the pose and come back into Star Pose before you switch sides.

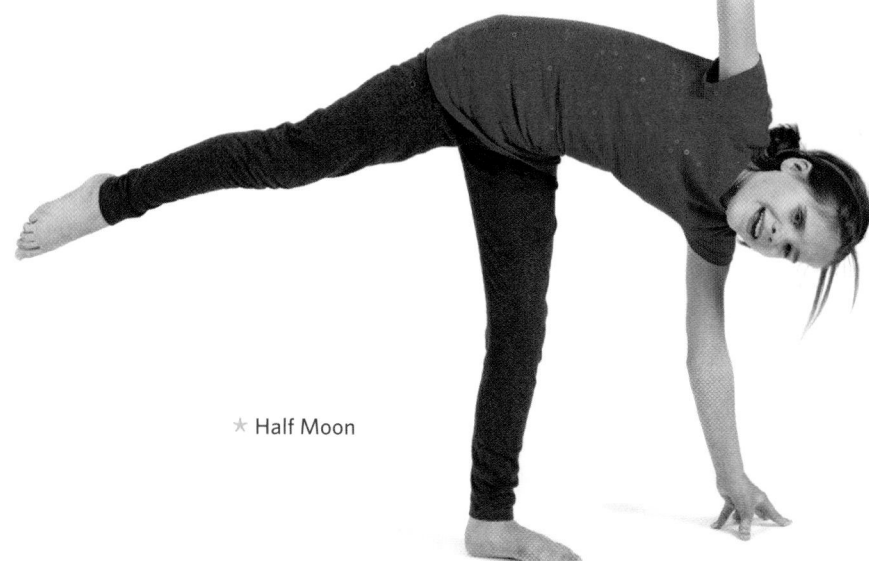

★ Half Moon

Benefits

Promotes circulation, brings fresh oxygen-rich blood to the brain

Builds confidence

WHAT TO DO

Handstand can cause fear as it is sometimes the first experience children have with going upside down. Try these ideas to help ease your child into the pose. First, ensure your child has the upper body strength required for holding the pose by practicing Ladybug Handstand (also known as Spiderman Pose). Have her come to a wall in Down Dog Pose with her heels on the floor near the wall. Have her lift one foot at a time up to "walk" on the wall like a ladybug (or Spiderman, etc.) Another option for building confidence is to use the Picture It Tree Visualization (Chapter 9) to have your child imagine herself in the pose. Help with affirmations such as "I am doing it!" or "I am confident and strong!" Always practice in front of a stable, clear wall and be sure to spot your child.

WHAT TO SAY

Come into Down Dog Pose, with hands a few inches from the wall. Tiptoe your toes closer and closer to your hands until your shoulders are over your wrists. Kick one leg up at a time, keeping your legs straight and your arms strong. Once your legs are up

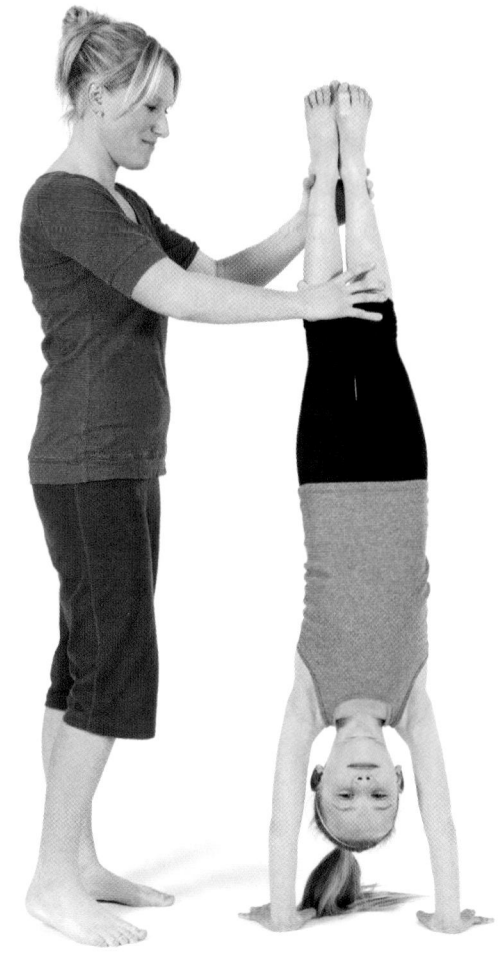

★ Handstand

against the wall, squeeze your feet and legs together and upward. Look at the floor beneath you. Play around with taking your feet off the wall. When you are ready to come down, bring one leg down to the floor at a time.

HAPPY BABY POSE

Benefits

Stretches and opens the hips, hamstrings, glutes, and groin

Soothes the lower back

WHAT TO DO

For a fun and beneficial variation of this pose, have your child stretch out one leg, then the other, as babies would do.

WHAT TO SAY

Lie down on your back. Wrap your first two fingers around your big toes or the outsides of your feet. Pull your feet back so that your knees come in toward your armpits. Ga, ga! Are you a happy baby?

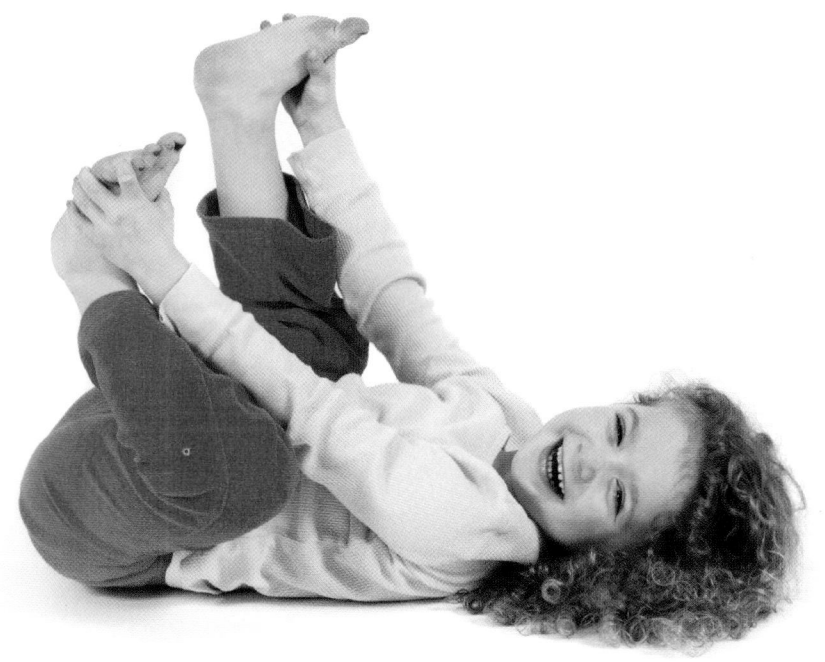

★ Happy Baby Pose

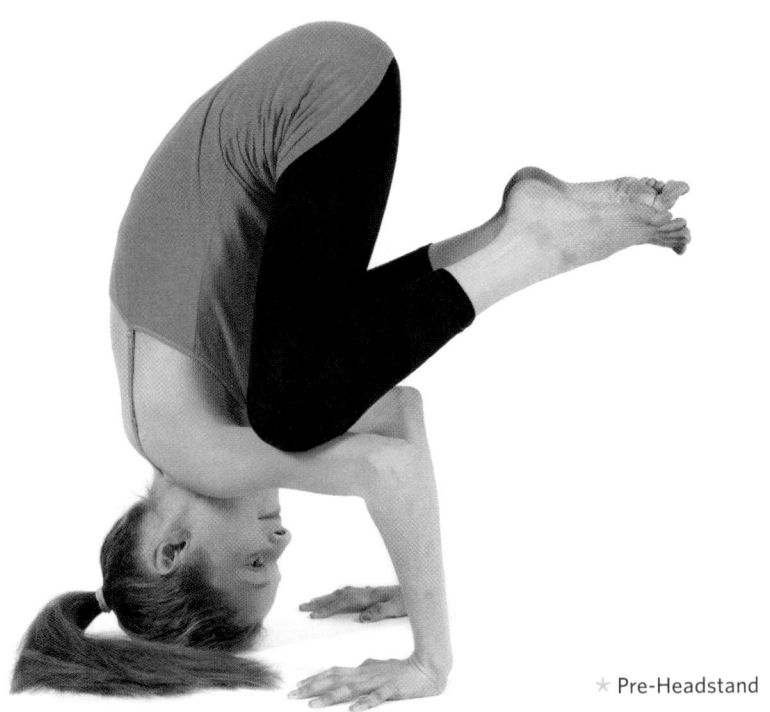

★ Pre-Headstand

PRE-HEADSTAND AND HEADSTAND

Benefits

Promotes balance and poise

Energizes entire body

Delivers freshly oxygenated blood to the brain

Builds confidence

WHAT TO DO

Poses with any weight put on the head and neck are not appropriate for most children under 6. To ensure your child has the upper body strength necessary for holding herself in a Headstand (see sidebar), begin by teaching her Pre-Headstand. Be sure your child comes onto the crown of her head, rather than her forehead. To ensure your child can be successful and safe, start by practicing near a wall. Always spot your child for safety.

WHAT TO SAY

Come into Table Pose in front of the wall. Back up so your hands are about a foot away from the wall. Be sure your fingers are facing forward and are spread wide. Lean forward and place the crown of your head on the floor in front of your hands to form a triangle shape with three equal sides. Now, tuck your toes and straighten your legs like you do in Down Dog. Keeping your arms and shoulders strong, begin to walk your feet up closer to your hands until you are completely upside down. Feel the weight of your body evenly distributed on your hands and head. Gently lift your right knee onto the back of your right arm and then your left knee onto the back of your left arm. You're in Pre-Headstand!

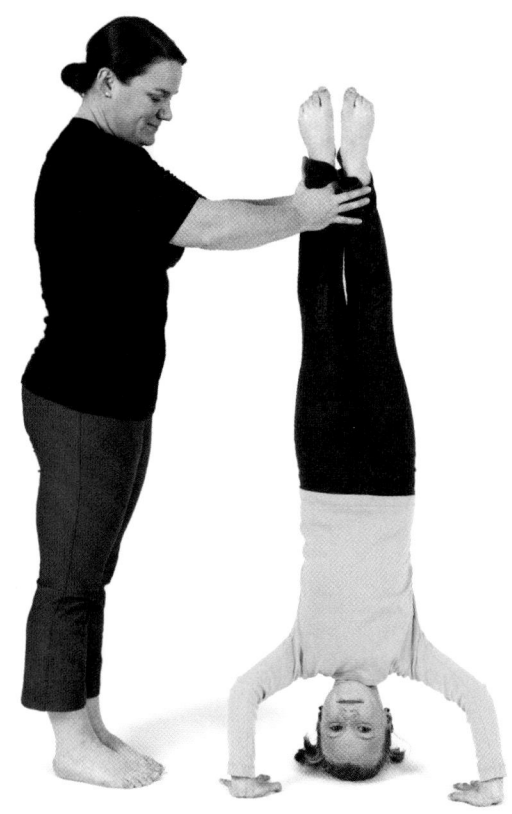

★ Headstand

Headstand

From Pre-Headstand, use your belly muscles to pull your knees up off of your arms and into your body. Pressing your legs together, straighten them to the sky using the wall behind you for support, as needed. Now you're in Headstand!

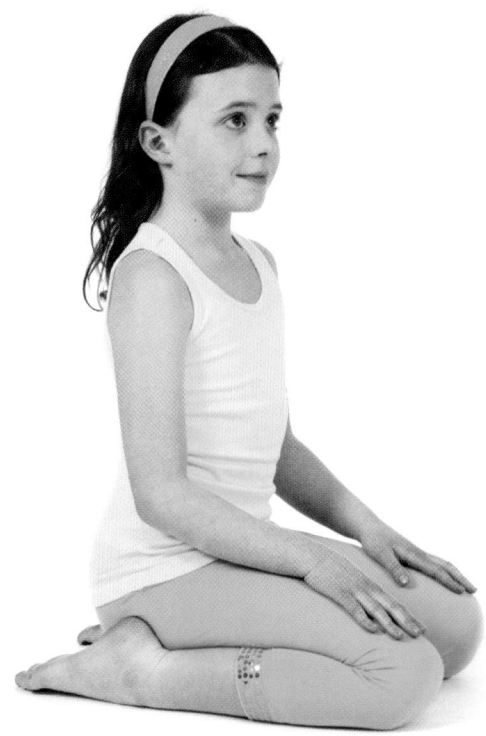

★ Hero Pose

HERO POSE AND THUNDERBOLT POSE

Benefits

Calms the body and encourages deep breathing

Stretches thighs and quadriceps

 Helps relieve stomach issues

WHAT TO DO

For children who are challenged to sit upright in Easy Pose, Hero Pose can provide a nice alternative. Be sure the tops of your child's feet remain flat on the floor and that she does not "W-Sit." (If your child has any knee or back issues, skip Thunderbolt Pose.)

WHAT TO SAY

Begin by kneeling with your knees together. Slide your shins and feet out to the sides slightly and then nestle your bottom between your heels. Sit up tall and rest your hands on your thighs. Breathe . . .

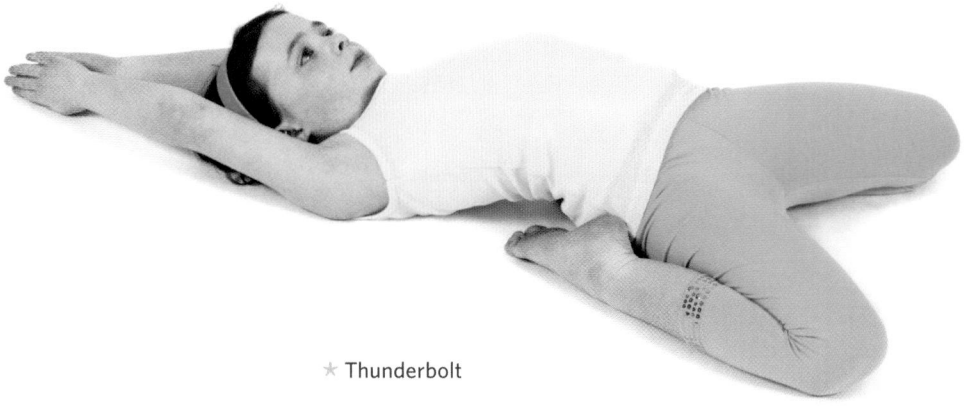

★ Thunderbolt

Thunderbolt

Lean back and reach your hands for the floor on either side of your feet. Begin to bend your elbows and carefully lower yourself back and down to the floor. Raise your arms over your head. You are a thunderbolt! Stay here for a few deep breaths. When you are ready, bring your arms back down to your sides and press into your elbows and forearms to rise back up out of the pose.

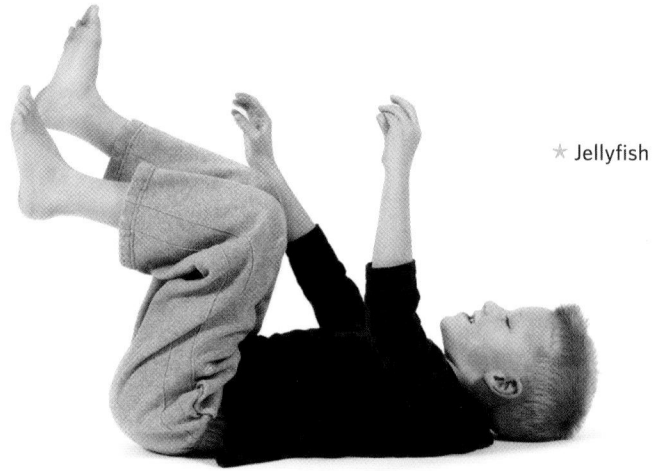

★ Jellyfish

JELLYFISH

Benefits

Calms and restores

Builds core strength

WHAT TO DO

Jellyfish is a peaceful, calming pose that can make for a nice transition to relaxation. Encourage your child to lengthen his limbs while flowing in Jellyfish Pose so that he strengthens his core muscles.

WHAT TO SAY

Lie on your back. Lift up your arms and legs to become tentacles. Let them flow and sway as they would in the ocean. Just float and flow with no particular place to go.

Partner Variation

Octopus. Create an octopus with eight tentacles by lying down side by side with your child. Collect small objects that can be picked up off the floor using the toes.

Now feed the octopus by using your arms to draw food into your mouth (small opening between the waists of your two bodies—point to it). Bring the object up with your hand and challenge your child (and yourself) to pass it around from hand to foot, touching every tentacle before dropping it into the octopus mouth!

KING DANCER

Benefits

- Improves balance and focus
- Stretches the shoulders and chest
- Strengthens the ankles and legs
- Encourages poise and posture

WHAT TO DO

[handwritten: → adaptive yoga]

This is a challenging balance pose. Have your child come to a wall first for support, practicing the pose on each side as she builds confidence in the pose.

WHAT TO SAY

Start in Mountain Pose and find a focus point. Shift your weight to your left foot and raise your left arm for balance. Slowly reach back with your right hand to grab the outside edge of your right foot. Find your balance and breathe . . . need more of a challenge? Press your foot into your hand as you arch your back and come forward. Keeping your eyes on your focus point, breathe in . . . breathe out. Can you hold King Dancer Pose for 3 to 5 full breaths? Let's see! Now switch sides.

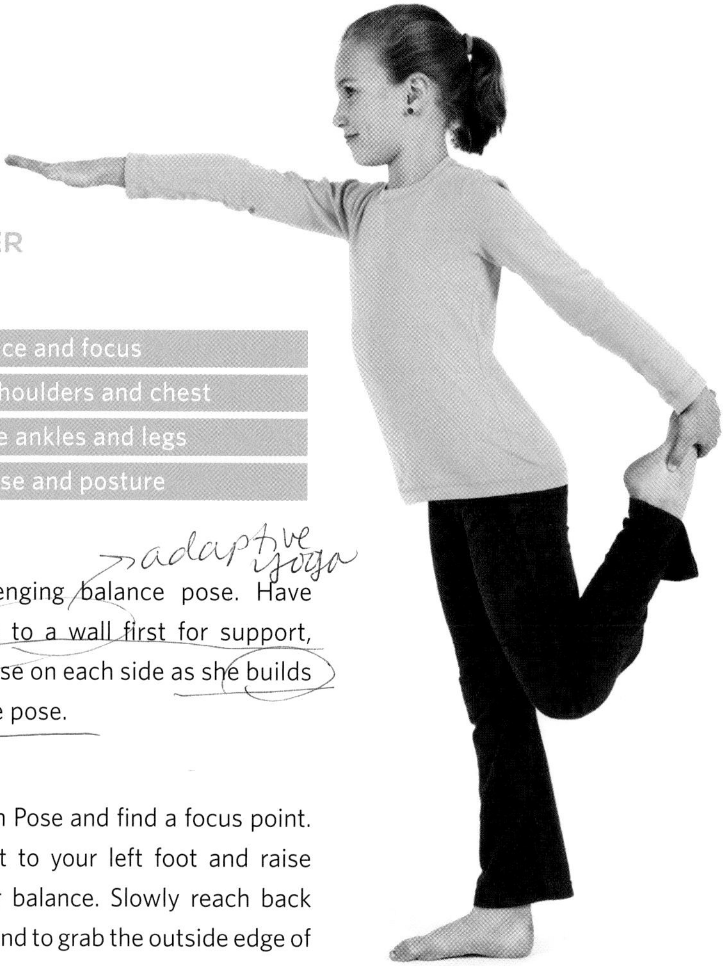

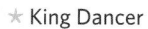

★ King Dancer

KING DANCER VARIATIONS

- **Double Dancer.** Stand facing each other in Mountain Pose. Reach same side arms up and press your palms together, then reach back for your opposite foot. Balance here together for five breaths. Switch sides.
- **Hop and Stop.** While in King Dancer, begin to hop in place. Then stop. Can you maintain your balance? You can if you hop with control. Use a focus point to help you.

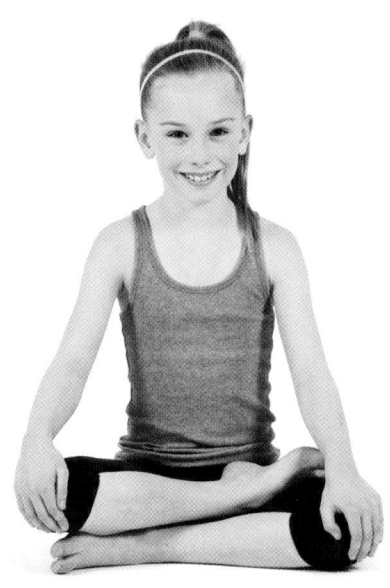
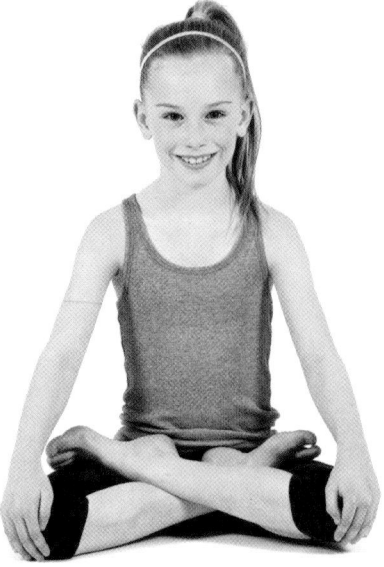

★ Half Lotus

★ Full Lotus

HALF LOTUS AND FULL LOTUS

Benefits

Improves posture

Stretches the ankles and knees

Improves attentiveness and focus

Opens the hips

WHAT TO DO

If your child has tight hamstrings and/or poor core strength, have her sit on a folded blanket or rolled-up yoga mat to bring her hips above her legs so that she can sit up straight. When practicing Half Lotus Pose, be sure your child switches legs, spending equal time on both sides. Unless your child is super flexible, be sure she practices Half Lotus to warm up before attempting Full Lotus Pose.

WHAT TO SAY

Start in Easy Pose. Draw your right foot up high onto your left thigh. The bottom of your foot should be facing up. Breathe here in and out slowly 3 to 5 times . . . release your right leg and shake your legs out. Switch sides and repeat. Now try Full Lotus. From Half Lotus Pose, draw your other foot up high onto your opposite thigh. Sit up tall, rest your hands on your knees, and breathe.

MERMAID

Benefits

Encourages poise and good posture

Cleanses internal organs, stimulates digestion

Opens the lungs

Stretches the hips and hamstrings

WHAT TO DO

Mermaid is a pose that encourages good posture and full spinal twist. Use this pose as a precursor to Pigeon. Encourage your child to lower her shoulders down from her ears while elongating her neck.

WHAT TO SAY

Sit with your knees both pointing to your right. Bring your right foot to the front of your left knee with your left foot tucked behind you. Place your hands on the floor on either side of your right knee. Now, pose like a mermaid sunning herself on a rock! Sit up tall with your chest open and look out over your left shoulder. Breathe for several breaths before switching sides.

MERMAID VARIATIONS

- **Splashing Mermaid.** Lean back to put your hands behind you on the floor. Keeping your feet "glued" to the floor, lift your knees up and switch them to face in the opposite direction. Swish them back and forth, "splish, splash!"

- **Swimming Mermaid.** Inhale deeply to sit up tall and fill your lungs with oxygen. Exhale, "Pssshhh!" as you bend forward from your hips to lower your chest to your thigh. Repeat by bringing your head up and down in a diving motion, moving with your breath. Switch sides by "splashing" over to the other side. Now, swim in the other direction!

★ Mermaid

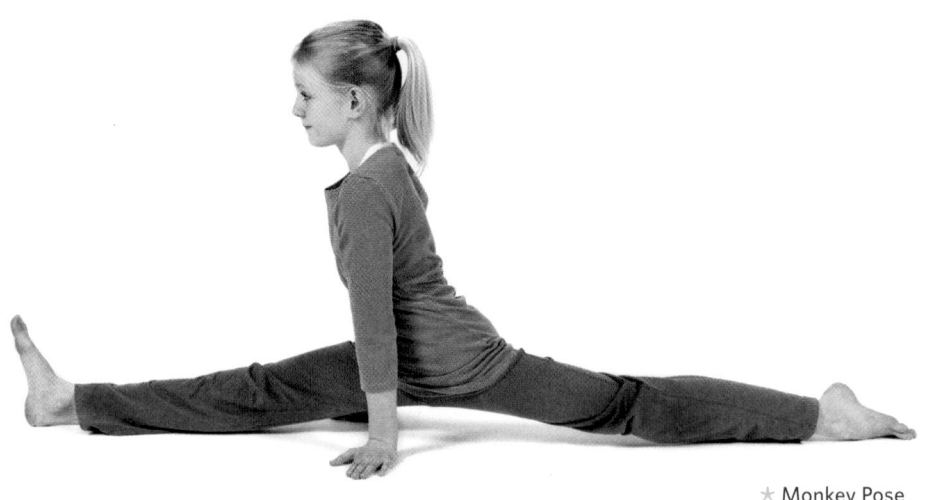

★ Monkey Pose

MONKEY POSE

Benefits

Stretches the hamstrings, thighs, groin, and hips

Strengthens the hamstrings and thighs

Stimulates abdominal organs

WHAT TO DO

To protect delicate knees, have your child practice on a yoga mat, carpet, or blanket. Also, placing blocks or books under the hands can help your child stay upright and adjust the amount of stretch she is experiencing. Try Pigeon Pose as a warm-up to Monkey Pose.

WHAT TO SAY

Start in a kneeling position. Bring your right foot out straight in front of you as you bring your hands down to the floor on either side for support. Begin to slide your left leg back as far as you can for a comfortable stretch. You're a monkey! Press into your hands to help you stay up straight. What does a monkey say when he's monkeying around? When you are ready, press into your hands and slide your left leg forward, then your right foot back to come back to a kneeling position. Sit or stand up to shake your legs out like a monkey before switching sides.

Benefits

Grounding, centering

Promotes good posture

WHAT TO DO

Mountain Pose is the foundation pose for all standing postures, and one that your child can use to center herself before attempting other poses. With Mountain Pose, children often mistake the pose as a stiff pose, rather than a strong, stable one. It is important that children be relaxed yet strong in the pose to reap its benefits.

WHAT TO SAY

Stand up tall and strong with your arms at your sides and your feet about hip-distance apart. Look straight ahead to find a focus point in front of you. Take a deep breath in and draw your shoulders up to your ears. Now exhale to round them back and down. As you exhale, imagine your feet are the base of the mountain, pushing into the ground with all of the weight of the mountain above it. Relax and breathe in and out normally 3 to 5 times.

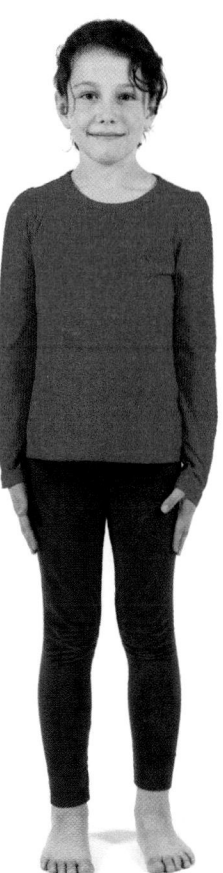

★ Mountain Pose

Stable Mountain or Tin Soldier?

Children often get "stiff" while practicing Mountain Pose—keeping their shoulders up near the ears and forgetting to breathe. To help them engage in the pose without tensing up, try this. Nudge your child's shoulder as you say, "Are you a mountain or a tin soldier?" If she's being a tin soldier, she will likely lose balance and fall over. Playfully shake your child's shoulders to relax them, encouraging her to raise them up and down as she exhales. Breathe deeply with your child to model. Try nudging your child again so that she feels in her body that she's a stable, strong mountain.

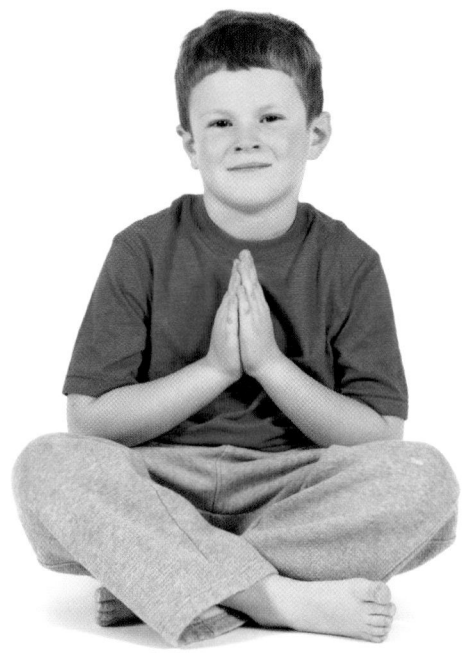
★ *Namaste* Pose

NAMASTE POSE

Benefits

Calming, centering

Balancing, integrates both sides of the brain

WHAT TO DO

Namaste Pose, otherwise known as *Anjali Mudra*, is commonly thought of as a prayer position, but in fact, it does not signify prayer. In India, pressing the hands together and saying, "*Namaste*," is a way of greeting or honoring someone. The word *Namaste* translates simply to mean "I honor you," or as one of my 4-year-old students translated it, "I see the beauty in your heart." As well, bringing the hands together in front of the heart and pressing the fingertips together helps center and focus the mind, so it is used often as part of various yoga postures and meditation exercises. Encourage your child to close his eyes when practicing *Namaste* Pose.

[handwritten annotations: "I see the image of God in you"; "image between"; "You look like Him too!"]

WHAT TO SAY

Bring your hands together in front of your heart. Press your fingertips together and your thumbs on your breastbone. Close your eyes and breathe . . .

OWL

Benefits

- Keeps legs limber
- Stretches the hips, inner thighs, and calves
- Aids digestion
- Improves balance
- Opens the chest and lungs

WHAT TO DO

Your child may want to balance on his toes, which is fine as it provides a balance challenge. However, to obtain the pose's full benefits, you'll want to encourage him to bring his heels to the floor. This is easier to do the farther apart the feet are placed. As well, a rolled-up yoga mat or blanket placed beneath the heels as a "'branch" can provide support.

WHAT TO SAY

Roll up your yoga mat or blanket. This is your branch! Stand in Mountain Pose with your feet spread apart, heels on your branch. Inhale deeply and reach back to hold your opposite elbows. Squat down to "perch" on your branch. "Hoo! Hoo!" Balance on your branch and breathe in and out for 3 to 5 breaths.

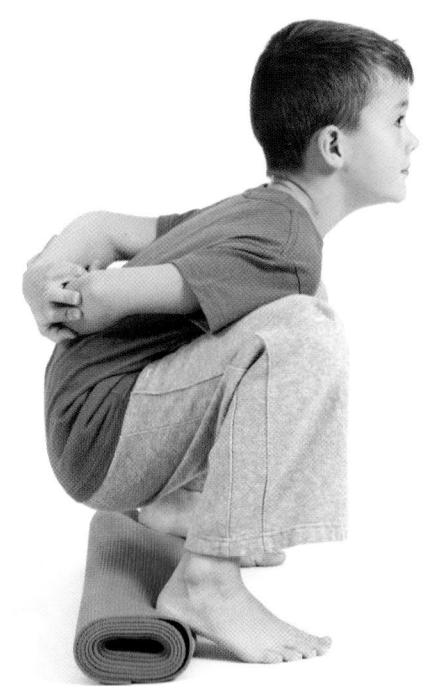

★ Owl

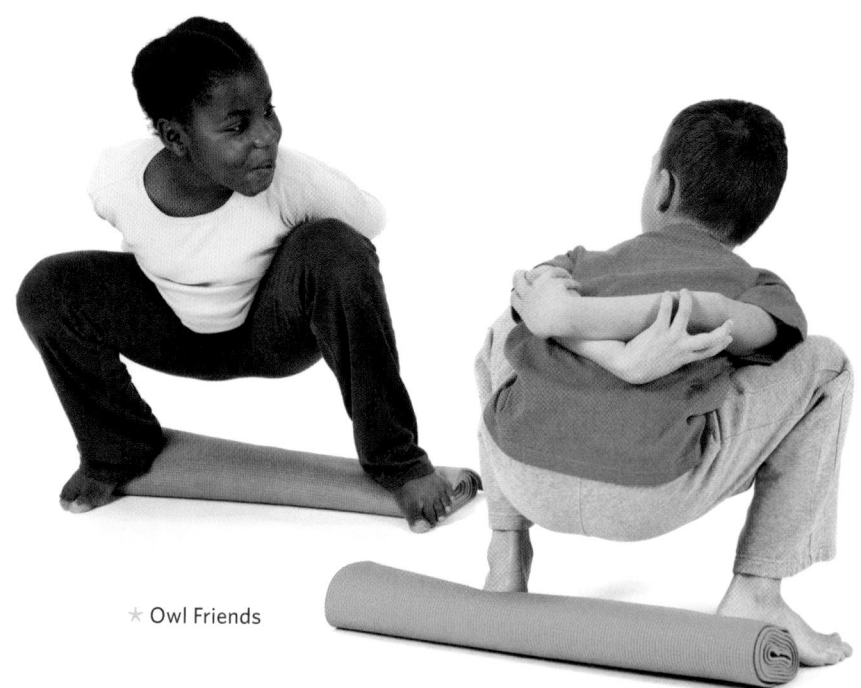

★ Owl Friends

OWL VARIATIONS

- **Owl Friends.** Perch on a branch beside your child facing in the opposite direction. Turn your heads to look at one another. "Hoo Hoo!" Now, turn to the other side. "Hoo Hoo!"
- **Owl Ears.** Owls have amazing hearing. Sit in silence on your "branch" for one minute. Share the sounds that you heard when the minute is up.

PIGEON

Benefits

Opens hips
Stretches glutes, groin, and hamstrings
Stimulates internal organs
Elongates the back, improves posture

WHAT TO DO

For children with tight hips, don't worry about their shin being square to the front of their mat. They will still gain some benefit even if their shin is slightly angled or not angled at all. This pose can stress the knee joint, so use caution, especially if your child has knee issues. For a deeper stretch, have your child try bending forward at the hips to lower her head down to rest on her arms on the floor.

WHAT TO SAY

Begin in Table Pose. Slide your right knee forward toward your right hand. Angle your right knee to the right and slide your shin forward a bit. Extend your left leg out behind you, keeping your hips squared to the front. Puff out your chest like a proud pigeon. Breath in and out for 3 to 5 breaths. Press into your hands and slide your leg back into Table Pose. Rest in Child's Pose for a moment before switching sides.

PIGEON VARIATIONS

- **Pecking Pigeon.** From Pigeon Pose, inhale to puff your chest. Exhale and bend in your elbows to lower your chest toward your thigh. Bob your head to peck for food! Repeat several times until your belly is full. (Parents, "feed" your pigeon by tossing pretend breadcrumbs down in front of your child.)
- **Partner Pigeon.** Come into Pigeon Pose facing each other. Connect hands above, look into each other's eyes, and breathe . . . don't forget to switch sides!

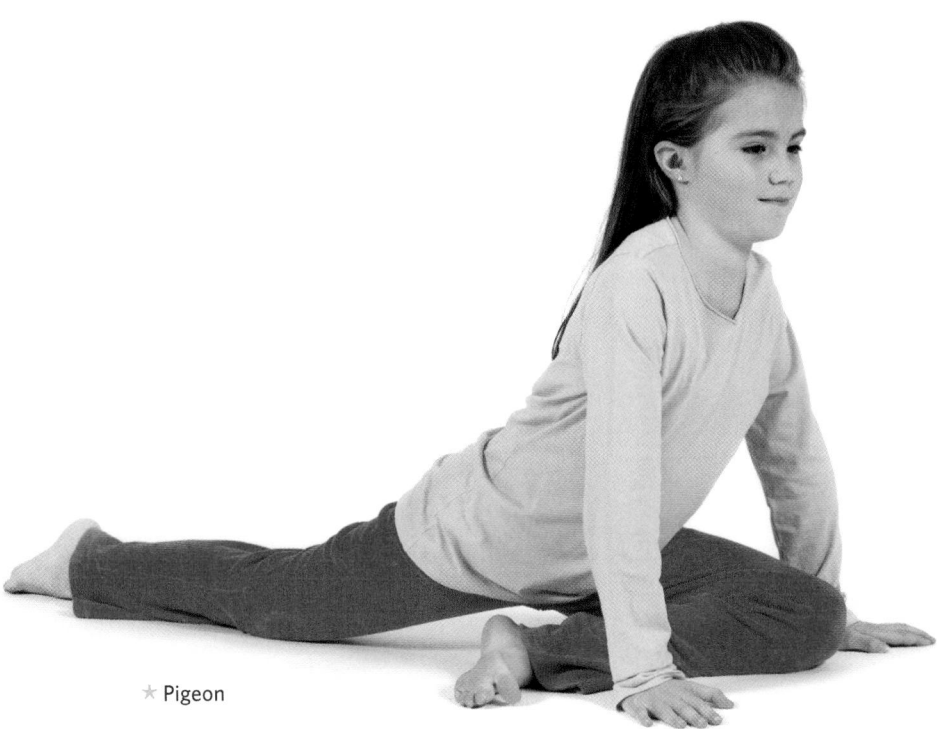

★ Pigeon

Benefits

Hip opener

Stretches the ankles, knees, upper thighs, lower back, and glutes

Builds core strength

WHAT TO DO

Double Pigeon is a wonderful hip opener. If your child has tight hips and/or poor core strength, have her sit on a folded blanket or mat so that her sitting bones are on the blanket and her legs and ankles are stacked on top of each other on the floor. Have her sit like this, switching sides after a minute or two, while watching TV, reading, or hanging out, a few times a week. To deepen the stretch, have your child walk her hands out in front of her shins while folding forward at the hips. Be careful, though. Even the smallest movement will add a lot of intensity to the stretch.

WHAT TO SAY

Start by sitting in Easy Pose. Now bring your right ankle up onto your left knee and slide your left ankle out slightly so that is lined up beneath your right knee. As you look down, do you see an upside-down triangle in the middle of your legs? Now sit up tall with your hands on your knees and breathe with me. In . . . and out . . . in . . . and out. Stretch out your legs and shake them out. Switch sides.

Rock the Baby

From Double Pigeon, take your hands around your foot and knee of your top leg to draw your shin up and in closer to your body. Gently rock from side to side to release tension in the muscles being stretched. Go ahead, sing "Rock-a-bye Baby." You know you want to! Release your leg and switch sides.

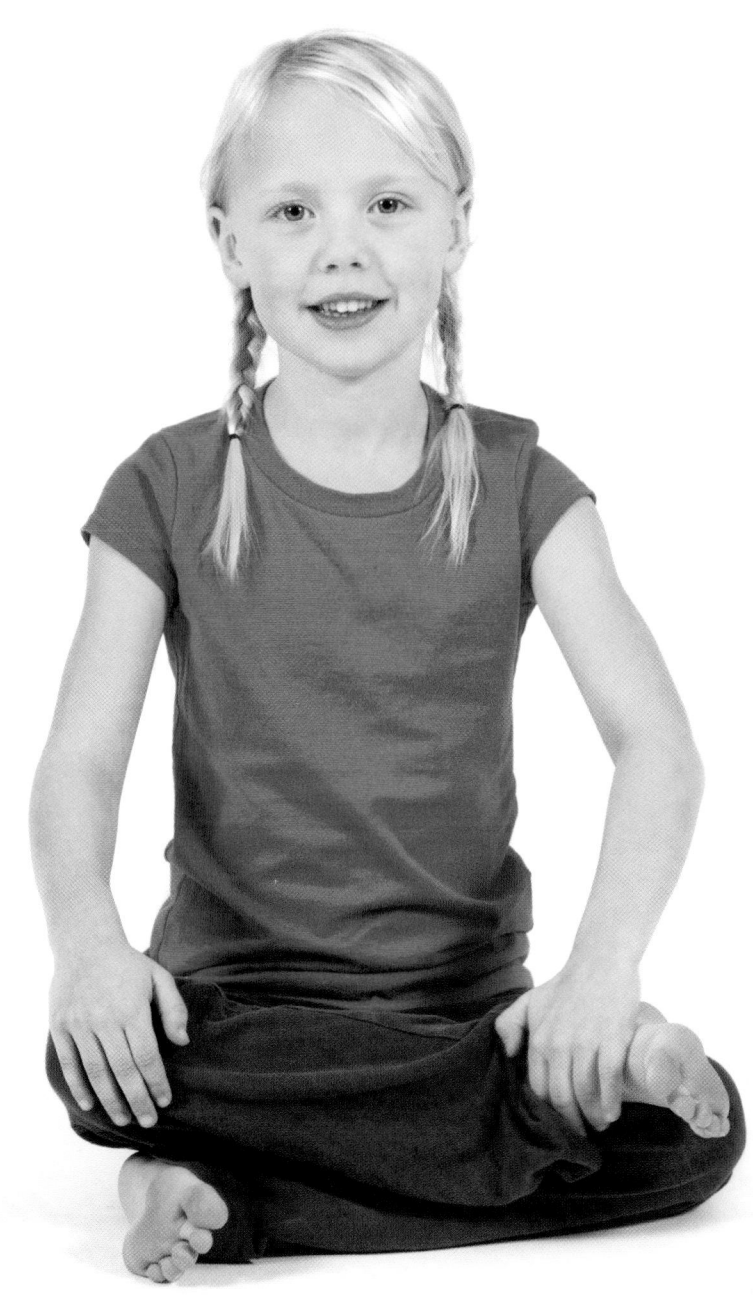

★ Double Pigeon

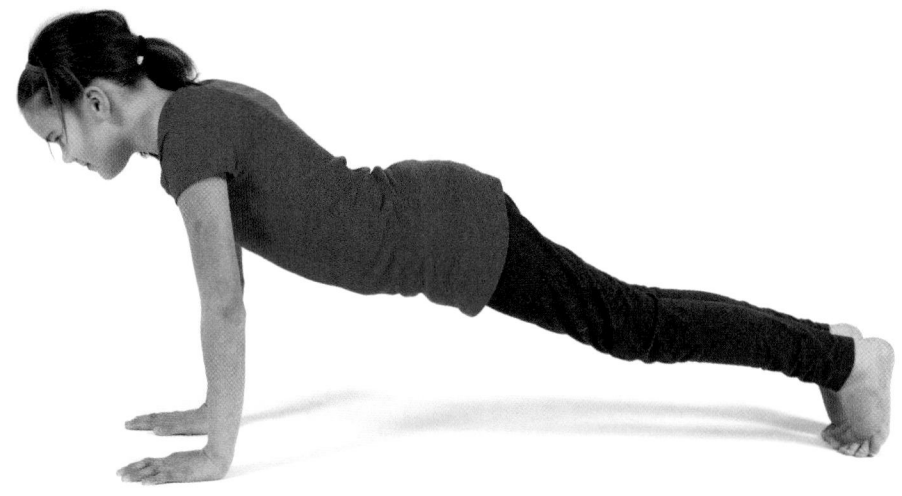

★ Plank Pose

PLANK POSE

Benefits

Strengthens arms, shoulders, wrists, legs, and core

Promotes a long spine, good posture

WHAT TO DO

→ tap to engage

To keep her midsection from sagging in Plank Pose, encourage your child to have strong arms and to pull in her belly muscles to engage her core. Does your child's Plank Pose look more like a Down Dog position? Say, "Try to make a straight line with your body. Good!" It can also help to use a mirror or take a digital photo so that your child can see what she looks like in the pose. Then have her try it again, noting the improvements. This will build her confidence while improving her body awareness.

WHAT TO SAY

Begin in Table Pose. Move your hands and body forward a bit and lift your head and chest. Curl your toes under and lift your knees off the floor. Try to straighten your body into a long, strong plank. Keep your neck long as you look at the floor in front of you. Breathe in and out for 3 to 5 breaths, and then return to Table Pose. Rest in Child's Pose, then stretch out to Plank Pose once again. You did it!

Benefits

Stretches the shoulders and spine

Stimulates abdominal organs

Rejuvenates, relieves stress and exhaustion

WHAT TO DO

Skip this pose if you or your child suffers from neck pain or injury. In general, to protect the delicate neck, encourage your child to come into Plow Pose slowly and mindfully. Your child's toes may or may not touch the floor overhead. It does not matter, so do not force him to do so. As well, once in the pose, ensure he keeps his head centered and gazing straight as opposed to turning his head and neck.

WHAT TO SAY   *& shoulder stand*

Begin in Candle Pose. Ensure your neck is long and your shoulders are down away from your ears. Inhale deeply. Exhale and slowly lower your legs behind you. Lower your arms to the floor to support the pose. Keep your head and gaze straight ahead as you breathe and relax in the pose. When you are ready, gently come out of Plow Pose by slowly lowering your legs to the floor. Rest here for a moment before sitting up or moving on to another pose.

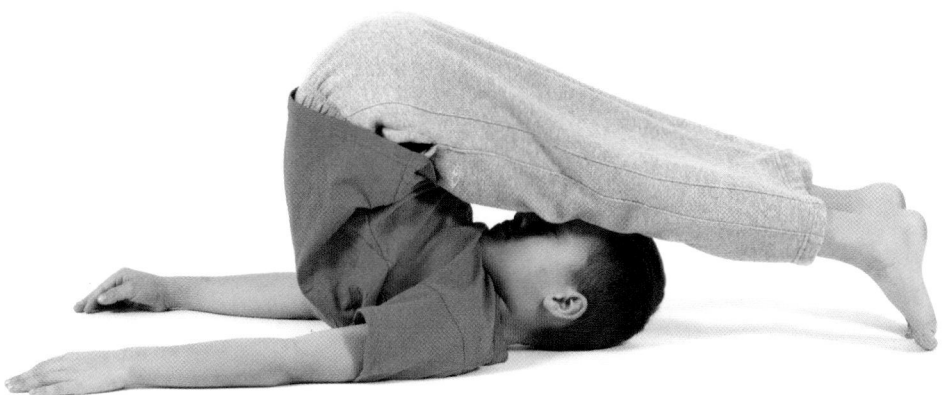

★ Plow Pose

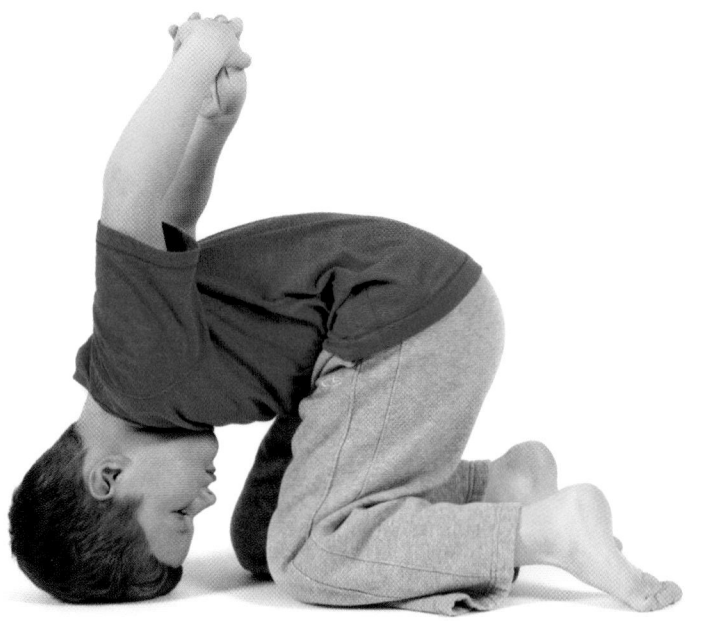

★ Rabbit Pose

RABBIT POSE

Benefits

Stretches the back, neck, and arms

Brings fresh oxygen to the brain

Stimulates digestion

WHAT TO DO

Have your child first balance a book on his head so that he can physically feel what part of his head should be pressing into the floor when practicing Rabbit Pose. To protect the top of the head, have your child practice on a folded yoga mat or blanket. To protect his neck, be sure your child keeps his head stationary.

WHAT TO SAY

Begin in Table Pose. Fold forward to bring your forehead close to your knees. Tuck your chin and place the top of your head gently on the floor. Reach back to clasp your hands behind you. Arch your back to the sky as you roll onto the crown of your head, raising your arms behind your head. Breathe and relax here for 3 to 5 breaths. Slowly roll back and release your feet. Come down to rest in Child's Pose.

RAG DOLL

Benefits

Calms the nervous system

Rejuvenates, relieves fatigue

Stretches the whole back side of the body, neck to heels

Helps improve concentration

Stimulates internal organ function, improves digestion

WHAT TO DO

Your younger child may need encouragement to stay in this pose. One idea is to have her count her toes. Alternatively, you might place a beanie buddy between her feet, asking your child to tickle the doll's belly as she reaches forward for her toes. Encourage slightly bent knees in this pose, with more of a bend if your child has tight hamstrings. *beanie babies (stay where you put them)*

WHAT TO SAY

Start in Mountain Pose with your feet about hip distance apart. Inhale deeply as you bring your arms up to the sky. Exhale and bend at your hips to hang forward like a floppy rag doll. Gently nod your head "yes" and "no" until all the tension is released from your shoulders, neck, and head. Let your arms be loose and relaxed. Try swinging them a bit from side to side like a gorilla before coming to settle down again at the center. Relax and breathe here, releasing a little more into the stretch with each exhale. Ahhh. When you are ready, start to tuck your tailbone and inhale to slowly roll back up into Mountain Pose.

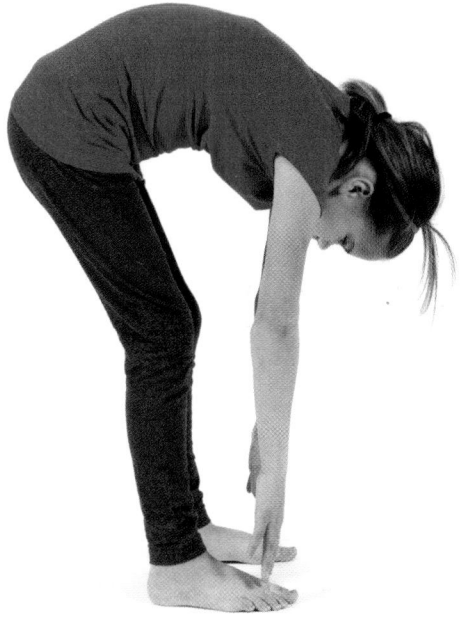

★ Rag Doll

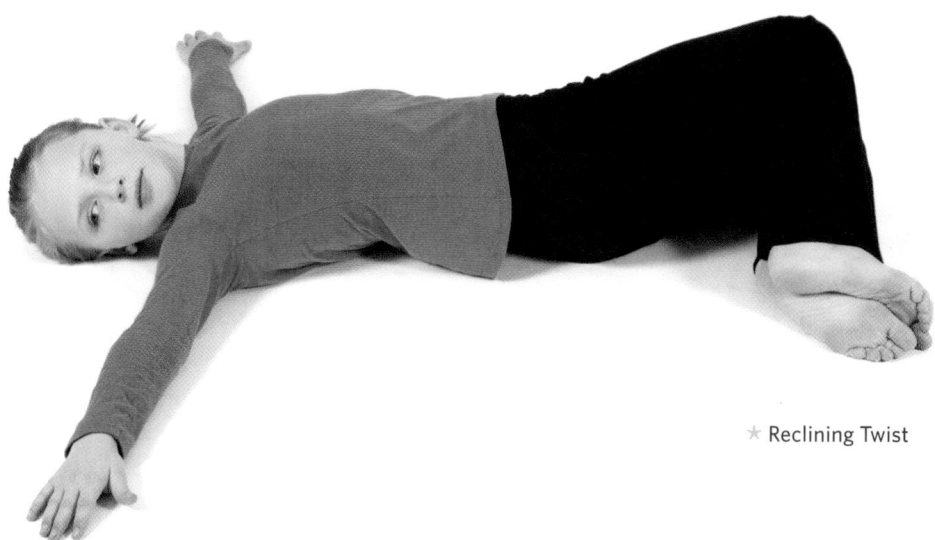

★ Reclining Twist

RECLINING TWIST

Benefits

Tones internal organs, improves digestion

Open the lungs

Stretches back and neck muscles

WHAT TO DO

Reclining Twist is restorative and restful, serving as a wonderful transition to relaxation. Encourage your child to keep her shoulders on the floor while twisting to ensure the benefit of a full spinal twist.

WHAT TO SAY

Lie down on your back. Place your feet flat on the floor, knees bent. Extend your arms wide out to your sides. Breathe in deeply. Breathe out and drop your knees to your left side as you turn your head to look out over your right shoulder. Shoulder check! Are your shoulders both on the floor? Good. Rest here for a couple of breaths. When you're ready, inhale your knees back up and switch sides.

ROADRUNNER

Benefits

WHAT TO DO

Roadrunner (or High Lunge) can be entered easily from Table Pose, Down Dog, or Rag Doll. Encourage your child to check his front knee to ensure it's over or slightly behind his ankle. His back leg should be strong and straight.

WHAT TO SAY

Begin in Rag Doll (or Table or Down Dog, see previous). Bend your knees and bring your hands to the floor. Take a big step back with your left foot. Good! Now adjust yourself so that your hands are placed on either side of your front foot. Your back leg is straight and strong with your toes tucked under. Knee check! Your front knee should be just over or behind your ankle. Great. Now keep your neck and back long and find a focus point in front of you. Breathe in and out slowly for 3 to 5 breaths. Switch sides.

ROADRUNNER VARIATIONS

- **Ready, Set, Go!** Lower the back knee slowly down to the floor. Say "Ready!" Bring the knee back up and say, "Set!" Now, say, "Go!" as you jump and switch your legs. Repeat five times or more.
- **Balance Challenge.** (For older children:) Sit up tall and take your hands off the floor to rest them on your knee.

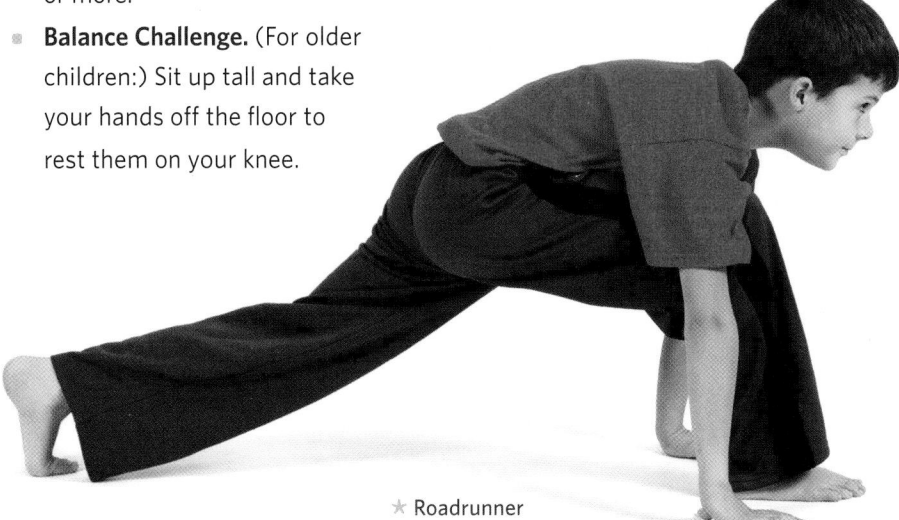

★ Roadrunner

SANDWICH POSE

Benefits

Calms the nervous system
Rejuvenates, relieves fatigue
Stretches the whole back side of the body, neck to heels
Helps improve concentration
Stimulates internal organ function, digestion

WHAT TO DO

If your child has tight hamstrings, place a folded blanket or yoga mat under her hips so that her sitting bones are on the blanket and her legs are stretched out on the floor in front of her. The tighter the hamstrings, the higher the hips should be off the floor (for super-tight hamstrings, try using a bolster or stack of books). As well, your child can also keep her knees slightly bent. This will lessen the strain on her lower back. In general, encourage your child to fold from the hips rather than at the waist.

WHAT TO SAY

Start in Easy Pose. To make the first slice of bread, straighten your legs out in front of you. Point your toes to the sky. Now, inhale and reach your arms up above your head to create the second slice of bread. Exhale as you fold forward, bending from your hips. Reach your hands toward your shins or feet to make your sandwich. Continue to breathe slowly and deeply. Try releasing into the stretch a little more with each exhale.

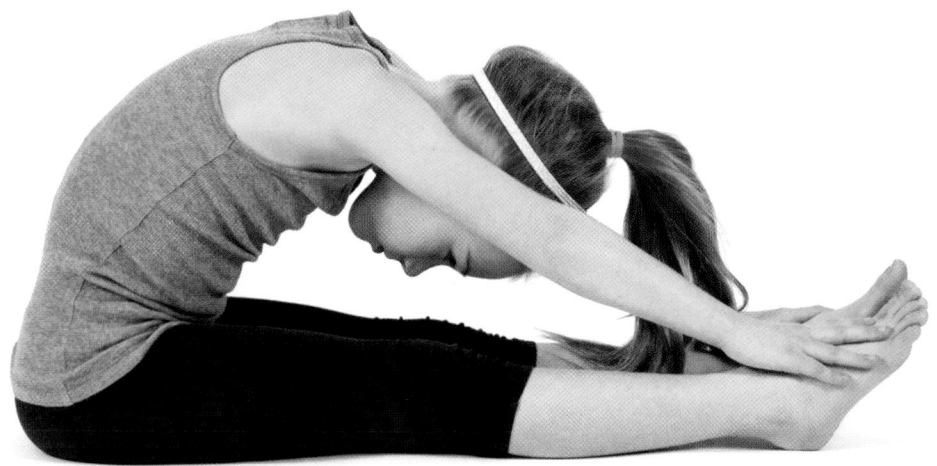

⋆ Sandwich Pose

Make It a PB&J

For extra fun, make your sandwich a PB&J! From Staff Pose, turn to your left and scoop some pretend peanut butter out from the jar beside you (choose another if allergic). Spread it all over your face, your arms, your belly, everywhere! Now turn to your right side and scoop some pretend jelly from the jar beside you. Remember, spread it everywhere! Now press both slices of your "bread" together, by folding forward. Press your hands together to make your "knife" to cut your sandwich in half! Drag the knife between your legs, from your feet to your waist. Now spread your legs apart—there are your two halves! Fold over each leg to eat both halves of your sandwich. Yum!

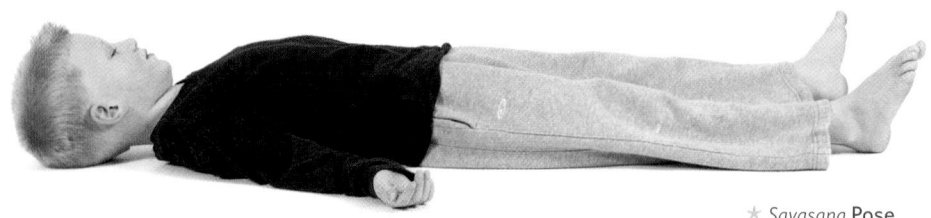

★ *Savasana* **Pose**

SAVASANA POSE

Benefits

Relaxes the body, lowers blood pressure
Calms the mind
Restorative

WHAT TO DO

For some children, this pose can be scary. Cover your child with a heavy blanket to give a sense of warmth and safety. A lavender-scented eye pillow (Chapter 3) can be comforting, too. Have your child focus on a spot on the ceiling to help her relax (a smiley face sticker on the ceiling is good for this purpose). If your child is still having trouble resting in *Savasana* Pose, use Crocodile Pose or Child's Pose instead. See Chapter 9 for many transitions to and variations of relaxation positions, as well as visual imagery exercises to practice.

WHAT TO SAY

Lie down on your back and stretch your body out long. Now, let your arms relax down at your sides, palms facing up. Allow your feet to flop out to the sides. Close your eyes if that's comfortable for you. Good. Now, breathe in nice and deep through your nose, expanding your chest and belly with air. Exhale out loud, "Haaaa . . . " Good. Do that again two more times and with each exhale, feel your body get heavy and relax down into the earth. Rest here in *Savasana* Pose for a few minutes. I will tell you when . . .

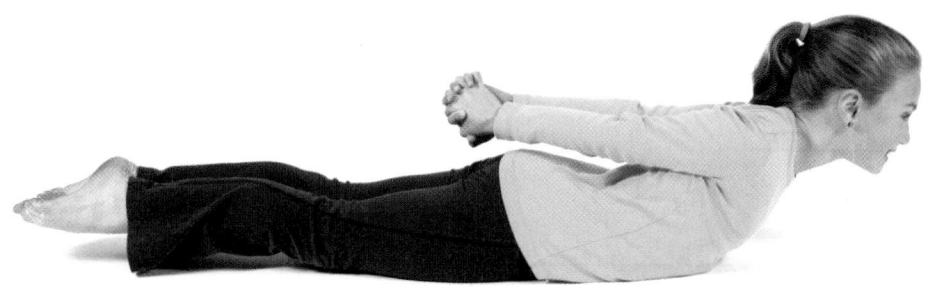

★ Shark Pose

SHARK POSE

Benefits

Opens chest and lungs

Stretches the shoulders and arms

Strengthens the core and lower back

WHAT TO DO

Have your child begin by lying on her belly, arms by her sides and palms facing the floor, and head facing the floor and a straight spine. As your child lifts off the floor, keep her from overextending her back by telling her to keep hers straight by keeping her gaze toward the floor. Say: "As you come up keep your neck long and your eyes to the floor—help keep your shark spine straight!" This pose isn't so much a backbend as it is an exercise to lengthen the spine.

WHAT TO SAY

Begin on your belly. Clasp your hands behind your back to make your shark fin. Breathe in and lift up your arms, legs, and chest all at the same time. You're a swimming shark! Breathe in and out here one more time and relax back down to rest in Crocodile Pose. Oh boy, here comes the shark again . . . (Repeat 3 times.) Now, let's rest in Child's Pose.

Benefits

Massages internal organs, helps with digestion
Improves flexibility of the spine
Improves circulation
Promotes calm

WHAT TO DO

If your child has tight hamstrings and/or poor core strength, have him sit on a folded blanket to lift his hips above his legs so that he is able to sit up straight. As a result, he will benefit from a full spinal twist when practicing this pose. With good posture, there should be little weight placed on the hand on the floor.

WHAT TO SAY

Start in Easy Pose. Sit up tall. Reach your right hand over across your left knee, and rest your left hand on the floor behind you. Good. Now, sit up nice and tall and take a deep breath in. Exhale as you turn your torso and neck to gaze behind you. Breathe in and out here for 3 to 5 breaths. Release and switch sides.

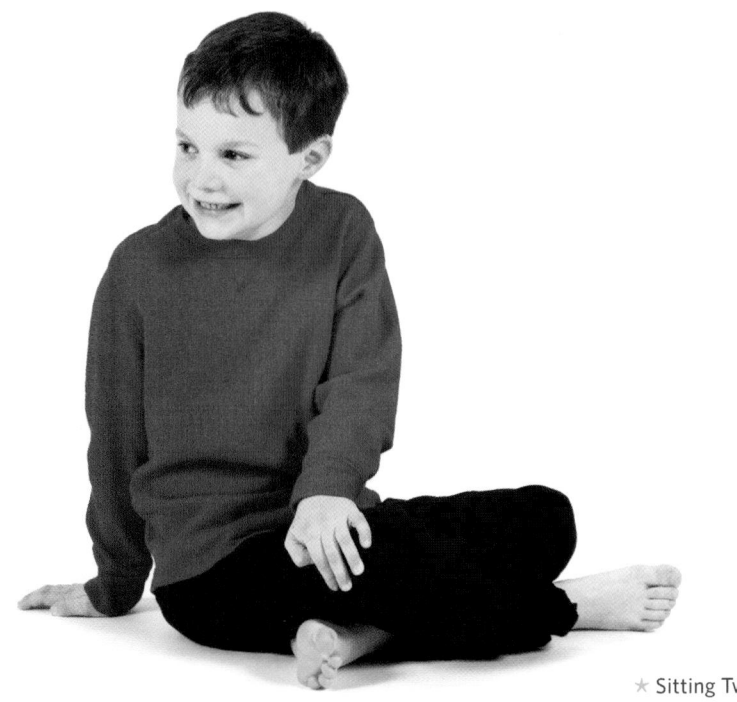

★ Sitting Twist

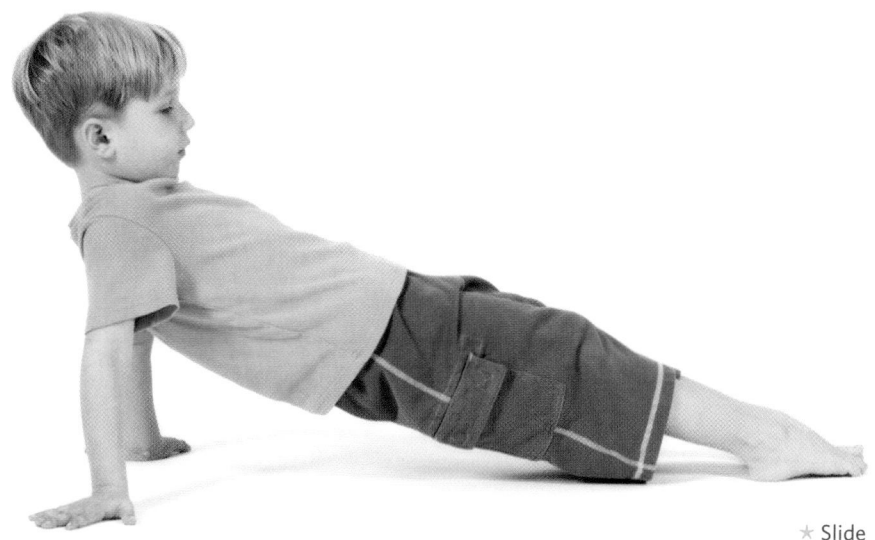

★ Slide

SLIDE

Benefits

- Strengthens arms, shoulders, legs, and core muscles
- Stretches the shins and feet
- Opens the chest and lungs
- Lengthens the neck and spine

WHAT TO DO

This pose is a challenging, full-body strengthener. Very young children or those with poor core strength may benefit from starting with Crab Pose. Encourage your child to use strong arms to keep his shoulders away from his ears. His core should be engaged. This will prevent him from sagging in the middle.

WHAT TO SAY

Begin in Staff Pose. Put your hands on the floor behind you, fingers pointing forward. Good! Keep your legs nice and straight and point your toes. Now, lift your hips up high off the floor. That's right. Use your belly muscles to hold your body up, straight and strong! Breathe here in and out three times. Lower your bottom to the floor and rest for a moment before trying it again. (Repeat 3 times.)

Benefits

Opens chest, lungs, and throat

Strengthens shoulders, arms, and lower back

Engages speech muscles

WHAT TO DO

Sphinx Pose is a gentle backbend that even the youngest of children can practice safely and successfully. This pose strengthens the upper body and opens the throat while strengthening the muscles important for speech development. Encourage your child to push down into his forearms, bring his shoulders away from his ears, elongate his neck, and push out his chest.

WHAT TO SAY

Lie down on your belly. Straighten your legs, keeping the tops of your feet flat on the floor. Elbow check! Are your elbows right underneath your shoulders? Adjust them and straighten out your forearms so they are pointing forward. Now, use strong arms and shoulders to really open your chest and pull your shoulders down away from your ears. Good. Lengthen your spine and neck and look straight ahead at a focus point. Breathe here in and out three times. When you are ready, gently come to rest in Child's Pose.

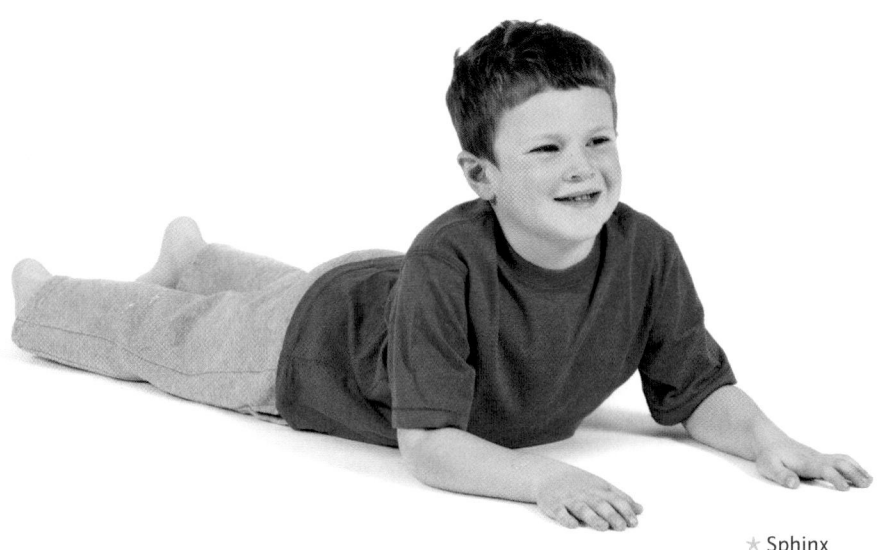

★ Sphinx

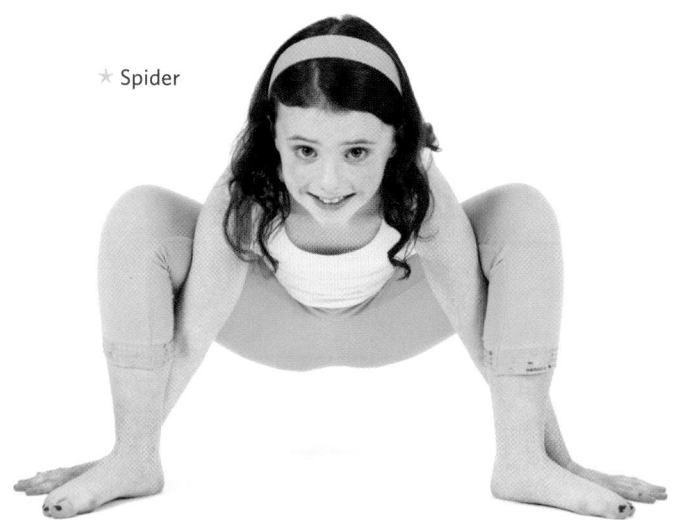

★ Spider

SPIDER

Benefits

Keeps legs limber

Stretches the hips, inner thighs and groin

Aids digestion

Improves balance

WHAT TO DO

Even though your child may be tempted to balance on her toes in Spider Pose, encourage her to bring her heels to the floor, which is easier with the feet placed farther apart.

WHAT TO SAY

Start by standing with your feet a little wider than hip-distance apart. Squat down by bending your knees out to the sides until your bottom almost reaches the floor. Can you bring your heels to the floor? Good. Bring your hands to the floor between your feet and slide them around the outsides of each of your feet. You're a spider! Look up and give me a spider face as you breathe in and out three times.

TRY THIS

- **Walking Spider.** "Walking" in Spider Pose requires mindful movements and good balance. Try it. Lift up your right hand and foot and step forward, then your left. How far can you spider walk?

- **Spin a Web.** Keep your hands on the floor and move your bottom up and down to weave your web. Where do you feel the stretch? (hamstrings)

Benefits

Stimulates internal organs, digestion

Improves posture

WHAT TO DO

If your child has tight hips and/or poor core strength, place a folded blanket or yoga mat under her hips so that her sitting bones are on the blanket and her legs are folded in front of her on the floor. This pose provides even the youngest children a fun opportunity to twist the spine and use the breath productively.

WHAT TO SAY

Sit in Easy Pose. Bring your elbows out to your sides and rest your fingertips on the tops of your shoulders. Inhale deeply through your nose. Exhale and twist from side to side as you make a sprinkler sound: "Pssh, pssh, pssh, pssh." When you are out of water, stop twisting for a moment to fill up your sprinkler hose by taking another deep breath in through your nose. Exhale and twist back and forth, once again. "Pssh, pssh, pssh."

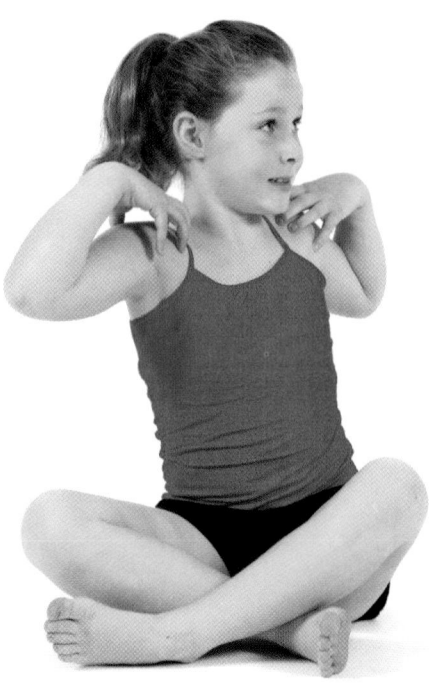

⋆ Sprinkler

Shake and Freeze

Once you are soaked with water, stand up and shake it off to music. Start with your head, shaking each individual part of your body until your whole body is shaking. When the music stops, freeze where you are!

Benefits

Strengthens the back, shoulders, and core muscles

Improves posture

WHAT TO DO

If your child has reduced core strength or tight hamstrings, place a folded blanket or yoga mat under her hips so that her sitting bones are on the blanket and her legs are stretched out in front of her. If your child's hands cannot comfortably reach to press into the floor, try putting a book or magazine under each hand, choosing items of equal height.

WHAT TO SAY

Sit on the floor with your legs extended out in front of you. Press your hands into the floor at the sides of your body. Good. Now, make your legs strong and flex your feet so that your toes are pointing toward the sky. Sit up tall and breathe . . .

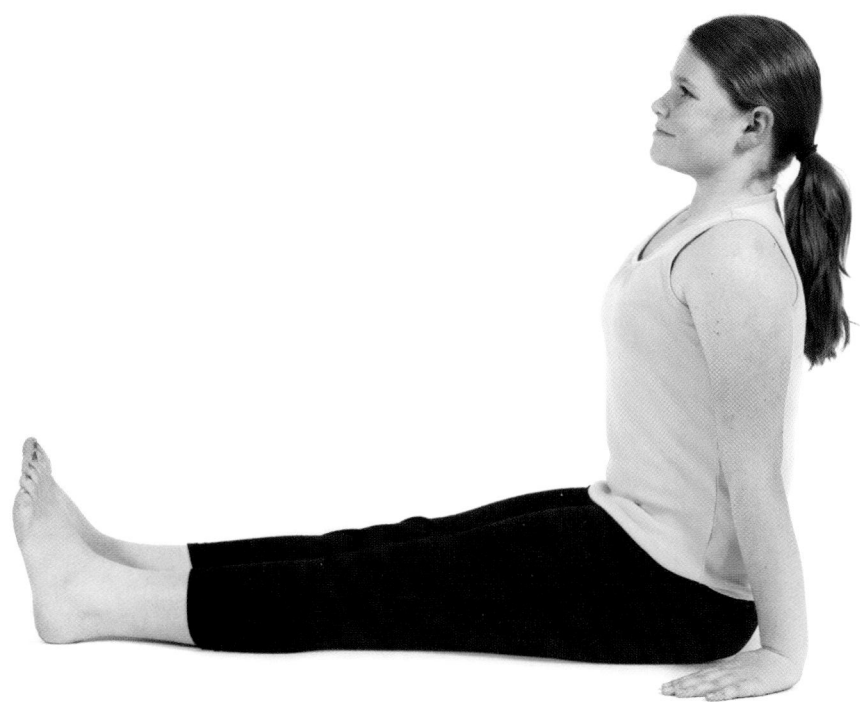

★ Staff Pose

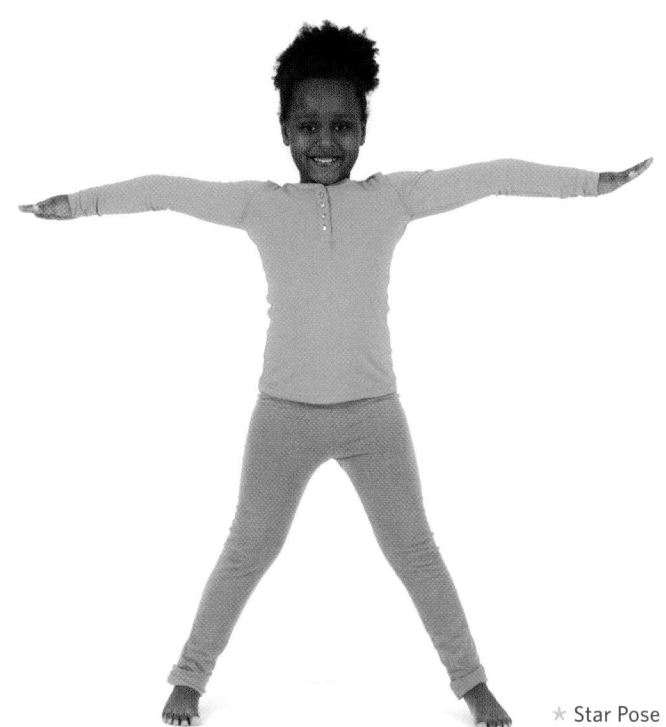
★ Star Pose

STAR POSE

Benefits

Strengthens and tones the entire body

Lengthens the spine, improves posture

WHAT TO DO

Star Pose (or Five-Pointed Star) seems simple enough, but holding the pose correctly for any length of time is actually quite challenging. Encourage your child to engage *all* the muscles of her body to maintain the pose.

WHAT TO SAY

Start in Mountain Pose. Hop your feet apart and stretch your arms out straight to each side. How many points do you have? Let's count them: . . . 1, 2, 3, 4, 5 (start with the head and point to each extremity, one by one). Good. Now stand up tall, lifting your head to the sky. Press your feet into the floor and stretch your arms out to your sides. Shoulder check! Are your shoulders up near your ears or relaxed and low? Yes, exhale and relax them down away from your ears. How long can you hold Star Pose? Let's breathe in and out here for 10 seconds . . .

STAR POSE VARIATIONS

It's easy to get creative with Star Pose. Try these engaging variations:

- **Twinkling Star.** "Twinkle" by keeping your arms and legs straight as you rock back and forth from one foot to the other. Go ahead and sing "Twinkle, Twinkle Little Star" while rocking! For a balance challenge, start and stop music, challenging your child to freeze (typically on one foot) when the music stops!

- **Folded Star.** Inhale to reach your arms back, opening up your chest. Exhale and fold forward. Grasp the outside edges of your feet or ankles. Your older child can grasp her big toes with her first two fingers. Breathe in and out three times before moving into Twisty Star.

- **Twisty Star.** From Folded Star, place your right hand on the floor between your legs. Inhale and lift your left arm up to the sky. Look up toward your hand. Breathe here in and out three times before switching sides.

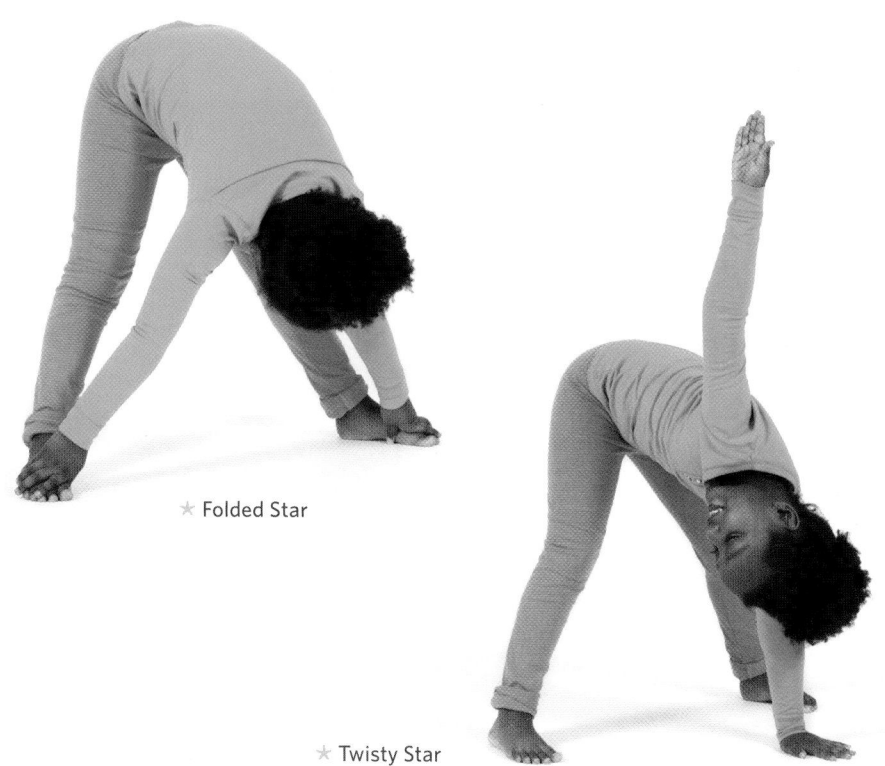

★ Folded Star

★ Twisty Star

Benefits

Restorative

WHAT TO DO

Starfish Pose is a wonderful position to use during relaxation or as a transition rest between other poses during a yoga session. For comfort, have your child lie down on a yoga mat, carpet, or blanket when practicing Starfish Pose. Add some magic by adding the Sea Scarf activity in Chapter 9.

WHAT TO SAY

Lie down on your back. Come into Star Pose lying down. Gently close your eyes. Imagine you are a starfish sunning himself on a rock in a tide pool. Inhale and reach your arms and legs out long and straight, tensing all of the muscles in your body. On your exhale say, "Haaaa," allowing your starfish body to relax onto the rock. Rest here for a minute, breathing in and out slowly and evenly.

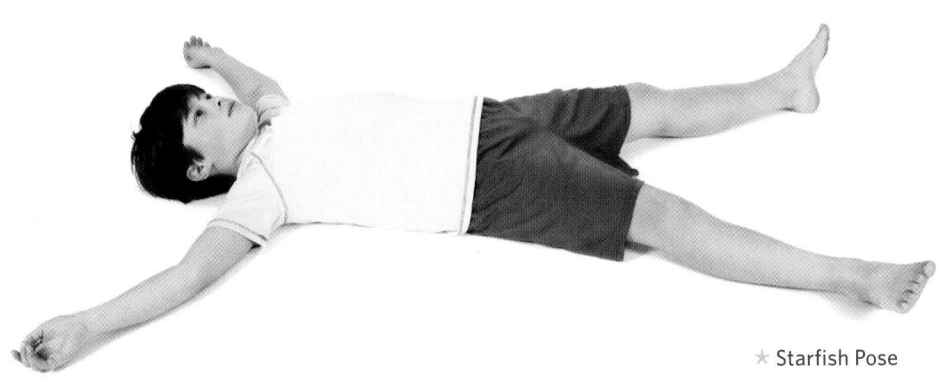

★ Starfish Pose

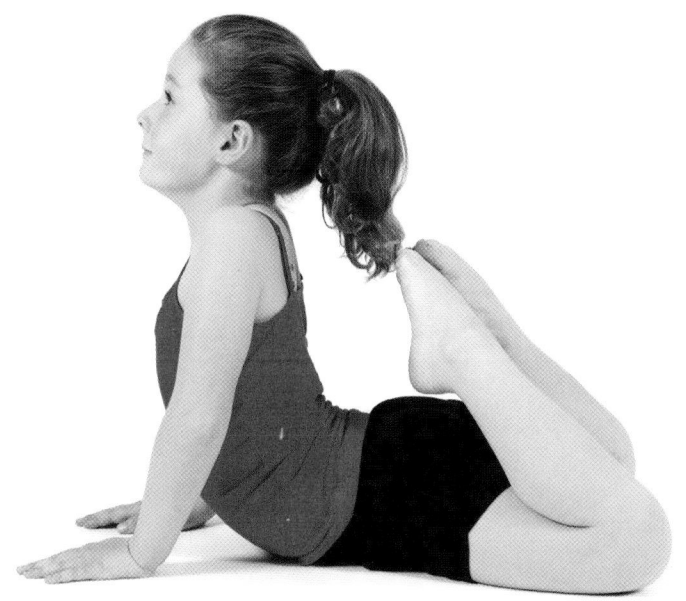

★ Swan

SWAN

Benefits

| Opens the chest |
| Strengthens the wrists and arms |
| Stretches the spine, back, and thighs |

WHAT TO DO

Some children may be able to touch their head to their feet, but that is very much dependent upon flexibility and leg versus torso length. Be sure your child understands that our bodies are all built differently and her effort attempting this and all poses is much more important than looking like what is depicted in photos.

WHAT TO SAY

Start in Table Pose. Lean forward on your hands as you bend your knees and lift your feet up in the air. Good! Keep your arms straight while lengthening your back and neck, opening up your chest. Stretch back to reach your toes toward your head. You're a beautiful, graceful swan! Breathe in and out three times before coming to rest in Child's Pose. Try it again if you'd like!

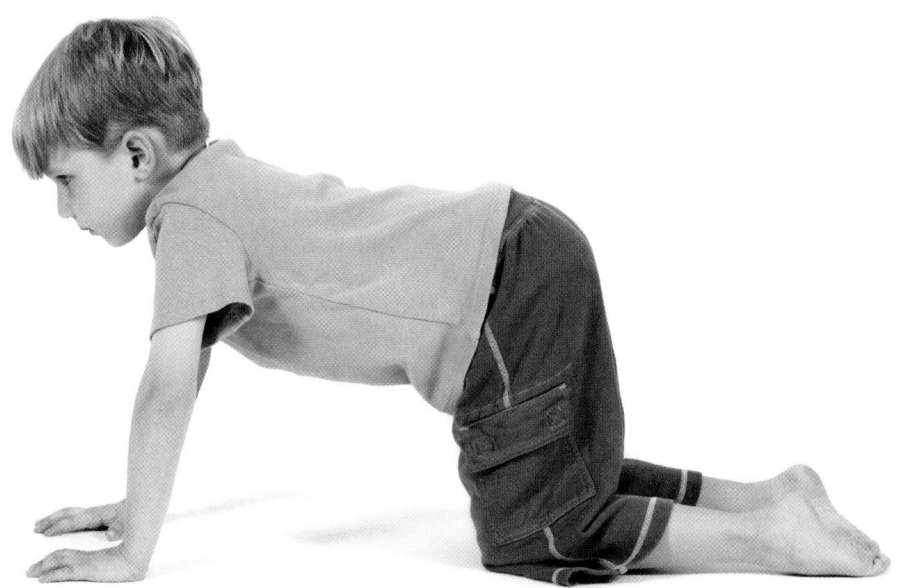

★ Table

TABLE

Benefits

Strengthens wrists, arms, shoulders, and core

Lengthens the spine and the muscles of the back and neck

WHAT TO DO

To protect arms and wrists, steer clear of this and other weight-bearing poses if your child has suffered recent arm or wrist injuries. To encourage your child to maintain a strong, flat back in Table Pose, try practicing in front of a mirror or take a digital photo and show it to him. If there are adjustments to be made, have him try again and take another photo until he succeeds.

WHAT TO SAY

Come onto your hands and knees with the tops of your feet flat on the floor. Be sure your hands are placed on the floor directly below each of your shoulders and your knees are directly beneath your hips. Spread your fingers wide. Good. Notice your midsection now. Can you keep your back long, strong, and flat, like a table? Breathe in and out three times while holding Table Pose.

Set the Table

To encourage your child to maintain a flat, strong back when practicing Table Pose, try setting the table! Create a place setting with a fork, knife, and spoon. Put a paper or plastic plate on his back. Pretend to eat from the table, lifting and lowering utensils, cutting up food, etc. Giggles are sure to happen, making this a seriously fun challenge in body control!

TREE POSE

Benefits

Promotes focus and concentration

Improves balance

Stretches the inner thighs and groin

WHAT TO DO

Focus, concentration, and balance can be difficult for some children. With practice, Tree Pose offers an opportunity to enhance those skills and builds confidence.

WHAT TO SAY

Begin in Mountain Pose with hands together in *Namaste* Pose. Find a focus point with your eyes. When you are ready, shift your weight to your left foot and turn your right knee out to the side. Rest your right heel on your left ankle, keeping your toe on the floor (version 1). If you are feeling balanced here, try lifting your right foot up to rest on the inside of your calf (version 2). Slowly grow your arm branches up to the sky. Your arms should be straight with your shoulders relaxed down away from your ears. You can bring your hands together over your head to make a pine tree or keep them apart as an oak tree. (Older children can try version 3: Bring your right foot up into your thigh.) Balance in Tree Pose for 3–10 slow, deep breaths or for as long as you are able.

"baby" tree
"mom" tree
"dad" tree

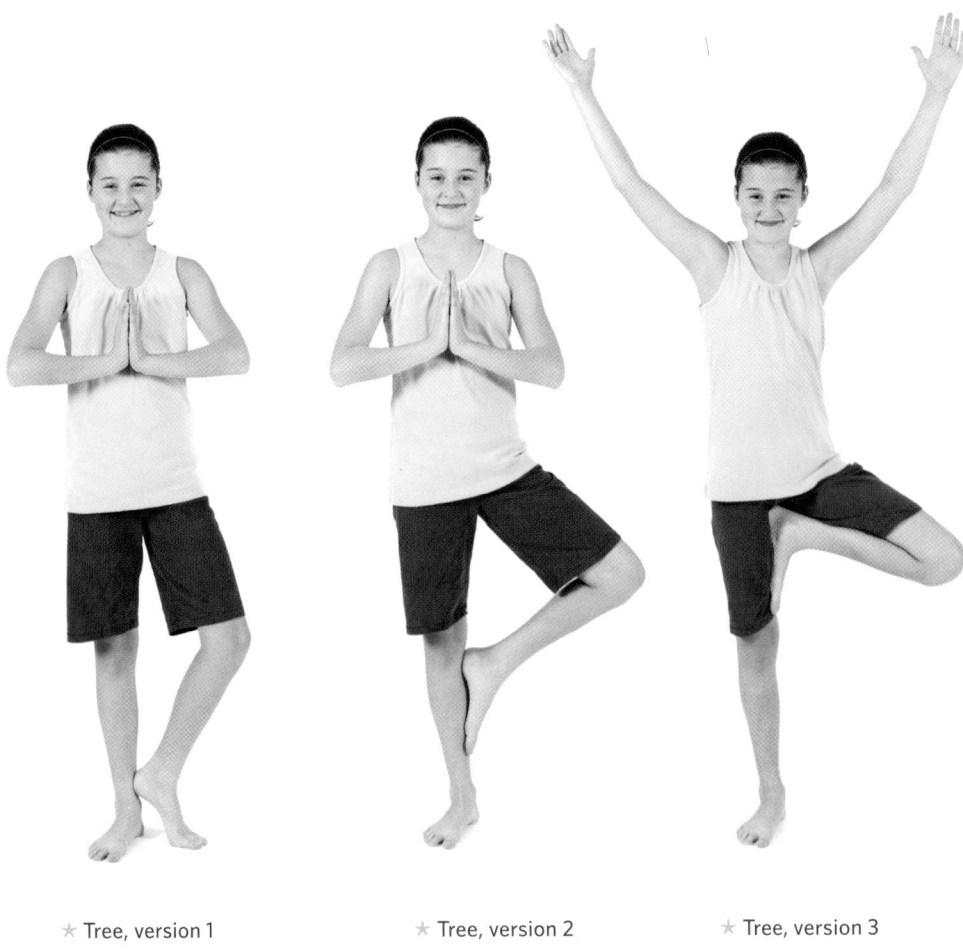

★ Tree, version 1   ★ Tree, version 2   ★ Tree, version 3

TRY THIS

- **Sprout Some Leaves or Fruit.** Bring your arms up overhead and out to the sides as branches. Sprout some leaves or fruit by spreading out your fingers. "Pop, pop, pop!"
- **Sway Your Branches.** Sway your branches in the wind while keeping your "roots" grounded deep into the earth.

let a bird land on your branch

TRIANGLE

Benefits

Stretches and strengthens the legs, arms, back, and waist

Opens the chest and lungs

Elongates the spine

Improves balance and endurance

Stimulates internal organs, digestion

WHAT TO DO

Oftentimes, children will bend forward to come into Triangle Pose, rather than sideways. To help your child "feel" the side bend, have her first practice coming into the pose with her back against a wall. To help your child lengthen her stretch and expand her rib cage, put your hand just above her hand and have her reach up to touch it.

WHAT TO SAY

Begin in Mountain Pose. Jump your feet out nice and wide and turn your right foot out to the right. Stretch your arms out to the sides. Inhale deeply to stand up tall. On your exhale, reach your right arm out while slowly bending sideways. Reach for your right shin with your right hand while raising your left arm up to the sky. Check to be sure you are bending sideways, rather than forward by imagining your body is the PB&J squeezing out from between two slices of bread. Try gazing up to your left hand. Stay for 3 to 5 breaths. Bend your right knee slightly and rise back up to standing, arms outstretched. Switch sides.

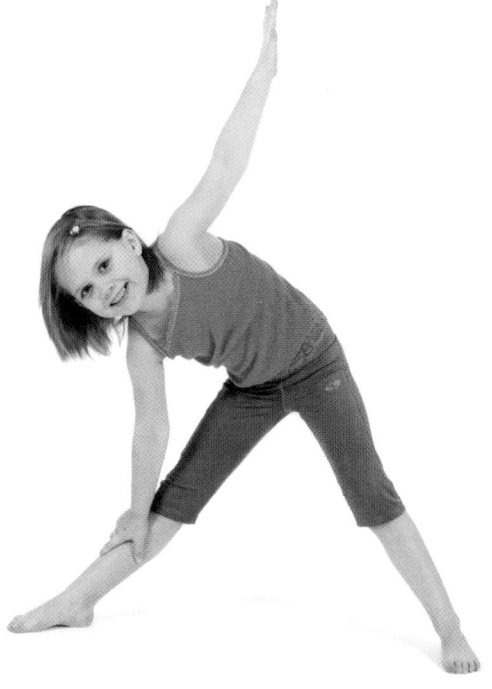

★ Triangle

TRIANGLE POSE VARIATIONS

- **How Many Triangles?** Between the legs, the two feet form the base and the top hand forms the point, the hand on the knee and the shoulder form the base and the waist forms the point. Can you find more?
- **Do the "Triangle Teapot Song."** (Chapter 8)
- **Play Pose Tag.** (Chapter 7)
- **Town Clock.** Put a clock on your "steeple" by pointing your finger and moving just your forearm all the way around while counting from 1 to 12 o'clock.
- **Triangle Partners.** Face each other and come into Triangle Pose holding hands above.

TURTLE POSE

Benefits

Stretches the hips, back, groin, and hamstrings
Lengthens the spine and neck
Stimulates internal organs, digestion

WHAT TO DO

An alternative for younger children or those with tight hips and hamstrings is to start in Butterfly Pose. Direct your child to slide his feet forward a bit so that he can fold forward to slide his hands and arms underneath his legs. He can then lay his arms out flat or wrap them around his feet to create his shell.

WHAT TO SAY

Begin in V-Sit Pose with your legs spread wide. Fold forward and place the palms of your hands on the floor and slide them under each leg. Hide in your shell by bowing forward, head down. Peek out of your shell by bringing your head up and out. Stay in this position, but bring the bottoms of your feet together to produce a new kind of turtle shell!

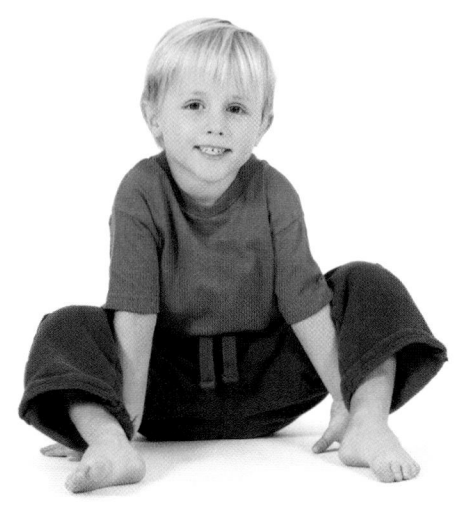

★ Turtle

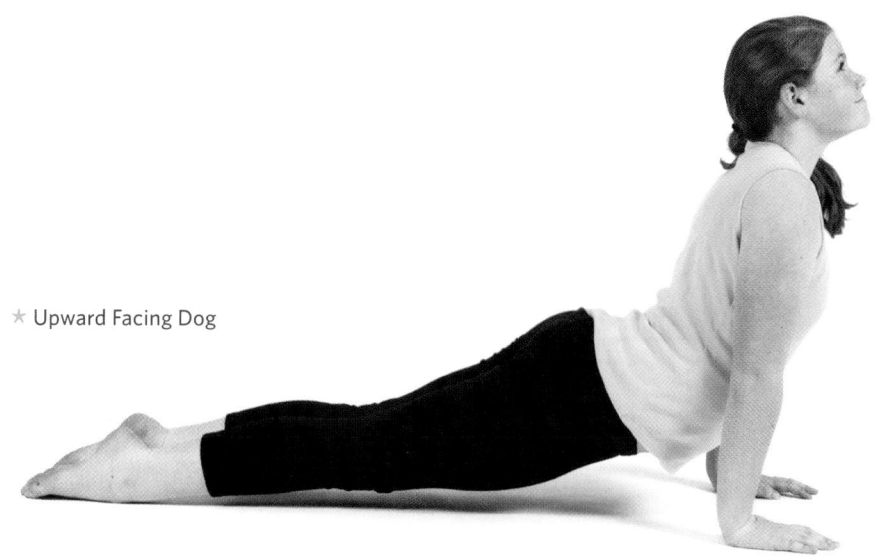

* Upward Facing Dog

UPWARD FACING DOG

Benefits

Strengthens the spine, arms, shoulders, and wrists

Opens the chest and lungs

Improves posture

WHAT TO DO

Your younger child may not have the strength to lift her entire body off the floor, so her Upward Facing Dog may look a bit more like Cobra. It's okay! As your child becomes stronger and more coordinated, her alignment will naturally improve with your encouragement.

WHAT TO SAY

Start by lying down on your belly. Place your hands on the ground alongside your chest, fingers spread wide. Be sure your elbows are tucked in close to your sides. Good. Now, stretch out your legs behind you. Press down into the tops of your feet and into your hands. With strong arms and shoulders, lift your body off the floor. That's it! You're in Upward Facing Dog. Body check! The only parts of your body touching the ground should be the tops of the feet and your hands. Good. Lengthen through your neck and spine and breathe . . . stay here and breathe in and out three times before lowering yourself back down to the floor. Rest in Child's Pose.

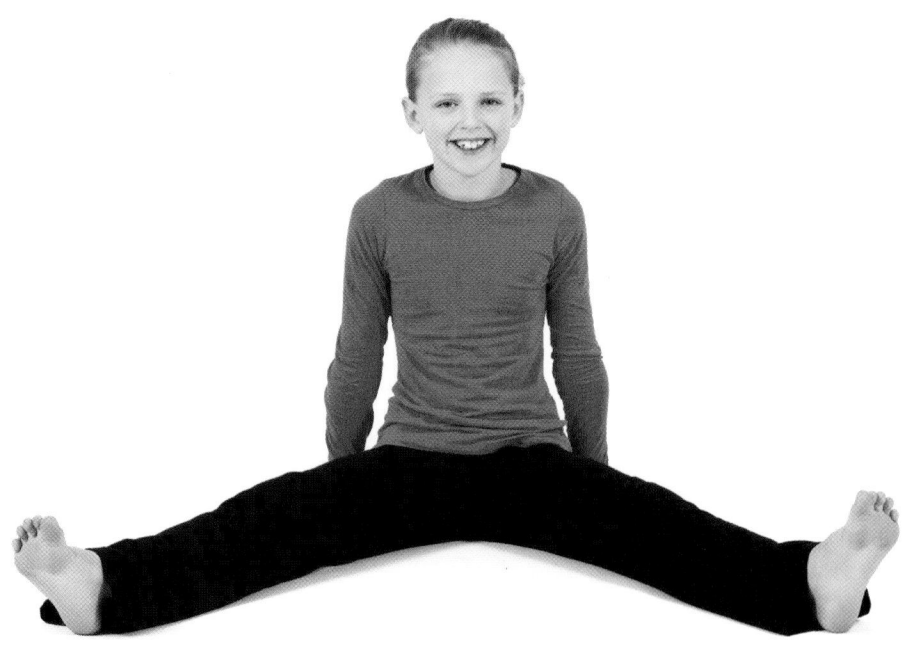

★ V-Sit Pose

V-SIT POSE

Benefits

Builds core strength

Improves posture

Stretches hamstrings

WHAT TO DO

If your child has tight hamstrings, place a folded blanket or yoga mat under her hips so that her sitting bones are on the blanket and her legs are stretched out on the floor in front of her. The tighter the hamstrings, the higher the hips should be off the floor (for super-tight hamstrings, try using a bolster or stack of books under the hips). As well, your child can also keep her knees bent a bit. This will lessen any strain on her lower back.

WHAT TO SAY

Start in Staff Pose and press your hands into the floor at your sides. Spread your legs apart from one another to create a "V" shape. Open up your chest and use your belly muscles to sit up tall. Breathe here in and out 3 to 5 full breaths.

Sitting Tree Fold

From V-Sit Pose, draw your left foot up into your right thigh. Now, inhale your arms up to the sky. Turn your body to face out over your right leg. Exhale and fold forward from your hips, reaching out over your right leg. Stretch out here for three breaths. Inhale your arms back up, then exhale them down to your sides. Switch legs and repeat.

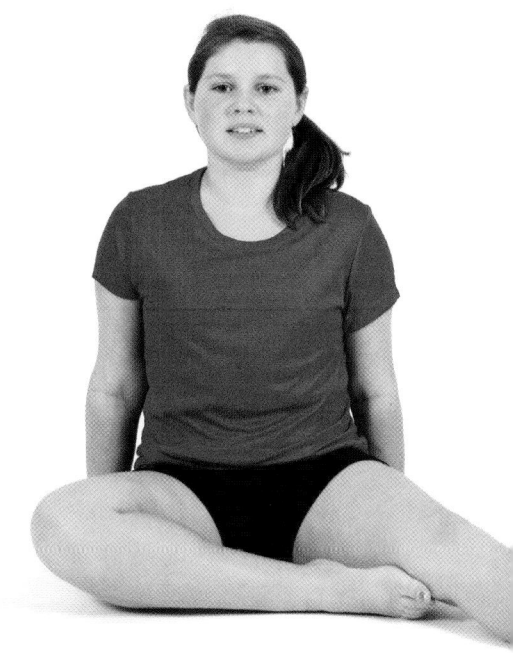

★ Sitting Tree

WARRIOR SERIES (WARRIOR I, II, AND III)

Superhero series

Benefits

Strengthens the entire body
Improves balance
Imparts boldness, personal power, confidence
Promotes focus and concentration

There are three basic variations of the Warrior Pose. After your child has mastered each of them, practice them in the following sequence. *Warrior vinyassa flow*

WARRIOR I

WHAT TO DO

In Warrior I and II, the front knee is bent and the back leg is straight. Often, as children learn the pose, the bend in the knee is lost. Say, "Knee check!" to help your child remember to keep the bend.

WHAT TO SAY

Start in Mountain Pose. Take a big step back with your right foot. Keep your hips facing forward. Bend your left knee so that your thigh is parallel to the ground. Back leg stays straight. Raise your arms up to the sky and breathe! Say: "I am strong!" Come back to Mountain Pose and switch legs.

WARRIOR II

WHAT TO DO

In Warrior II, the hips open to the side, but the legs stay in place with the front knee bent and back leg straight. A quick "Knee check!" will remind your child to check his alignment without feeling corrected. As well, encourage your child to relax his shoulders down away from his ears. Strong warriors don't shrug their shoulders!

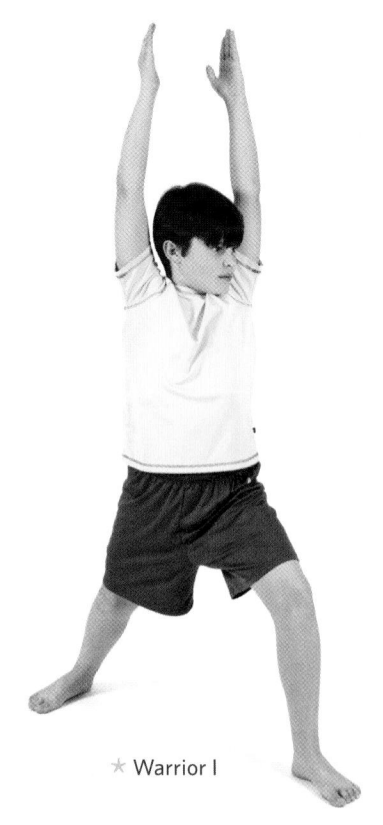

★ Warrior I

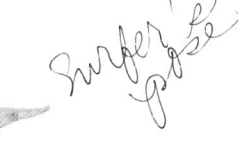

WHAT TO SAY

From Warrior I, open your hips to the side. Keep your left leg bent over your ankle. Bring your arms straight out to the sides so that they are parallel to the ground. Turn your head to your left to look out over your fingertips. Say: "I am powerful!" Proceed to Warrior III.

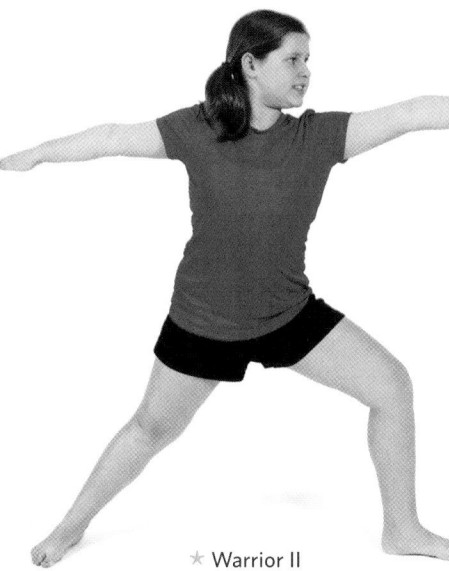

★ Warrior II

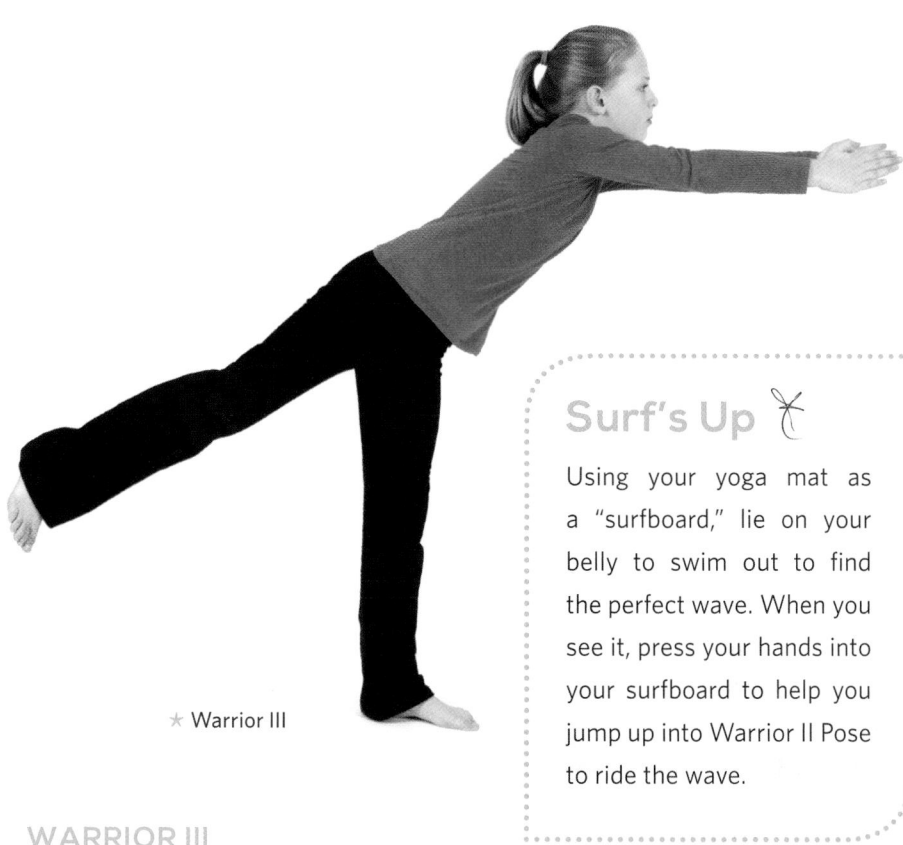

★ Warrior III

Surf's Up

Using your yoga mat as a "surfboard," lie on your belly to swim out to find the perfect wave. When you see it, press your hands into your surfboard to help you jump up into Warrior II Pose to ride the wave.

WARRIOR III

WHAT TO DO

With Warrior III, it is important to keep the standing leg straight, foot firmly planted into the ground. This contributes to the sense of "power" in this pose. If your child is open to it, try holding her standing foot and press it firmly into the ground to help her "feel" the power of connecting herself to the ground. Say, "A strong base makes a strong Warrior!"

WHAT TO SAY

From Warrior II, turn your hips forward once again. Putting your weight on your left foot, begin to straighten your left leg. Stretch your arms out in front of you. Once balanced, pick up your right foot and stretch it back behind as you reach forward. Good! Keep both legs active and strong as you balance in Warrior III. Say, "I am brave!" Mindfully return to Mountain Pose and shake it out. Repeat Warrior III or the entire Warrior Sequence on the other side.

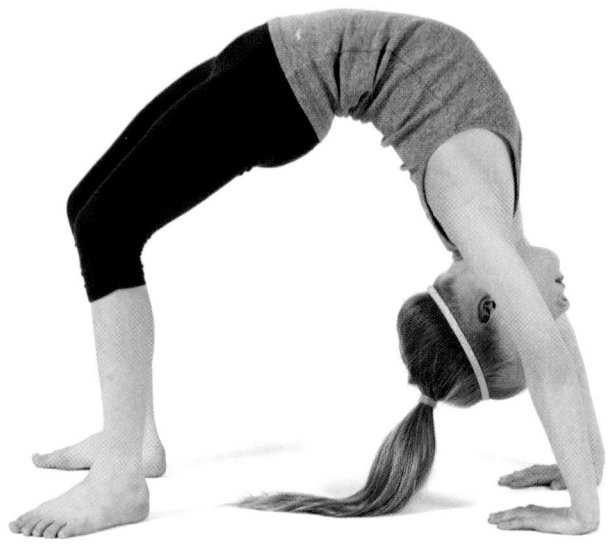

★ Wheel

WHEEL

Benefits

Improves flexibility of the spine

Builds strength in every muscle of body

Opens chest and lungs

WHAT TO DO

Due to the strength and coordination needed to successfully and safely practice Wheel Pose, it is not recommended for children under 5 years old. At any age, make certain your child is strong enough to hold herself up in the pose before attempting it. *Do* spot your child at all times. *Do* encourage your child. *Do not* allow your child to lift up and then rest on her head. Try practicing Lizard on a Rock (see More Partner Poses) first as a supported backbend, or have your child practice over a large ball with your assistance.

WHAT TO SAY

Begin by lying down on your back. Place your feet flat on the floor about hip-distance apart. Bring your arms up over your head and place your hands, palms down, next to your ears. Press your elbows toward each other. Push into your hands and feet to lift your body up off the floor. Keep your legs parallel to each other. Try and straighten your arms and legs, curving your body into an upside-down "U." Breathe in and out here. When you are ready, bend in your elbows and lift your head as you slowly lower yourself back down to the floor.

MORE PARTNER POSES

Partner Poses have been presented as sidebars for many of the poses in this chapter, but there are many more to try! Partner and group poses provide an opportunity for the whole family and even friends to get involved and engage with each other. You'll depend on each other for physical support, have fun negotiating the poses together, and in some cases, make the poses more challenging!

ELEVATOR

Benefits

Promotes trust and teamwork

Builds confidence

Builds leg strength and promotes balance

WHAT TO DO

Elevator Pose requires two similar-sized people, so if your child is significantly smaller than you, invite friends or other family to come and join the fun. This pose is most successful when both partners trust one another because it requires each to lean back with straight arms in a supported chair pose, trusting that the other person will not let them go. You'll know when you've got it as the elevator will start to move smoothly with little effort from either partner. Face each other holding hands. Step back until both of your arms are straight and you can lean back away from each other, chests open. When you're both ready, bend your knees to come down at the same time. Then come back up together.

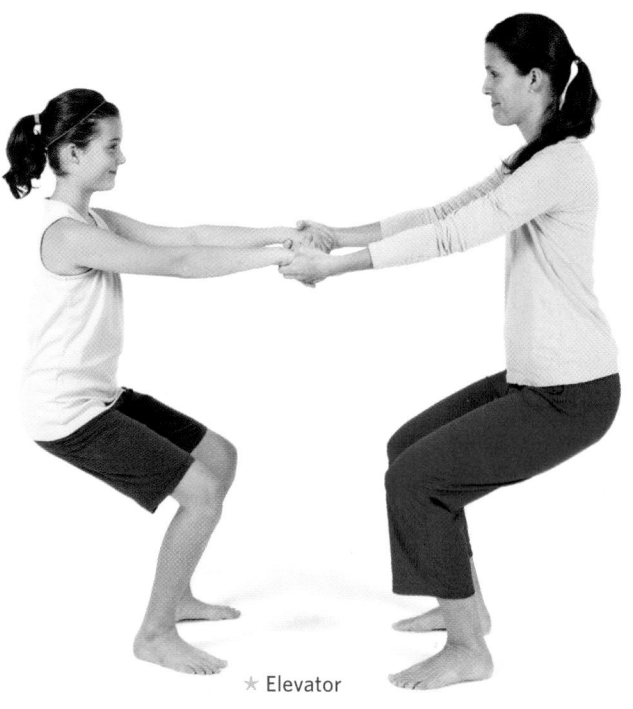

★ Elevator

WHAT TO SAY

Face me and hold my hands. Step back until your arms are nearly straight. Lean back slightly using the grip of your hands and my weight to keep you upright. Keep your feet flat on the floor. We're going to bend our knees to lower the elevator at the same time. Good! Now, let's come back up. We're an elevator, moving smoothly up and down.

HUDDLE POSE

Benefits

Connects and calms

Stretches shoulder and upper back

Opens the chest and lungs

Relieves neck tension

Nurtures

WHAT TO DO

Note that Huddle Pose works best with a parent and child who are not significantly different sizes. Kneel down to face your child and come into Child's Pose together with your arms extended. Be sure to give each other a little massage as you relax and breathe in the pose.

WHAT TO SAY

Let's kneel down and face each other. Place your hands on my shoulders and I'll put mine on yours. Good. Let's back up a tiny bit so that our arms are nice and straight. Let's take a deep breath in together . . . and now let's bend forward to exhale and come into Child's Pose with our arms extended. Ahhh. Can we massage each other's shoulders and upper back from here? Thank you!

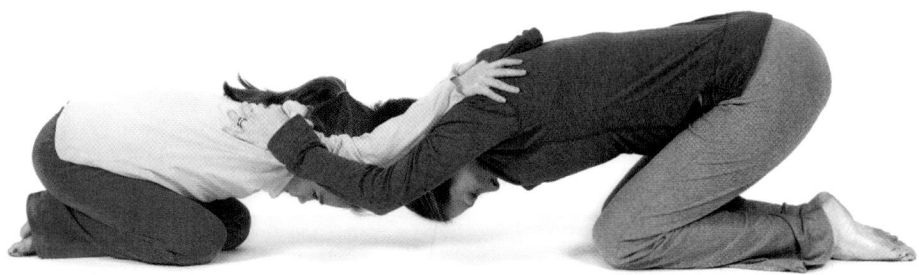

★ Huddle Pose

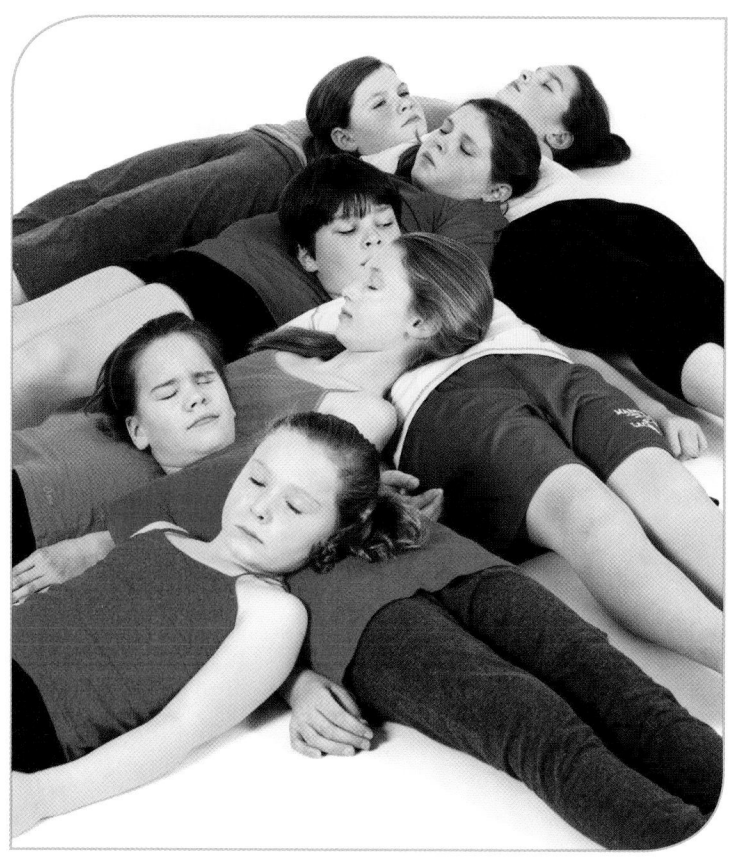

★ Human Zipper, group

HUMAN ZIPPER

Benefits

Promotes connectedness teamwork (in a group)

Brings awareness to the breath

WHAT TO DO

To form your "zipper," have your child lie down with the back of his head resting on your belly. Encourage your child to match his breathing with your breathing, keeping it deep and calm. After a few minutes switch so that your head is resting on your child's belly. Alternatively, this pose can be practiced with a group (see photo). One person lies down, the next lies down so that his head rests on the first person's tummy. The third person lies down with her head on the second child's tummy, and so forth and so on, until all children are lying down in a descending, alternating, zigzag pattern. Be sure to take a digital photo to show the group!

WHAT TO SAY

Lie down and rest your head on my belly. Close your eyes and let's just relax and breathe here together. Do you feel my belly rising and falling? Try to match your breathing with mine, inhaling as my belly rises, exhaling as my belly falls. Good! (After a minute . . .) Shall we switch so that my head is on your belly now?

LIZARD ON A ROCK

Benefits

Opens chest and lungs

Builds confidence with Wheel Pose

Promotes teamwork and communication

WHAT TO DO

This pose provides a safe, supported introduction to Wheel Pose. The rock is in Child's Pose, and the lizard does a backbend (Wheel Pose) over the rock. Make sure to stress that whomever is performing the lizard sits down gently and quite low on the back of the person performing the rock. The lizard then slowly rolls back and puts her arms overhead to reach the floor, eventually coming into a supported Wheel Pose. To come out of the pose, the rock and the lizard need to communicate clearly! "Rock" should say, "Okay, I'm ready . . . 1, 2, 3." On three, rock arches her back like a cat and gently sits up to roll lizard up and off. "Lizard" should be able to stand right up! Important: Because you are in the pose and unable to help direct your child, it is important to recruit a third person, preferably an adult, to serve as a leader and spotter to ensure safety and understanding of the instructions.

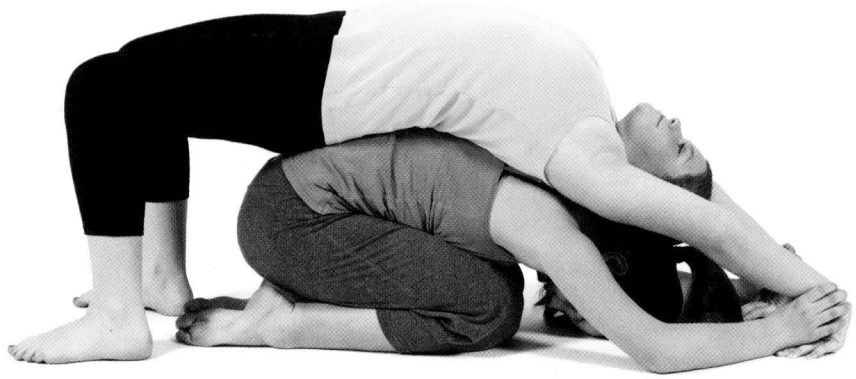

★ Lizard on a Rock

WHAT TO SAY

Leader/Spotter: Okay Rock, come on down into Child's Pose, with your hands on either side of your head. Good. Lizard, go ahead sit down low on Rock, facing away from her. I'm going to spot you so that you can roll back into Wheel Pose. Awesome. Rock, go ahead and reach for Lizard's wrists, and tug them out slightly to give her a nice stretch! Wow, you are a beautiful lizard relaxing and sunning itself on a rock! Ready to come off now? Rock, when you are ready, let go of Lizard's wrists and count to three. On three start to arch your back like a cat and sit up slowly. As you do, Lizard will roll up to standing. When you're ready . . . nice! You did it!

PARK BENCH

Benefits

Stretches hips and thighs (bench)

Relieves tension in lower back (bench)

Encourages good posture (sitter)

WHAT TO DO

In this position, one person is the "bench" and the other sits on the bench. Typically, the smaller person (especially if a very young child) should be the sitter and the older, larger person, the bench. The person sitting should be careful to sit gently on the lower part of the bench's back.

WHAT TO SAY

I will come into Child's Pose to become the park bench. You get to sit and relax on the bench! Face away from me and be sure to sit down low on my back. Good! Let's breathe here together for a while. Ahhh. (If approximately the same size or with an older child, say: Let's switch now.)

★ Park Bench

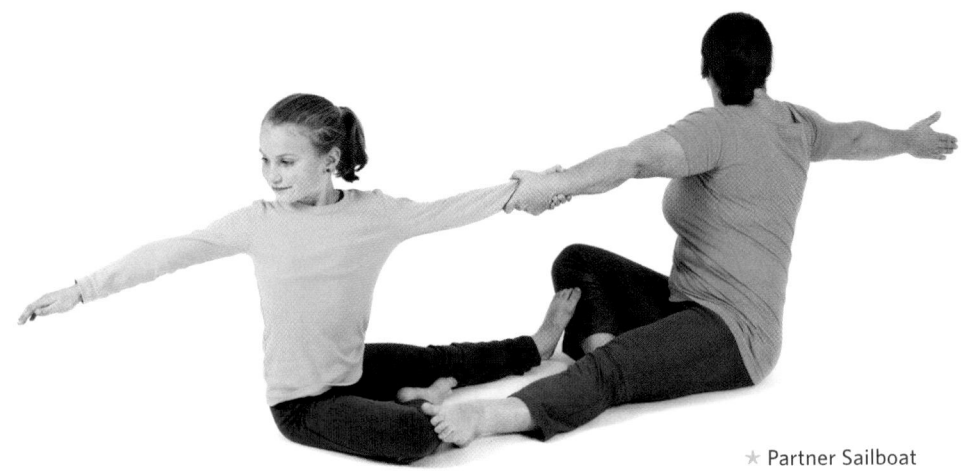

★ Partner Sailboat

PARTNER SAILBOAT

Benefits

Stretches back muscles and hips

Massages internal organs, helps with digestion

Improves flexibility of the spine

Promotes calm

Enhances connection

WHAT TO DO

If you or your child has tight hamstrings or poor core strength, sit on a folded blanket to elevate your hips before attempting this pose. This will help ensure proper, upright posture in this pose. When "sailing," try pulling away from each other for a deeper stretch.

WHAT TO SAY

Let's sit down in Staff Pose, facing one another. Let's both pull our right feet into our left thighs. Good. Now, connect your left foot to my right knee and I'll connect mine to yours. Let's reach out our left arms and grasp onto one another's forearms. Let's inhale to sit up nice and straight. Now, let's exhale and twist out to our right, reaching our "sails" (right arms) out behind us. Great! Smooth sailing from here! Let's breathe here in and out, in and out, for five breaths. Good. Let's switch legs and arms to sail in the opposite direction!

Benefits

Stretches arms and shoulders

Enhances connection

Stretches hips and hamstrings

WHAT TO DO

Puppy Friends is a standing variation of Down Dog. Face each other and place your hands on one another's shoulders. Take a step back and bend forward at your hips. Encourage your child to relax her head and neck and push her hips back to flatten her back. If either of you feels a strain in your lower back, bend your knees slightly.

WHAT TO SAY

Stand facing me, and place your hands on my shoulders. Take a step back and bend forward with me so that our heads come down to relax between our arms. Our legs and arms should be straight, and our backs should be flat. Where do you feel the stretch? (shoulders, arms, hamstrings, and calves) Let's breathe in and out together three times. Release into the stretch a little more with each exhale. Breathing in . . . and out . . .

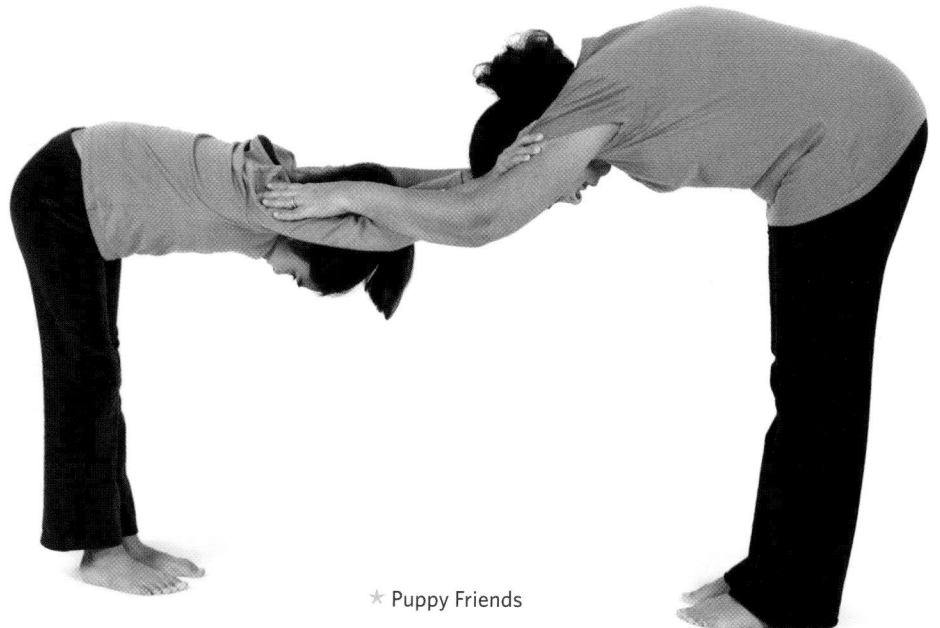

★ Puppy Friends

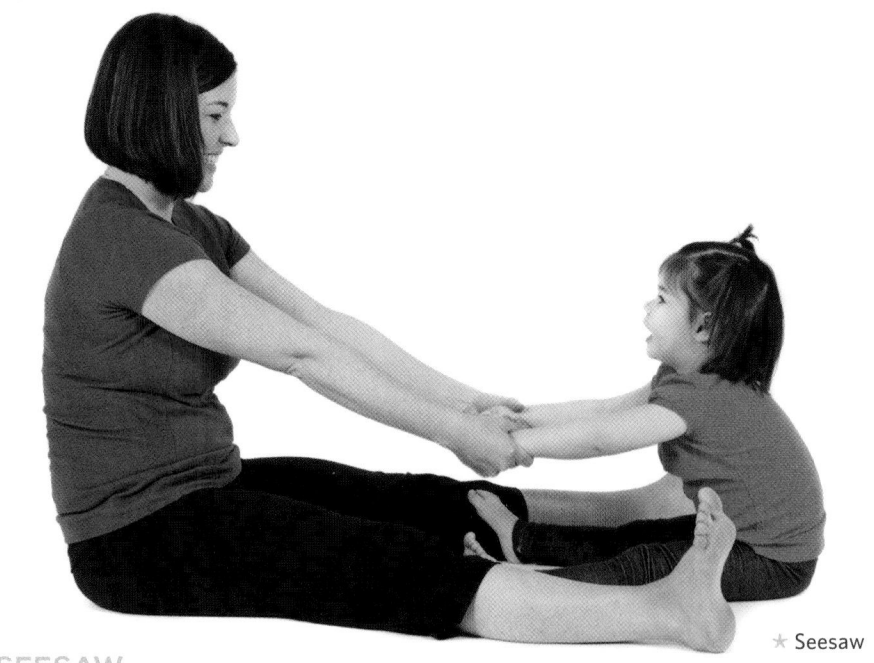

★ Seesaw

SEESAW

Benefits

Stretches hamstrings, glutes, and hips

Encourages connection

WHAT TO DO

If you or your child has tight hamstrings or poor core strength, sit on a folded blanket to elevate your hips before attempting this pose. This will help ensure proper, upright posture in this pose. Depending on flexibility and size, your feet may be touching, or your child's feet may come to the inside of your longer legs. Either way, be sure both partners can sit up tall holding hands with their arms straight out in front. As you pull gently back and forth to "seesaw," continue to encourage good posture—chest open, back flat. For super-tight hamstrings or to protect a delicate lower back, it's always okay to bend the knees a bit.

WHAT TO SAY

Sit across from me in V-Sit Pose. Let's sit up tall and hold hands. Now, I will gently pull you forward as I lean back. Try to keep your shoulders back and your chest open. Good! Now you pull me by leaning backward. Ahhh. To older children: Inhale up and exhale forward. Let's go back and forth, moving with our breath . . . pull gently back and forth.

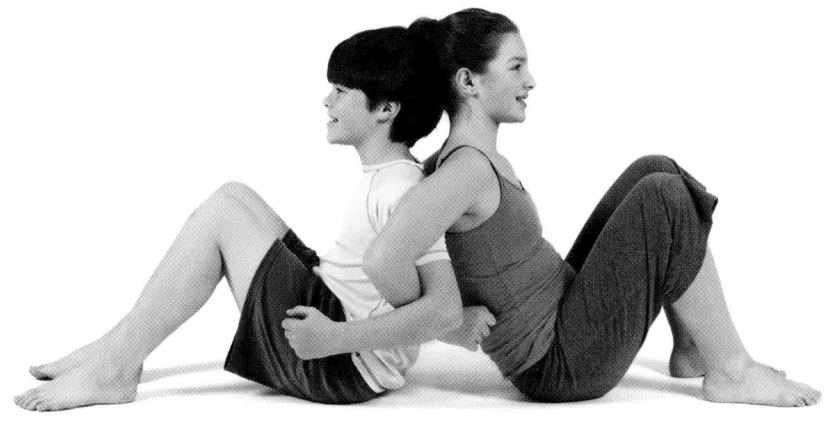

★ Submarine

SUBMARINE

Benefits

Empowers

Promotes teamwork

WHAT TO DO

Submarine is another name for the classic "Back-to-Back Standing" challenge we all faced in PE class. It requires two similar-sized partners, so it's perfect for a larger child and smaller parent or two siblings or friends. The trick is to press back into the head and shoulders as opposed to leaning forward to try to stand up!

WHAT TO SAY

Let's sit on the floor back to back, and hook elbows. With our feet flat on the floor, let's begin to push back into each other's head and shoulders, and work together to push up to standing.

SUNFLOWER

Benefits

Builds core strength

Promotes cooperation

WHAT TO DO

Sunflower requires a group, with each person representing one flower petal. Once everyone gets the hang of this foundational sequence, encourage them to use their imagination to create new and different types of flowers. For example, if everyone connects hands overhead, it's a simple Lotus Flower. Connect the feet and hands and roll backward to create a two-tiered Lotus Flower. Continue to move and connect in various ways to create other beautiful symmetrical shapes. Be sure to use a digital camera to record the creations!

WHAT TO SAY

Let's sit in a circle and come into Staff Pose so that our feet are in the center of the circle. See the little circle between our feet? That's the center of our sunflower. Now let's inhale our arms up and exhale to reach forward to close up our "petals," making sure that we are folding from our hips, rather than our waist. Extend out through our hands, reaching for our shins or feet, and pushing back in our hips, bending our knees a bit if that's more comfortable. Good! Now, the sun comes out and the sunflower opens up. Inhale to lift our arms up to the sky. Exhale and come to lie down on our backs, arms still overhead. A beautiful open-petal sunflower! Sun is setting . . . petals begin to close up again. We use our belly muscles to pull ourselves back up, reaching our arms way up to the sky as we inhale. Now we exhale and close our petals, folding forward again. Let's continue this flow a few times . . . can we go faster? How about in a wave, opening and closing one after the other?

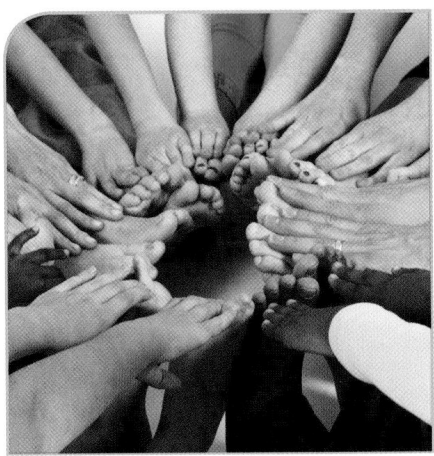
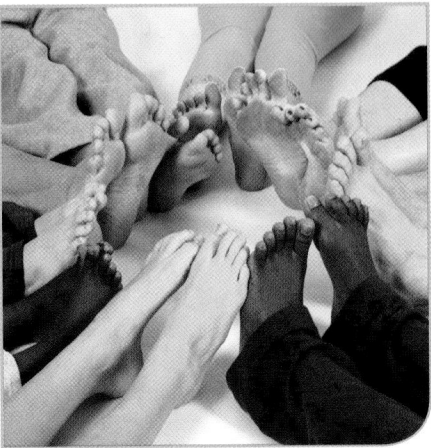

★ Sunflower, closed   ★ Sunflower, open

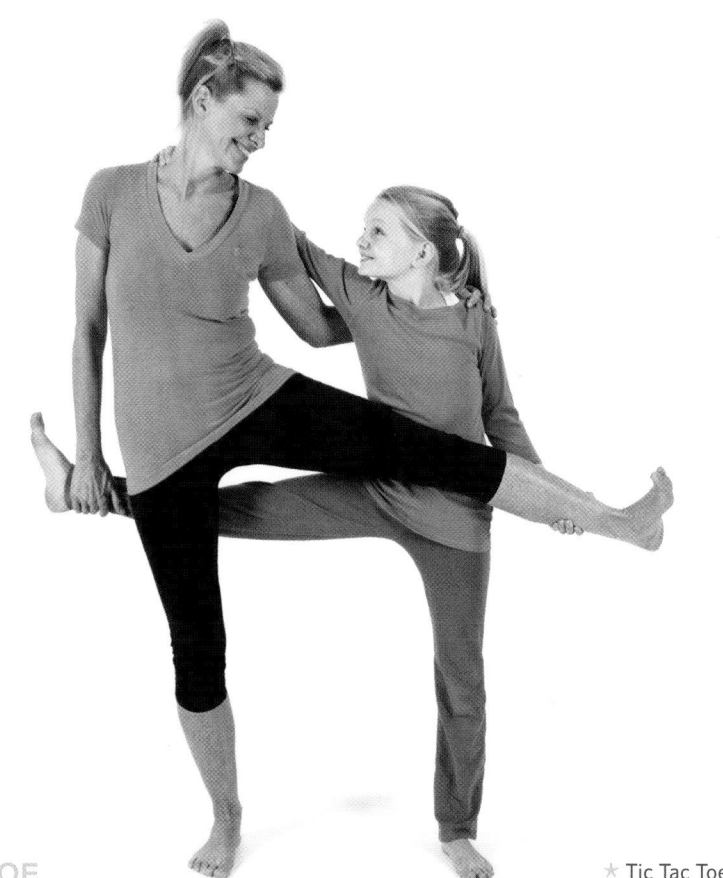

TIC TAC TOE

★ Tic Tac Toe

Benefits

Stretches the inner thigh

Promotes balance

Builds trust

WHAT TO DO

Tic Tac Toe pose requires two similar-sized partners, either a taller child and shorter parent or two siblings or friends of similar height.

WHAT TO SAY

Stand to my left and let's anchor ourselves by putting our arms around each other's shoulders. Lift your right leg up behind me so that I can grab it with my right hand. Good! Now, I'm going to lift my left leg in front of you so you can hold it with your left hand. Are we balanced? Great! Let's see if we can release each other's shoulders and extend our arms out to create our Tic Tac Toe board. We did it! Let's turn around to switch sides.

Benefits

Massages internal organs, helps with digestion

Improves flexibility of the spine

Promotes calm

Encourages connectedness

WHAT TO DO

Back-to-Back Twist is appropriate for any size parent and child; however, to reach around to one another's knees will require partners to be of the same approximate height and arm length.

WHAT TO SAY

Let's sit back to back in Easy Pose and start with some Back-to-Back Breathing (Chapter 5). Good. Let's breathe in and sit up tall. As we exhale, let's reach our left hand across to our right knee and our right arm out straight to reach around for each other's left knees. Breathe with me here for three breaths and then we'll switch sides.

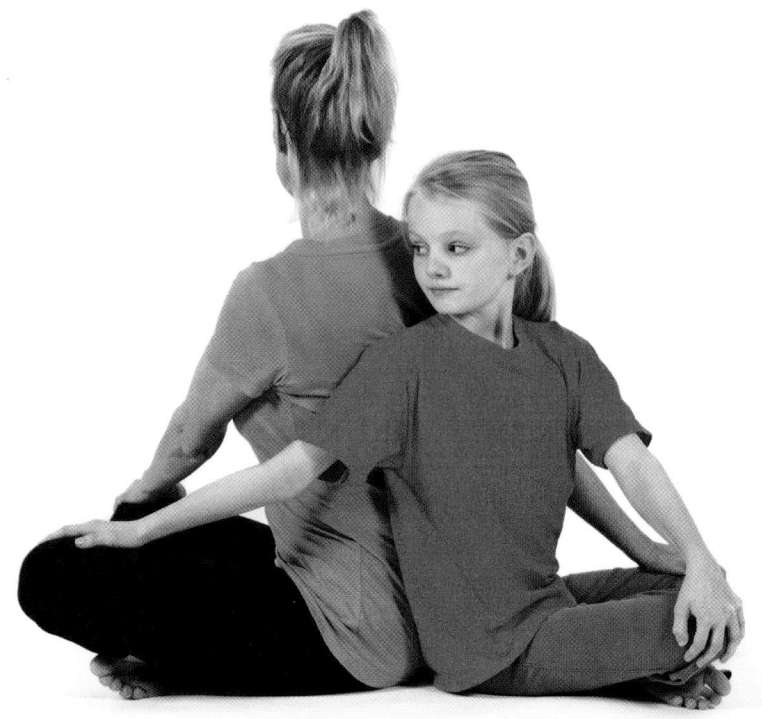

★ Back-to-Back Twist

CHAPTER 7

Family Yoga Games

BRINGING THE FAMILY TOGETHER

How often do you and your family really get a chance to "hang out" together? To spend quality, valuable time together—talking, listening, laughing, and playing? It used to be that dinnertime was "sacred"—a time when families could regroup and end their days together in a meaningful way. Now work schedules creep later into the day, and busy after-school schedules make family dinnertime a miracle if it happens at all! But it's extremely important for families to spend time together somehow, and if you make it fun, it becomes a lot easier to make it a priority in your lives.

Family yoga games are a great way for you and your child to extend your yoga practice to encourage a sense of community and togetherness—as well as strengthen family bonds. With these games, you can build trust and inspire confidence in your child and his or her yoga practice as you work together as a team. These noncompetitive games offer everyone a chance to connect, contribute, and share their special abilities, making all feel stronger as individuals and family members.

You can incorporate these games into your yoga sessions, or you can set aside a time for these family yoga games every week, or even every day. With this special time set aside for connection and play, your family will become stronger. And if you invite others—friends, neighbors—your "family" becomes a lot bigger! Note that these activities are fairly noncompetitive and most are relevant for ages 4-12 years, though you'll want to use your best judgment and understanding of your own child to determine appropriateness.

ALPHABET SOUP

Benefits

Pose practice

Enhances memory skills

Promotes speech and sound practice

Builds confidence

WHAT TO DO

You can play this game with your child alone, or invite as many others to play as you wish. Players should be able to read or at least be learning letter sounds. To play, you will need refrigerator magnet letters or die-cut letters and a bag or other opaque container to reach into. Choose a number of poses your child has already learned and put the first letters of those poses into the bag. Have your child take turns pulling out a letter. Your child then tries to think of a pose that begins with that letter and demonstrates it for you.

WHAT TO SAY

Reach in and grab a letter from the bag. What letter did you get? (For pre-readers: What is the letter sound?) Can you think of a pose that begins with that letter (sound)? You can? Yes! Let's practice that pose together.

CREATE-A-POSE

Benefits

Fosters creativity

Promotes teamwork and cooperation

WHAT TO DO

For this game, have your child create a new yoga pose and perform it for you (invite other family members to create an audience). Be sure she names the new pose and decide together if it would make sense to add this new pose to your favorite pose list (made-up poses are always the best ones!). For a group version, work together to come up with a pose (see photo). The group then performs the pose together. You can also incorporate one or more props. Have fun with it! To commemorate everyone's success, take a digital photo and start a "new pose" journal, adding new poses and photos as you play this game over time.

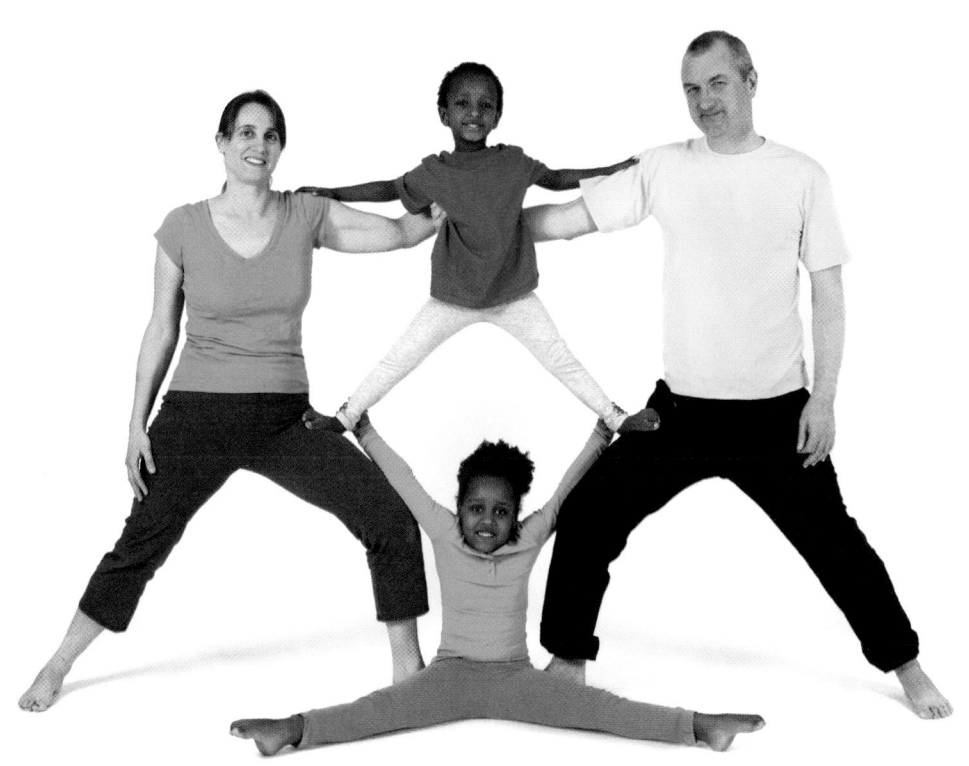

★ Create-a-Pose, group

WHAT TO SAY

If you could create a yoga pose, what would it look like? What is your favorite yoga pose? Can you make it different? Create your own yoga pose and show me!

POSE TAG

Benefits

Encourages practice of individual poses

Promotes teamwork

Energizes

WHAT TO DO

Gather a group of at least three players, preferably more. One player is chosen to be "It" and he chooses a pose that tagged players must freeze in. He also gets to choose what his untagged friends must do to free the tagged player. One example: the "It" player could choose Triangle Pose. If a player is tagged, he must freeze in Triangle Pose and perhaps can be released when an untagged player slides under his legs. For Tree Pose, it might be tickling the player. For Crab Pose, it might be sliding under his back. Once a player has been freed, he can join back in the game. You should begin by being "It" to make sure everyone gets tagged evenly. The object is to keep the game going, so the more players get unfrozen by other players, the longer the game can go on—a great feat of teamwork! Optional: Time the person who is "It." After time is up, count how many players are still frozen in the chosen pose. Keep a tally and compare at the end.

WHAT TO SAY

I am going to be "It." When I say "Go!" run around the room away from me so that I don't tag you. If I tag you, you must freeze in Triangle Pose. The only way you can be unfrozen is if someone else runs between your legs. If you see someone frozen help them out, but don't get caught!

GRATITUDE BALL

Benefits

Promotes connectedness
Lifts mood
Encourages mindful reflection
Promotes appreciation of the "small things"

WHAT TO DO

You will need a beach ball or yoga ball for this exercise. Gather a good-sized group of four or more people. Have everyone stand (or sit) in a circle. Start to bounce (or roll) the ball around the circle. When someone catches the ball, he or she says something for which he or she is grateful. That person then bounces the ball to someone who has not yet had a turn. Encourage everyone to think of 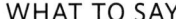 an original blessing, and not to repeat a blessing they have already heard. Some ideas to ponder might be "something nice someone has done for you," "what you are grateful for outdoors in nature," etc. After exhausting ideas, encourage your child or the group to reflect on the exercise and how they feel.

WHAT TO SAY

Lets get in a circle. I am going to bounce this ball around the circle. If you catch it, say something for which you are grateful. For example, I might say, "I am grateful for my family." When you have finished, bounce the ball to someone else who hasn't had a turn. Try not to repeat what someone else said, even if you agree! You want to think of all in your life for which you are grateful. You might think about a time someone did something nice for you or said something kind. You might appreciate a certain person or place. Let's begin!

HOOP CIRCLE GAME

Benefits

Promotes teamwork
Builds coordination
Encourages problem solving

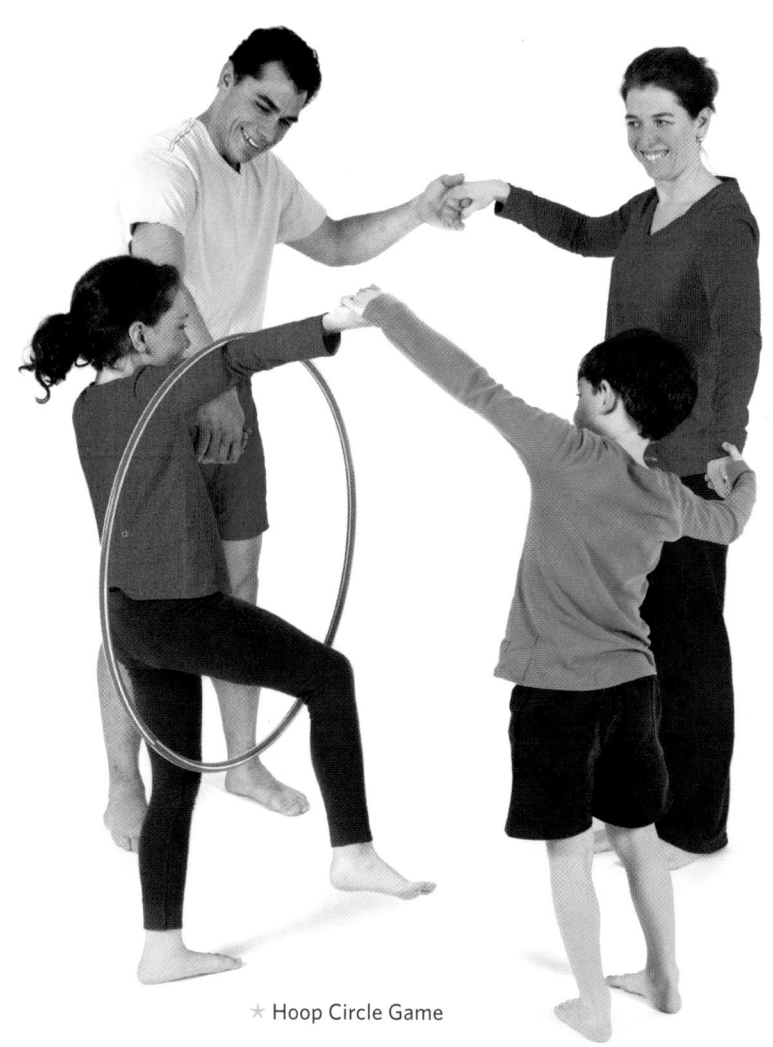

★ Hoop Circle Game

WHAT TO DO

Gather a hula hoop and a group of four or more people. Begin by having everyone stand in a circle. Have everyone pretend to paint glue on their hands before holding hands with the people on either side. Link the hula hoop through your arm before holding hands with the person next to you. Challenge the group to get the hoop all the way around the circle without anyone letting go of hands. The trick of course is to climb through the hoop and bump it over your head to the next person, but see if the group can figure it out before you show them! Once the group gets the hang of it, you can add more hoops to the game for extra fun!

WHAT TO SAY

Lets get in a circle. Paint some sticky, pretend glue on each of your hands. Good! Now, everyone hold hands. Your hands are glued together so don't let go! We need to pass this hula hoop all the way around the circle . . . *yes*, we can do it. I wonder how. Any ideas?

POSE RACES

Benefits

Encourages no-stress, fun competition

Enhances pose practice

WHAT TO DO

Many poses can be "raced" from one end of a room to the other—Crab, Tree, Eagle, Staff Pose, Table, King Dancer, Mountain—just to name a few. Demonstrate for your child how to "race" in the pose. For example, for Tree Pose, you may hop on one leg across the room while in the pose. Stage pose races with your child by marking a start and finish line. Invite others and have relay races! For extra fun, add props such as paper plates on the backs of the "tables." Be sure to play several rounds of races, perhaps changing out the pose with each race.

WHAT TO SAY

You remember [name of pose], right? Lets race in [name of pose]! When I say "Go!" start. On your mark, get set, go! (For relay races:) When I say "Go!" start. When you reach the finish line, tag the next person who will then race back to the start. The team who gets back to start first, wins!

FOLLOW ME DANCE

Benefits

Engages creativity

Energizes

Improves mood

Promotes support and connection

WHAT TO DO

For this game, find some fun, upbeat dance music and some open space. Gather a group of four or more people. Have everyone form a line. The person at the start of the line begins a dance, perhaps even stopping to do a yoga pose as she weaves around the room. Everyone follows the leader, copying whatever moves the leader makes. When the leader is ready for a break (you may need to provide a reminder), she breaks away from the front to come to the back of the line. The next person in line takes the lead with a new dance or yoga move. The line snakes around the room, similar to a conga line but without touching each other. Continue until everyone has had a turn as the leader.

WHAT TO SAY

Who likes to dance? Lets find out! Let's get into a line, one behind the other. I am going to play some music. The person at the front of the line, show us your dance moves! Everyone behind the leader, copy the leader's moves! When the leader is ready for a break, go to the back of the line. The person at the front of the line is the new leader. Let's do this until everyone gets a turn!

STICK TOGETHER

Benefits

Promotes focus and concentration

Builds teamwork and connectedness

Mindful and meditative

WHAT TO DO

Stick Together can be played by two people or with a group in sets of partners. You will need one or two wooden dowels for each set of partners. Dowels should be approximately ¼ inch in diameter and approximately 18 inches long. Play quiet, slow-tempo music to set the mindful tone of this activity. Have partners face each other and hold the stick between their palms and begin to move. For older children, the stick could even be held between the tips of their index fingers. The goal is for partners to work together to move mindfully so as not to drop the stick. Encourage silence during this activity to promote nonverbal communication and "listening." To increase the level of difficulty, add another stick for the pair to hold between their other palms or index fingers. Following the activity, ask your child or the group about their experience.

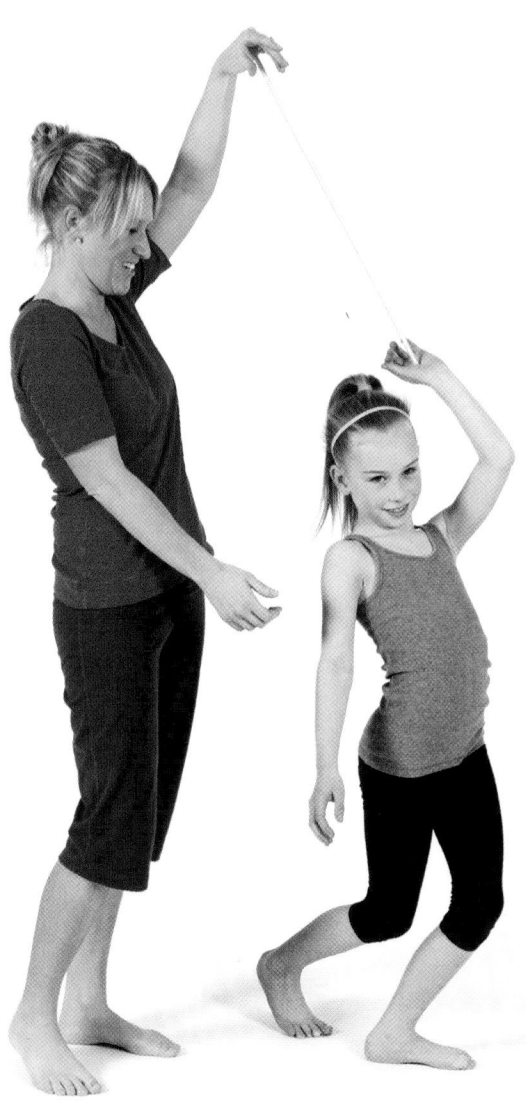

WHAT TO SAY

Face your partner. Hold up opposite hands. If you are holding up your right hand, your partner should be holding up his left. Good. Hold the stick between your raised palms. When I say "Start," begin to move to the tempo of the music, slowly and mindfully. The more mindful and slow your movements, the more you'll be able to keep the stick between you. If you do drop it, just pick it up and start over. Ready?

★ Stick Together

TRUST CIRCLE

Benefits

- Builds trust
- Improves connection
- Builds confidence

WHAT TO DO

This game requires a group of at least six people. This is a game of trust, support, giving, and receiving, and can be anxiety-provoking for some. But once everyone is comfortable, they'll be smiling! Have everyone stand in a circle, shoulder to shoulder, with one leg forward and the other leg back to form a solid stance. One child stands in the middle. Keeping his body and legs strong and straight and his arms

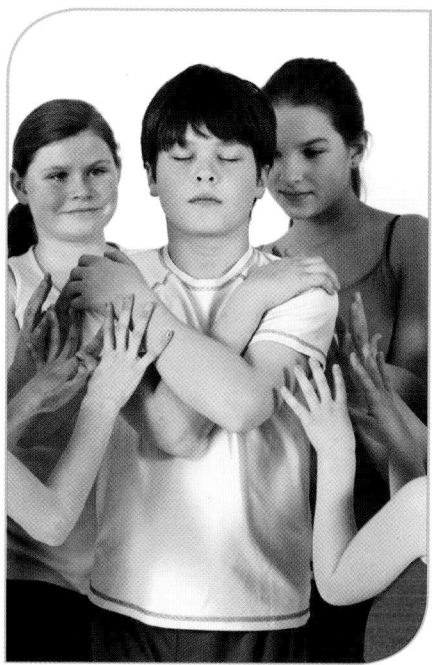

★ Trust Circle

crossed over his chest, the child in the middle "falls" forward, back, or to the side. The rest of the players catch him and gently nudge him over in the opposite direction. Following the game, encourage sharing. What did it feel like to fall? And, to catch? What did you notice?

WHAT TO SAY

Everyone stand in Mountain Pose in a circle. Now come stand shoulder to shoulder, with one leg forward and the other leg back. Now someone come to the center. Lean back or forward as the others catch you. Good! Can you try closing your eyes?

WEB OF CONNECTION

Benefits

- Creates a sense of community
- Encourages family bonding
- Promotes family appreciation

WHAT TO DO

You will need a spool of yarn or thick string for this exercise. This game is for at least four (preferably more) players ages 4 and up. First, have everyone sit in a circle. The object is to pass the yarn from one person to the next, but what makes it an especially wonderful community-builder is to have the children share something about themselves, something for which they are grateful, or something they appreciate about the person to whom they are passing the yarn. As the yarn is passed, each person should wrap it once around the end of his or her finger to secure it. Also, be sure the yarn is passed across the circle, not around it. When everyone has received the yarn, it should go back to the start person. Now, you have a "Web of Connection!" For groups of children 6 and older, direct them to stand up and slowly work together as a group to figure out how to unravel themselves. (Yes, it is possible, but let them figure that out! Hint: Have them follow the direction of the yarn they are holding.) Once unraveled, everyone should be in a wide open circle. Most likely, the starting person will end up facing out, but that's okay!

WHAT TO SAY

Let's sit in a circle. We are going to pass around a ball of yarn so that in the end we are all connected. When it's your turn and you receive the ball of yarn, wrap the yarn around your finger to hold your place. Then, you'll pass the ball of yarn to someone else. When he or she catches it, express what you appreciate most about him or her. After everyone has had a turn, we will have a web of connection—and then we'll see if we can unravel ourselves!

WHAT AM I?

Benefits

Inspires creativity

Builds communication skills

Promotes working memory and reasoning skills

WHAT TO DO

For this game, it's best if players are 5 years or older, and have some knowledge of yoga poses already. Write the name of a familiar yoga pose on a sticky note and stick it on your child's forehead. Make sure she hasn't seen the pose name as the object of the game is to guess the pose. If you have pose cards

(Chapter 3, The Basic Props), you can use those as well by attaching the pose card to her forehead with a small piece of tape. Have your child ask Yes or No questions to answer, "What am I?" With older children, you have the option of allowing a limited number of questions. This game is especially fun when practiced with two or even three players playing at the same time asking questions to determine what they are. The first player to guess correctly, wins!

Some examples of Yes/No questions are:

1. Am I an animal?

2. Is my pose a standing pose (sitting pose, balance pose, etc.)?

3. Are both of my feet touching the ground in the pose?

4. Did we practice this pose today?

WHAT TO SAY

I'm going to stick a pose card onto your forehead so that I (we) can see it but you can't. No peeking! Your job is to guess what you are by asking us Yes or No questions. Once you figure it out, perform your pose!

YOGA PLAY OBSTACLE COURSE

Benefits

Builds coordination

Focuses attention

WHAT TO DO

Everyone loves an obstacle course and this game can be played with one or an entire group of players! Create an obstacle course starting with yoga mats spread around the room. Place a yoga pose card at the front of each mat. Fill in the spaces between the mats with other fun obstacle course activities such as using yoga blocks to make stepping stones. Have a hula hoop station and/or make a hopscotch out of hula hoops. Make an eye pillow toss area using a bucket, bin, or basket set about 8 feet from a line where eye pillows are tossed. Make paths from one mat to another using unrolled yoga straps that players have to "balance" across as if on a high wire. Get creative! Once the obstacle course is created, have each player begin on the mat of their choice, doing the relevant yoga pose for at least 3 to 5 breaths. Play fun, upbeat music and begin!

WHAT TO SAY

I have created a yoga obstacle course for you! Can you complete it? (Explain the course you've designed and how to complete it.) When you hear the music, begin!

ASSEMBLY LINE

Benefits

- Builds teamwork
- Promotes pose practice
- Builds planning skills

WHAT TO DO

For this game, gather a group of at least four players. This game is best for older children who have built up enough of a practice to have a few favorite poses. Have players form a line and come into their favorite yoga pose. Set up a basket a few feet away from the last person. Give the person at the start of the line an item to pass that will be thrown into a basket at the end. Staying in some form of their yoga pose, each person takes and passes the item to the next person until it reaches the end of the line, where it is tossed into a basket or other receptacle. Using body parts other than hands is encouraged. Items continue to get passed until the game is through or players change poses. This game is fabulous for getting things put away!

WHAT TO SAY

Lets form a long line, one after another. Everyone come into your favorite yoga pose. I am going to give you a [item name] to pass to each other, starting with the person at the front of the line. You must stay in your yoga pose while you pass the object. Don't lose the pose! The last person tosses the item into the basket!

INTUITION GAME

Benefits

- Builds observation skills
- Develops perceptive insight

WHAT TO DO

For this game, gather a group of three or more players. Have one person leave the room. While that person is away, another person hides a flat object such as a card, feather, etc., (so it is not visible to the naked eye) behind him or under his mat. The first person returns to the room and tries to determine who has the object. Encourage players to listen "inside" to their intuitions, looking carefully at everyone's face and nonverbal cues to pick up clues to determine who has the object. Make sure no one gives it away by looking in the direction of the person with the object!

WHAT TO SAY

Someone is going to hide this object. [Player's name], please go to the next room. (Give the object to someone to hide and call in the player.) [Player's name], try to guess who has the item under his mat. Who looks suspicious? Is anyone smiling? Use your intuition to tell you who's hiding something!

I PRACTICED YOGA TODAY . . .

Benefits

Promotes memory

Encourages pose practice and review

WHAT TO DO

This is a simple review game that will help your child remember and practice the poses you've taught him or her. Start by saying, "I practiced yoga today and I learned/did [pose name]." Then, demonstrate the pose with your child. Encourage your child to add on by saying, "I practiced yoga today and I did [pose name you stated here]" and then state another pose learned at a previous session. Encourage your child to say and *do* the poses. Reflect on your practice.

WHAT TO SAY

Can you tell me what you learned today? Say after me: "I practiced yoga today and I learned/did . . . " What did you learn? What pose did you do? Good! Now what pose did you learn last time we did yoga together? I practiced yoga, too, and I did . . .

Benefits

Energizes
Focuses attention
Promotes coordination

WHAT TO DO

This game is a fun take on the old classic, "Musical Chairs." Bring together a group of six or more players. Begin by arranging everyone's mat (or other placeholders) in a circle. Place a yoga pose card at the front of each mat. Play music and direct the players to walk around the circle of mats. When the music stops, players must find a mat as quickly as possible and come into the pose on the card on that mat. Repeat the game until everyone is exhausted (seriously, this game could go on forever if the kids have anything to do with it!). I usually do not have children be "out," but if you choose to play that way, it would be the last person to come into a pose that would be "out." If you do choose to play the "you're out" version, have the child who is out conduct the next round, taking charge of the start and stop of the music. For extra fun, the person in charge of the music can also choose the mode of circling the mats, e.g., hopping, walking backward, side-stepping, skipping, tippy toes, dancing, etc.

WHAT TO SAY

Gather around the circle of mats. Notice that each mat has a yoga pose card at the front. When the music comes on, start to walk around the mats. When the music stops, jump on a mat and do the yoga pose on the card on that mat. (For the "out" version:) Whoever finishes their pose last, is out, so hurry! The last person standing wins.

PASS IT ON

Benefits

Fosters communication skills
Encourages community building
Promotes mindful listening

WHAT TO DO

Have everyone sit in a circle holding hands with their eyes closed. The first player squeezes the hand of the person to the left, but does not say in which direction the "squeeze" is going. The squeeze then gets passed all around the circle. This can be tougher than it sounds! The squeeze can easily get "lost" as it is passed around because it takes focus and concentration from the entire group to make the squeeze go around the circle successfully. To make this game more complicated, try passing a "pattern" of squeezes (for example, long/short/short squeeze). Another variation is to pass an unspoken sentiment such as peace, love, respect, happiness, etc., with the squeeze.

WHAT TO SAY

Everyone sit in a circle holding hands. Close your eyes. I am going to squeeze the hand of the person next to me, but I will not say which one. When you feel the squeeze, let it pass through you and use your other hand to pass the squeeze to the next person. We must keep the squeeze going in one direction! Can we do it?

PICK A POSE GAME

Benefits

Inspires creativity

Encourages pose review

WHAT TO DO

For this game, you'll need a deck of Pose Cards (Chapter 3, The Basic Props) or animal toys—beanie buddies, animal figurines, or even a deck of animal cards. You can play this game alone with your child, or invite a group. This game is great for children of any age! First, have everyone come into a circle. Place the items you've gathered in the middle of the circle (or in an opaque bag), cards facing down. Call on players to flip over a card or choose an animal toy and then demonstrate the pose associated with that animal. If there is no pose for a chosen animal, the player gets to make one up!

WHAT TO SAY

I am going to place these pose cards face down on the floor in the center. When I call your name, choose a card or toy from the center. Now demonstrate the pose associated with the animal! Can you? If there is no pose for that animal, make one up!

Benefits

Promotes focus and listening skills
Encourages memory
Encourages pose practice

WHAT TO DO

This is a variation of the traditional "Red Light, Green Light" game and is best played with three or more players. The leader stands at the end of the room with her back to the rest of the players. She calls out a yoga pose—this is the pose players must freeze in when she says "Red Light!" When she says "Green Light!" players slowly and quietly creep toward her. When she says "Red Light!" players must freeze into the predetermined yoga pose. The leader turns around to try to catch someone still moving. If she does, that person must take three large steps backward. The winner is the player who reaches her to tap her on the shoulder first. He then becomes the leader. For this game, it's wise to choose the players moving the "most"—otherwise, it can be a very long time before someone wins!

WHAT TO SAY

Line up across the room. When I say "Green Light!" you can move quietly toward me. When I say "Red Light!" I will turn around and you must be frozen in [leader's choice] Pose. If you are still moving, I will call you out to take three steps backward. The first person to tap me on the shoulder becomes the new leader!

SHOW AND TELL

Benefits

Builds community among family and friends
Celebrates individuality

WHAT TO DO

Invite as many people as you can together in a room. Invite everyone to "show and tell" a talent of theirs. This can range from singing the national anthem to juggling to making a unique sound. Nearly anything goes!

WHAT TO SAY

Let's gather together to play Show and Tell. What are your talents? What can you do that's special? What would you like to do for us, just for fun? Let's take turns and share our unique talents with each other. Who'd like to go first?

STORY YOGA GAME

Benefits

Builds community
Encourages pose practice
Promotes storytelling skills
Supports sequential planning
Promotes creativity and imagination

WHAT TO DO

For this game, you will need several players or several partner pairs. Have players break into smaller groups (or partners). Each group creates a verbal or written yoga story (for an example of a yoga story, see Chapter 10, Mouse, Cat, and Dog Story) or maps out the story with yoga cards. One person becomes the narrator and begins to tell the story, starting with the first yoga pose. For example, "Once upon a time there was a **tree**," as she does Tree Pose. The second player adds onto the story, performing the next yoga pose, and so on. Have each player continue to tell the story, each part with his own pose demonstration. Keep in mind the story can be planned in advance as previously described *or* can develop organically as you move from player to player. If everyone playing is familiar with the yoga poses, it can be incredibly engaging and fun to allow the story to unfold naturally. Have fun with it!

WHAT TO SAY

Let's play the Story Yoga Game! Everyone get into a group (or partners). With your group or partner, make up a story using yoga poses. You can write it down, draw it out, or use yoga pose cards to provide yourself with a visual sequence for your story. Choose someone to start the story and demonstrate the first pose. The next person in the group will then pick up where he leaves off, telling the next part of the story and demonstrating that pose, and so on. When everyone has had a turn, finish your story and take a bow as a group.

TELEPHONE

Benefits

Builds focus

Promotes teamwork

Enhances listening skills

Encourages patience

WHAT TO DO

Telephone is a group game where a word, phrase, or sentence is whispered in one ear and then gets passed around the circle, whispered from ear to ear, until it has gone all the way around and back to the starting person. It can be hilarious to hear the ultimate word or phrase that comes out at the end! Ultimately, it is a game of focus and teamwork. The goal is to have the end phrase the same as it started. The longer the message, the tougher this game is. Gather a large group and have everyone sit in a circle. Have the first person send around a simple message such as "This is a fun yoga day." With younger children, start with a simple, one-word message. With older children, encourage the creation of longer messages. The longer the message, the sillier the results! In my experience, you may need to remind them to "keep it clean!"

WHAT TO SAY

Sit down in Easy Pose in a circle. Who's leading first? I want you to think of a word (or phrase or sentence) to send around the circle. Start with the person on your left and be sure to cup your hand around her ear so that no one else can see or hear what you are saying. Continue to pass the message around the circle from person to person as everyone else remains quiet and still in Easy Pose. Once the message reaches the last person, she should say aloud what is whispered to her. The leader then states the original message. Do they match up? Let's try another one! Who wants to lead?

YOGA FREEZE DANCE

Benefits

Energizes

Promotes listening and focus skills

Encourages family fun

WHAT TO DO

This is a fun game to get everyone energized and moving! The more players, the more fun the game, so gather as many people as possible. Find fun, upbeat music. As the leader, tell players that when you stop the music, they must freeze in a yoga pose of their choice (or you can choose the yoga pose for an extra challenge, changing it up each time as you call it out). The last child to freeze into a pose becomes the new leader (instead of being "out"). Last player left in the game is the winner.

WHAT TO SAY

Everyone gather around! We're going to play Yoga Freeze Dance! When I hit "play," dance around! I want to see you move! When I hit "pause," you must freeze in a yoga pose. The last person to freeze will become the leader!

YOGI SAYS

Benefits

Builds listening skills

Encourages focus and concentration

Promotes memory skills

WHAT TO DO

This game is played exactly the same as "Simon Says," but you will say "Yogi Says" instead of "Simon Says," and your commands will always be yoga poses or related activities. Be sure to explain that "yogi" means anyone who practices yoga, so we are all yogis! Gather a group of three or four players. The object of the game is to do whatever yogi says, but only when preceded by the words, "Yogi says . . . " Otherwise, the player is out. Alternate times when you precede your command with "Yogi says" and times when you don't so that players don't have expectations and can be surprised. You can have children take turns being "yogi."

WHAT TO SAY

I am "yogi" and I am going to give a command. Do the pose that I say to do. For example, when I say "Yogi says do Tree Pose!" do Tree Pose, but only if I say "Yogi says" first. If I don't say "Yogi says," do not do the pose. If you do the pose, you'll be "out" and can help me catch the others as they forget to listen for "Yogi says."

CHAPTER 8

Songs and Chants

YOGA AND THE POWER OF MUSIC

If you ever danced your heart out to an upbeat song, or played your favorite music while cleaning your home, you know about the power of music. Since ancient times, people around the world have used music, singing, and chanting to lift their spirits, connect with others, and heal themselves from the inside out. Studies have shown that music has the power to influence certain brain-wave frequencies that improve brain function. Listening to music has the ability to promote feelings of well-being, boost creativity, reduce pain, improve memory, and improve coordination.

Singing and chanting provide natural opportunities to activate the breath, as the act of singing forces us to inhale and exhale more deeply than in regular speech. Singing helps us regulate our breath, which can have a calming effect on our nervous system. With singing, we can inspire and motivate, connecting with others to build a strong sense of community. Singing with your child can be a powerful way for you to connect!

The repetitive nature of chanting produces a calming, grounding effect on the brain and body. Chanting produces a healing effect on the endocrine system, normalizing hormone production that balances our moods—which contributes to a greater sense of well-being.

For children especially, incorporating songs, chants, and music into yoga sessions adds much to the practice. It sets the tone, making the practice more enjoyable, and highlights the whole body/mind experience while promoting a deeper connection between you. Use the songs and chants in this chapter to build playful themes for your sessions, or vice versa. The song descriptions contain a note about which traditional tunes they can be sung to, but if you'd like to hear the original music accompanying the songs, they are all included on the CD I created with Sammie Haynes, *I Grow with Yoga: Yoga Songs for Children.* (You can purchase the CD online at *www.childlightyoga.com.*) The songs and chants are grouped into "Chants," "Opening/Closing Songs," "Pose Variation Songs," "Silly, Energizing Songs," and "Calming Songs," for your ease of use. Once you become familiar with the songs, don't be afraid to spontaneously call upon them at any time. If you notice your child is feeling a little anxious, is in a bad mood, or bouncing off the walls—choose one of these songs or chants from the appropriate category and watch how quickly your child's mood and energy are transformed—along with your own!

Music and the Body

Music has a powerful effect on your child's state of being. To bring the point home, play 30 to 60 seconds each of three different styles of music (preferably without lyrics), for example, African drumming, classical, or a heavy metal riff. After each segment, allow time for your child to observe the effects of each piece on his state of being. You might ask, "As you listened to the music, what happened in your body? Did your breathing change? How? What were you thinking about—what was happening in your mind?" Discuss the observations together. Music truly has the power to change your body!

Chants

"Om" is often referred to as "the sound of the universe." Chanting Om is powerful for centering as it produces an energy that literally changes us physiologically. Chant a few rounds of Om with your child at the start of your yoga practice for focus, in the morning to clear the slate for a new day, or before bed for transitioning to restful sleep.

CHANTING OM

Benefits

Calms and centers

Promotes connectedness

WHAT TO DO

While in Easy Pose, your child should breathe in deeply and exhale the "Om" sound (Aaaaaaauuuoooommmm) as long as he is able before beginning another round. With an older child, you might try a staggered start, where your child begins a round of Om, then you begin another round slightly after, and so there is a constant Om sound in the room for as long as possible. When finished, be sure to check in with your child about his experience and discuss.

WHAT TO SAY

Sit or stand up tall. Breathe in deep to fill up your belly and exhale out to the sound of Om, like this, "Aaaaaaauuuoooommmm," as long as you are able. Your turn . . . great! Now, let's close our eyes and try it again, chanting together for three full rounds of Om. Breathing in . . . "Aaaaaaauuuoooommmm" . . .

NAME CHANTING

Benefits

Calms and centers

Re-engages attention

WHAT TO DO

Name chanting is magical—an instant energy changer. When a child hears his name in this calm, sing-songy way, he stands up a little taller and his attention becomes quickly engaged. This is a great chant to use when energy is high or negative. You and your child sing each other's name three times, dragging out each syllable. For example, the name Jennifer would be sung, "Jeeee-niiiii-feeerrrrr," and repeated three times. Keep in mind, you can also use Name Chanting as a parent to sing your child's name with or without his involvement, to re-engage his attention or help shift his mood. Try rocking rhythmically from side to side as you sing to help set the tone.

WHAT TO SAY

Sit or stand up tall. We are going to sing each other's names three times. I'll sing your name first. "Ja . . . son . . . , Ja . . . son . . . , Ja . . . son . . . " Now, let's sing together. First, we'll sing your name again three times and then mine. Ready? . . .

Opening/Closing Songs

Using opening and closing songs to begin and end your yoga sessions with your younger child is a great way to create a sense of ritual in the practice. Singing "Hello There," your child will know it's yoga time and you'll be better able to help your child transition into the practice. Singing "Goodbye for Now," your child will know that practice is over, and will feel inspired from a sense of accomplishment!

HELLO THERE

WHAT TO DO

Begin sitting in Easy Pose with your hands pressed together in front of the heart in *Namaste* Pose (Chapter 6). Bow at "*Namaste.*" Repeat three times. When you first teach the song, explain the meaning of *Namaste* as "I honor you." You might note that in India, the term is also used as "goodbye" and "thank you."

> Hello there,
> This is the yoga way
> To greet each other we say
> *NA-MA-STE.*

GOODBYE FOR NOW

WHAT TO DO

Use the same tune as in the "Hello There" song. Sit in Easy Pose and press your hands together in *Namaste* Pose in front of the heart. Bow at "*Namaste.*" Repeat three times. Again, remind your child of the meaning of *Namaste* as "I honor you," as well as "goodbye" and "thank you."

> Goodbye for now,
> The time has come today,
> To end our yoga play . . .
> *NA-MA-STE.*

WHAT TO DO

With your child, begin by standing in Mountain Pose. Alternate lifting and lowering an arm and the opposite knee (a standing crawl motion) while chanting the following script.

Do the peace crawl (*lift right arm and left knee and down*)

Up and down (*lift left arm and right knee and down*)

Moving slow (*lift right arm and left knee and down*)

Without a sound (*lift left arm and right knee and down*)

Quiet my thoughts (*lift right arm and left knee and down*)

Focus my mind (*lift left arm and right knee and down*)

Let's crawl for peace (*lift right arm and left knee and down*)

A second time (*lift left arm and right knee and down*)

(Repeat and end with:)

You can crawl for peace (*lift right arm and left knee and down*)

Most any time! (*lift left arm and right knee and down*)

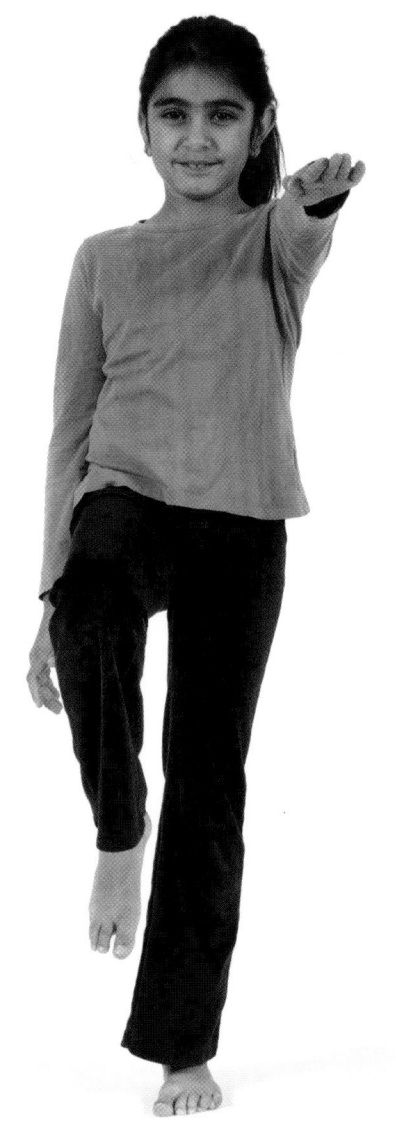

⋆ Peace Crawl

Pose Variation Songs

Connecting poses to songs is a way to really bring home yoga's whole mind/body experience. These songs connect movement to lyrics, creating fun practice that promotes learning and use of breath. Use these songs when you want to add an extra dose of fun to the practice, especially when your child needs a pick-me-up!

THE TRIANGLE TEAPOT SONG

WHAT TO DO

Sing this song to the tune of "I'm a Little Teapot." Start standing with legs apart, and move in and out of Triangle Pose to the words. Between the verses, have your child place his hands on his belly and breathe in deeply to refill his "pot." Repeat as often as you like, and switch sides by replacing "left" with "right"!

I'm a little teapot, short and stout,
Left is my handle, right is my spout.
When I get all steamed up, hear me shout,
Tip me over and pour me out!
I hang out here a while and look on up,
I wanna see who's drinkin' from that cup.
When I get tired, I stand right up,
And breathe in deep to refill my pot.

THE BUTTERFLY SONG

WHAT TO DO

Sing to the tune of "I'm a Little Teapot." Gently lift and lower your knees ("wings") while sitting in Butterfly Pose as you sing.

I'm a little butterfly, light and free.
I have wings . . . like a fairy.
Can you count (or, smell) the flowers that I see?
Close your eyes and fly with me!

ROW YOUR BOAT

WHAT TO DO

Sing this song to the tune of "Row, Row, Row Your Boat." Sing two or three times while in Boat Pose while "rowing" with your arms.

Row, row, row your boat,
Sing it if you please.
Keep your feet up off the ground,
And don't forget to breathe!

Silly, Energizing Songs

These songs are guaranteed to raise your child's energy, shake him up, and lift his mood. They're silly, fun, and inspire lots of dance. They're also great as warm-ups.

GO DO YOGA RAP SONG

WHAT TO DO

Use this song when your child needs a pick-me-up. Dance around to loosen up for the first two verses, then simply follow the movement cues in the lyrics. A favorite for all ages!

(Chorus:)
Go Do Yoga, Go-Go Do Yoga,
Go Do Yoga, Go-Go Do Yoga.

When you've had a bad day and you're feeling down,
Put a smile on your face with the Yoga Rap Song—Let's sing it!
(Repeat chorus)

Now, clap your hands and move your feet,
Just get your groove on—and move to the beat—You got it!
(Repeat chorus)

*Raise your arms right up into the sky, (Come into **Tree Pose**.)*
While you take your foot up into your thigh—Now hold it!
(Repeat chorus)

*Now sit on down in **Easy Pose**,*
Stretch your legs straight out, and clap those toes—Just clap 'em! *(Come into*
    ***Staff Pose** and tap your big toes together to the beat.)*
(Repeat chorus)

*Now, let's lie down and do the **Bridge**,*
Keep your shoulders on the floor and raise those hips—And hold it!
(Repeat chorus)

Get one foot up into the air,
Then switch and shake 'em like you just don't care—Alright!
(Repeat chorus)

Now stand on up, it's up to you,
Pick your favorite yoga pose, anything you choose—And do it!
(Repeat chorus)

Notice your breath and dis-po-sition,
Don'cha feel much better after those positions? Yeah!!
(Repeat chorus)

I GROW WITH YOGA (by Sammie Haynes)

WHAT TO DO

When you get to the second verse, slow down significantly so that your child has the chance to "be" the butterfly, turtle, frog, and bunny. Otherwise, try practicing this song with other family members or friends, with each person having his or her own role in the second verse. After the second version, everyone gets back up to finish the song as a group. Begin standing side by side and follow the lyrics for movement cues, noting the poses (found in Chapter 6) in bold to guide you. Makes a great transition to relaxation. Hold hands and take a bow as a "happy family" at the end.

(Chorus:)
I grow with yoga,
Yoga grows with me,
And when we grow together,
We're a **forest of trees**!

I grow strong like a **mountain**,
Tall and straight as a **tree**,
I blossom like a blooming **flower**,
I buzz, buzz like a **bee**!
(Repeat chorus)

I'm a **butterfly**, *I flap my wings,*
I'm a **turtle** in my shell,
I hop, hop, hop just like a **frog**,
As a **bunny**, I listen well!
(Repeat chorus)

I see the universe in you, (Sweep the arms to signify the universe.)
When we're both in that place, *(Cup hands one over the other and then switch.)*
The beauty in your heart shines through, *(Place hands over heart and then bring them out, palms up to the sky.)*
I say, *NAMASTE! (Bow with hands pressed together in front of the heart.)*
(Repeat chorus, ending with "We're a happy family!" *Hold hands and bow together.)*

WALKING, WALKING SONG

WHAT TO DO
Sing this song to the tune of "Frère Jacques." It is wonderful to use for transitions, e.g., when using yoga adventure stories or themes that require getting from one place to another. Begin by standing and follow the movement cues in the lyrics.

Walking, Walking, Walking, Walking,
Hop, Hop, Hop, Hop, Hop, Hop,
Running, Running, Running,
Running, Running, Running,
Now, let's stop, Now, let's stop!

Marching, Marching, Marching, Marching,
Hop, Hop, Hop, Hop, Hop, Hop,
Tippy, Tippy, Tip Toes, Tippy, Tippy, Tip Toes,
Now, let's stop, Now, let's stop!

THE WARM-UP SONG

WHAT TO DO
Sing this song to the tune of "Go In and Out the Window." Hold hands with your child and stand across from each other. Bend your knees to bounce up and down as you sing . . .

Let's stand up in a circle (3x),
And take a breath or two. *(Let go of hands and breathe slowly and deeply in and out three times, using the hands over the belly to demonstrate* **Balloon Breathing***.)*
Let's stomp our feet together (3x),

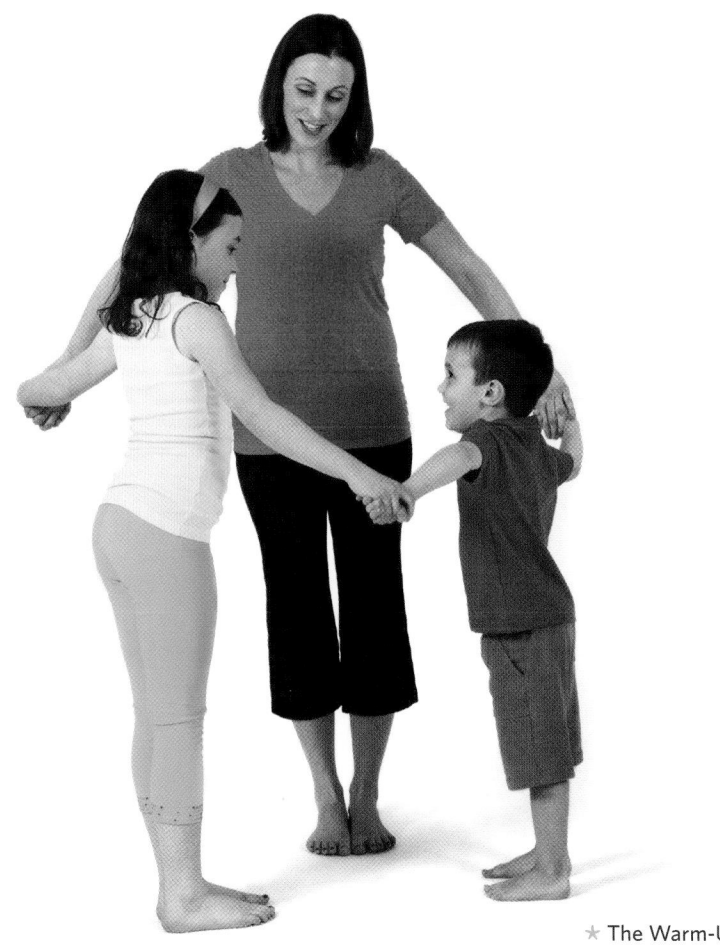

★ The Warm-Up Song

And jump so very high. *(Jump up and down a few times. Ask your child, "How high can you jump? Let me see!")*

(Reach up to stretch overhead with one hand and then the other as you sing . . .)

Let's reach up to the sky (3x),

Then down to **Rag Doll Pose**. *(Fold over and hang down in Rag Doll Pose for a few breaths. Encourage your child to be loose and floppy, breathing deeply.)*

(Come into Star Pose and then twinkle [Chapter 6].)

Let's twinkle like a **Star** (3x),

Now back to **Mountain Pose**. *(Take a few breaths in Mountain Pose.)*

Let's all sit down together (3x),

And touch our toes to nose. *(Fold forward sitting in **Butterfly Pose**, or lift each foot one at a time to touch toes to nose. Tickle your nose with your toes for a good giggle!)*

Calming Songs

When it's time to be calm, usually at the end of a session, or any time you notice your child is overactive, tense, or upset, use these songs to encourage peace and calm. Turn the lights down low to set the tone.

BIG WHITE STAR

WHAT TO DO

Sing this song to the tune of "Twinkle, Twinkle Little Star." Begin in Star Pose, while twinkling (Chapter 6) and follow the lyrics for other movement cues, noting the poses or movements in bold to guide you. Makes a great transition to relaxation.

Twinkle, *twinkle big white star,*
Can you see from up so far?
I like to be a big oak **tree**,
Just you watch and follow me.
Twinkle, twinkle big white star,
Let's do yoga a little bit more!
Twinkle, twinkle big white star,
Can you see from up so far?
Bring your right foot back behind,
Warrior is always kind.
Twinkle, twinkle big white star,
Let's do yoga a little bit more.
Twinkle, twinkle big white star,
Can you see from up so far?
Rag Doll Pose is always fun,
Take a breath before you're done. *(Breathe in and out deeply and slowly.)*
Twinkle, twinkle big white star,
Let's do yoga a little bit more.
Twinkle, twinkle big white star,
Can you see from up so far?
Bring your left foot to the back,
Warrior is coming back.

Twinkle, twinkle big white star,

Let's do yoga a little bit more.

Twinkle, twinkle big white star,

Can you see from up so far?

Let's lie down and take a rest, *(Transition down to* Savasana *Pose.)*

A rest, a rest, to feel our best.

Twinkle, twinkle big white star,

Let's do yoga forever and more!

IF I WERE... *christian version*

WHAT TO DO

From a standing position, use the movement cues in italics to guide you. As with all songs, feel free to add your own verses—for example, for Dolphin, you might use, "If I were a dolphin, I'd dive for you" and "If I were a bumble bee, I'd buzz for you," etc.

If I were the **sun**, *I'd shine down on you. (Reach for the sun, then fold over to bring down the sun.)*

If I were a **rose bud**, I'd open for you. *(Do Flower Pose, standing.)*

If I were a **puppy**, I'd wag at you. *(Do Down Dog Pose and lift your leg to "wag your tail.")*

But, since I am a child, I'll sing for you. *(Point to self, then face palm to floor to represent "child.")*

If I were a **star**, I'd **twinkle** for you. *(Do Star Pose, then twinkle.)*

If I were a **penguin**, I'd waddle to you. *(Stand up straight with arms stiff at sides, palms facing the floor. Waddle from side to side.)*

If I were an **eagle**, I'd soar to you. *(Do Eagle Pose, then "soar" by bringing arms and legs out like wings out to sides.)*

But, since I am a child, I'll sing for you. *(Point to self, then face palm to floor to represent "child.")*

And, since I am your child, I'll give you hugs too! *(Point to self, point to parent, then face palm to floor to represent "child." Give parent a* Big *hug!)*

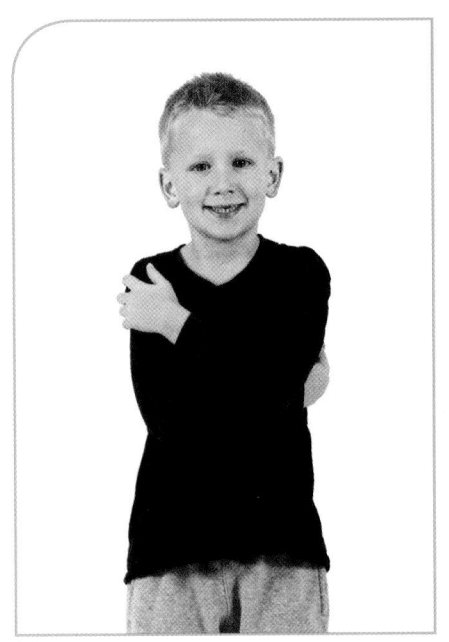
★ Hug

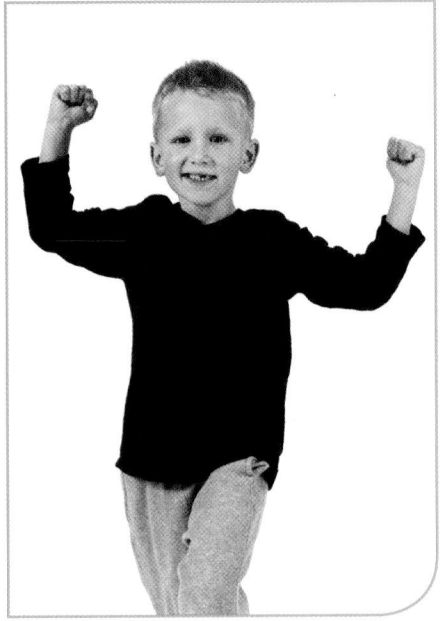
★ Showing Muscles

BREATH BY BREATH

WHAT TO DO

Sing to the tune of "The Garden Song" by David Mallet. This song consists of a lot of calm singing with just a few poses mixed in, so it's perfect to use as a transition to relaxation, nap, or bedtime. Come into the poses as they are sung to act out the song.

(Chorus:)
Breath by breath, pose by pose,
Gonna make this body grow,
I love yoga 'cause I know,
It feels so good inside. *(Give yourself a hug.)*

When I wake up, and I'm mad,
Not a good thought to be had,
Geyser pose always makes me glad,
'Cause it gets those grumpies out. *(Explode like a geyser, "pssh!")*
(Repeat chorus)

When I need some energy,
I reach up and breathe so deep,
Fold right over to touch my feet, *(Come into Rag Doll Pose.)*
And then I do it again. *(Do Rag Doll Pose again.)*
(Repeat chorus)

Sometimes I get the answers wrong,
I might feel down but not for long,
Warrior makes me feel strong,
And filled with confidence. *(Show your muscles!)*
(Repeat chorus)

LISTEN TO YOUR HEART

WHAT TO DO

The first verse is sung very quietly, in an almost whisper. The second verse is louder and stronger. Try patting your hands in your lap during the second verse on the "Yes," then continue to the beat to finish out the second verse.

Listen, listen to your heart, (Put hands over your heart and gently tap your chest.)
It says very important things,
What it tells you from the start,
Is the song you'll want to sing.
It says . . .
Yes I'm special, Yes I'm smart, *(Pat your hands on your legs to the beat as you sing.)*
Yes I'm strong, so says my heart,
I try my best and do my part,
Let's hear that song a-gain!
YES!
(Repeat both verses)

CHAPTER 9

Relaxation and Visualization

IMPORTANCE OF RELAXATION AND VISUALIZATION FOR CHILDREN

In our society, in general, children are deprived of quiet time. Opportunities for relaxation can provide a much-needed respite from an often chaotic, overstimulating world. In yoga, it is tradition to end practice with *Savasana* (Corpse or Dead Body Pose) as a way to bring the body and mind into full relaxation, but relaxation can be practiced any time. As the body relaxes, it has a chance to integrate the benefits of the practice. The inner focus inherent in relaxation activities slows brain waves, allowing the nervous system to find its way to balance. The mind is allowed time to rest and recharge. These quiet moments bring the body and mind to the present moment to experience peace, calm, and self-awareness.

Some children find it difficult to concentrate and sit still. Without stillness, the brain and body become increasingly unable to relax, focus, and learn. Quiet moments of relaxation help children develop a sense of peaceful well-being that supports their ability to focus, learn, and be aware of themselves and the people around them.

When you add visualization exercises as part of a relaxation practice, you provide an opportunity for your child to build skills in problem solving, creative and critical thinking, vocabulary, sensory release, and focus and attention. Through guided visualization, children can use their imaginations to become still enough to connect to their own inner wisdom. Tension is released, and children learn strategies for dealing with life's emotional challenges. Using creative imagery can give your child something to focus on, easing your child's way to relaxation. Your child can also be guided to bring his or her awareness, or energy, to various parts of his or her body. This is the practice of yoga at its best—the unifying of body and mind!

Preparing for Relaxation

To prepare for relaxation and visualization exercises with your child, follow these tips.

- Play relaxing background music, preferably without words if you are planning to use a visualization exercise.
- Turn the lights down low.
- Before any exercise, have your child lie down in *Savasana* Pose with feet shoulder width apart and arms comfortably to the sides, palms up. Encourage your child to close his eyes and relax his body. Guide your child to practice Balloon Breathing or to do Ocean Breath (Chapter 5).
- Some children are not comfortable resting on their backs, as they may feel vulnerable in that position. If your child is anxious lying on his back, ask him to lie on his stomach or side or cover him with a heavy blanket. Over time, he may feel comfortable and safe enough to come to lie on his back on his own.
- Some children have an especially difficult time lying still. Having the weight and warmth of a heavy folded blanket or two on top of their bodies can help ground them. Also, see Kid Roll-Up Pose (see exercise in this chapter).
- In general, if a transition or activity involves touching your child, be sure to let him know you are going to do so in advance and ask his permission.
- Following relaxation, discuss the experience of the activities with your child. Were they helpful to your child? What did he enjoy most? Why? What, if anything, did he not enjoy? Through these discussions and your observations, you'll learn together what is most effective and beneficial for your child (and you!). Together, you will inevitably discover your favorite relaxation transitions, poses, activities, and visualizations and will perhaps make them a ritual for relaxation time.

Transitioning Into Relaxation

One of the goals of relaxation is to draw your child's awareness inward and this can be achieved by bringing her attention to each part of her body through a progressive relaxation. Depending on the theme you choose, you can help your child transition into relaxation with a visualization exercise based on the theme. If, for instance, you are working with an ocean theme, you can say: "Now feel your body floating on the water. Feel the warm water on your back . . . " Speak slowly and calmly, and begin naming the body parts from head to toes: "Feel the water on the top of your head, the back of your head, your shoulders, your rib cage . . . " Leave a few seconds between each body part so your child has a chance to draw her attention to them.

If you are not using a "place" theme you might just say something like, "Feel your body relax, as if it's sinking into the floor. Feel the top of your head," . . . etc. (see the Tense and Relax exercise).

Once you are done guiding your child into relaxation, allow your child to continue resting comfortably. If your child's eyes are open or she is having trouble keeping still, try using one or more of the following tools. Sometimes, gently placing your warm hand on your child's abdomen or head, or both hands firmly on her feet, can help her to relax. If you see that your child's legs and arms are stiff, gently shake them, encouraging your child to allow her limbs to be like spaghetti (see Spaghetti Test exercise). Smoothing your fingers over your child's forehead can also work.

TRANSITION TO RELAXATION ACTIVITIES

The following are some transition-to-rest activities. Each activity described should be followed up with a time for rest and relaxation.

NOW, IT'S TIME TO REST

Benefits

Benefits
Calms
Teaches directional awareness
Integrates and organizes

WHAT TO DO

This is a simple series of mindful movements combined with a chant that encourages directional awareness while providing a fun way to transition to relaxation. It works well with very young children.

WHAT TO SAY

Read the following script:

North Pole, (Reach for the sky.)
South Pole, *(Reach for your toes.)*

East Coast, *(Bring one arm out to the side.)*
West, *(Bring the other arm out.)*
Give yourself a hug, *(Hug yourself!)*
'Cause now it's time to rest! *(Gently roll down to the floor to lie down.)*

NOW, IT'S THE END

Benefits

Calms
Promotes connectedness

WHAT TO DO

This is a simple chant and movement series to a familiar song, providing a fun way to transition into relaxation time. It works well as a transition from standing to sitting or reclining poses. Hold hands and walk in a circle while singing softly and slowly to help set the tone of transitioning to relaxation. When you are finished, each of you gently comes down to rest on your yoga mat and you say, "Now, it's the end!"

WHAT TO SAY

Ring around the rosie,
Yoga is my friend, (or, Love is what I send)
Inhale, Exhale
Now, it's the end!

MELTING

Benefits

Grounds
Calms
Promotes mindful movement

WHAT TO DO

Have your child think of something that melts (chocolate, ice cream, ice cube, butter in a pan, icicle, candle, etc.). Play appropriate "melting music" (anything by Steve Halpern, for example) and then have your child pretend he is that object or material melting—swaying and slowly dissolving down into a "puddle" to prepare for relaxation. Challenge your child to see how *slowly* he can melt. After all, melting takes time!

WHAT TO SAY

To help us transition down to a calming relaxation, let's think of things that melt. Yes, an ice cream cone does melt—great idea! Stand up on your mat to be an ice cream cone. What kind of cone are you? A regular or sugar cone? Okay. Set your cone firmly onto the ground so that we can pile on the scoops of ice cream. Let's see . . . how many scoops would you like? Okay, three! Press the scoops into the cone by hugging and squeezing yourself. Good! And maybe you can put some sprinkles on as well. Tap, tap, tap the sprinkles on top of your head, over your face, and all over your shoulders and arms. Now, close your eyes . . . as you breathe fully in and out, imagine the warm sun coming out and beginning to melt your ice cream cone body. Start to melt, moving very slowly swaying back and forth, then shrinking and dripping as you breathe all the way down to *Savasana* Pose. How slowly can you melt? Use the music as a guide to challenge your body to move slowly and mindfully. You're melting . . .

TENSE AND RELAX

Benefits

Promotes body awareness

Dissolves tension

Calms

WHAT TO DO

This activity is a form of progressive relaxation, working to bring awareness to each part of the body and then release tension from the body by consciously tensing and relaxing. For younger children, you can help them bring awareness to each body part by gently touching that area (with his permission) as you say it.

WHAT TO SAY

Lie down on your back. Let's breathe in and out together three times, as you settle your body into your mat. Good. Now breathe in and make a sourpuss face by scrunching up all the muscles in your face. Good! Exhale to release and relax all of your face muscles. Let your face muscles just melt and relax. Now, your neck and shoulders. Breathe in and bring your shoulders up to your ears; squeeze them tight. And exhale, relax them down. Ahhh. Now tense up your arms and squeeze your hands into fists. Tense, tense, tense and . . . relax. How about your belly . . . your legs . . . your feet and toes . . . your whole body . . . now, relax completely. Allow your whole body to melt now into the floor. Just relax and breathe normally . . .

SPAGHETTI TEST

Benefits

Promotes body awareness

Promotes calm

Enhances full-body relaxation

WHAT TO DO

This exercise is an old favorite in my classes. Children love the spaghetti test and I find it works with young and older children alike as an exercise to learn to be very still without being tense and stiff. As your child comes into her relaxation pose, lift and lower her "noodles" (your child's arms or legs) to test whether they are "cooked" yet. Your child may be quite stiff. If she is, just jiggle her limb gently while telling her to try and relax it, making it "loose and floppy as cooked spaghetti." Once your child gets the hang of it, remind her to try and make her whole body just as loose and relaxed as that noodle.

WHAT TO SAY

What is spaghetti like coming out of the box before it is cooked? Right, it's hard, stiff, and brittle. What is spaghetti like after it is cooked? It is floppy and jiggly! Are your noodles "almost cooked"? Let me test them!! (Pick up your child's arm or leg.) Oh! This noodle is a little stiff. Not done yet! (Jiggle your child's arm or leg gently.) Relax, now, and make this noodle loose as cooked spaghetti! That's right, good. Can you make your whole body just like that? . . .

YOGA WAND MAGIC DUST

Benefits

Promotes a sense of magic and wonder

Encourages relaxation

WHAT TO DO

See Chapter 3 on how to make a yoga wand. All children love the idea and magical sound of the yoga wand. The yoga wand contains magical dust that when shaken over us can help us to relax and rest. Have your child lie down on his or her back, and sprinkle "magic dust" on him with your yoga wand. When your child has been sprinkled with dust and is magically and peacefully resting, you can begin reciting a story or a visualization exercise.

WHAT TO SAY

Come into *Savasana* Pose and take some deep, relaxing breaths. Good. When I see your body still and silent, I will sprinkle you with the yoga wand "magic dust" ... know that the magic dust will help your body to relax and rest. And when I see that is so, I will know you are ready for me to begin the visualization ...

REST WITH BREATHING BUDDIES

Benefits

Improves breathing awareness

Calms

Engages

WHAT TO DO

Have your child choose a "breathing buddy" (a stuffed beanie doll) and lie down with the buddy resting on her tummy. The weight of the breathing buddy brings your child's awareness to her breath as she feels and sees the buddy moving up and down on her abdomen.

WHAT TO SAY

Lie down on your back. Place your buddy on your belly so that he can comfortably go for a ride rising and falling as you breathe in and out slowly and deeply. Good. Close your eyes now. Go ahead and start to practice your Balloon Breathing by breathing in, filling your belly all the way up, and then slowly exhaling to let out all the stale air. Did you feel your buddy moving up and down? Let's try it again ...

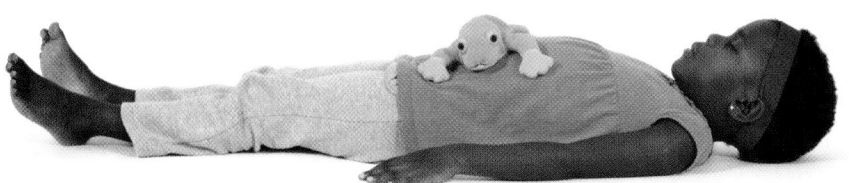

★ Rest with Breathing Buddies

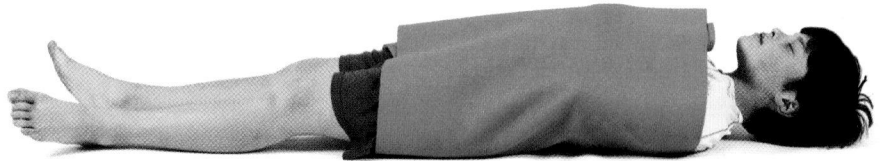

★ Kid Roll-Up

RELAXATION POSITIONS AND ACTIVITIES

The following positions and activities are especially beneficial to use for relaxation with your child.

KID ROLL-UP

Benefits

Nurtures

Calms and centers

Integrates and organizes

WHAT TO DO

Kid Roll-Up, which is essentially a big-kid variation of "swaddling," provides essential sensory input beneficial for soothing the nervous system, particularly for children diagnosed with Sensory Integration Disorder, autism, ADD, or ADHD. In general, it's a helpful position for a child who finds it challenging to still his body in relaxation. Have your child roll up tight in a yoga mat or heavy blanket folded lengthwise. Be sure his head and mouth are well above the top of the mat so that his breathing is not obstructed. Allow your child to rest on his back or tummy while in Kid Roll-Up, whichever is most comfortable for him.

WHAT TO SAY

Lie down on your back perpendicular to your yoga mat. Grasp the edge of the mat and begin to roll yourself up in it from one end to the other! Ta da! You are a kid roll-up! Lie on your back (or tummy), close your eyes, and settle into the safe, warm feeling of being held and hugged.

BALL SMOOSH

Benefits

Calms and centers

Soothes the nervous system

Integrates and organizes

Improves body awareness

WHAT TO DO

Have your child lie down in *Savasana* Pose or Crocodile Pose (Chapter 6). Using a Pilates or large yoga ball that is "smooshy" (not fully inflated), start at your child's feet and press the ball down on his feet, rolling the ball up and down your child's body and limbs. Bring the ball around to press the top of his head as well. Be sure to ask your child whether he is comfortable or would prefer a softer or firmer pressure. This deep pressure activity can be particularly grounding for children with ADD, ADHD, and Sensory Integration Disorder. For extra fun, have your child give you a ball smoosh, too!

WHAT TO SAY

Come to rest in *Savasana* Pose or Crocodile Pose. Here comes the ball smoosh. I'm going to start with your feet . . . how does that feel? Should I smoosh you more firmly or more softly? Bring your attention to each part of your body as the ball passes over it . . . your feet, right leg, hip, belly, chest, right arm, right hand . . . (When finished:) Rest here in *Savasana* Pose as you continue to feel all the parts of your body that the ball has touched.

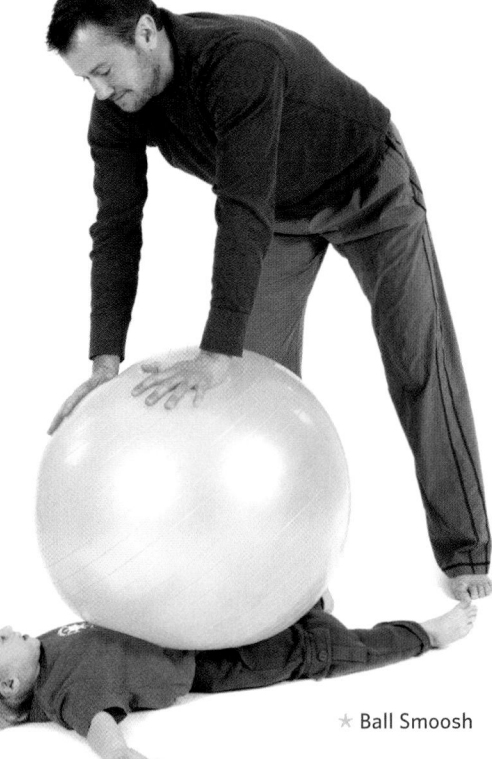

★ Ball Smoosh

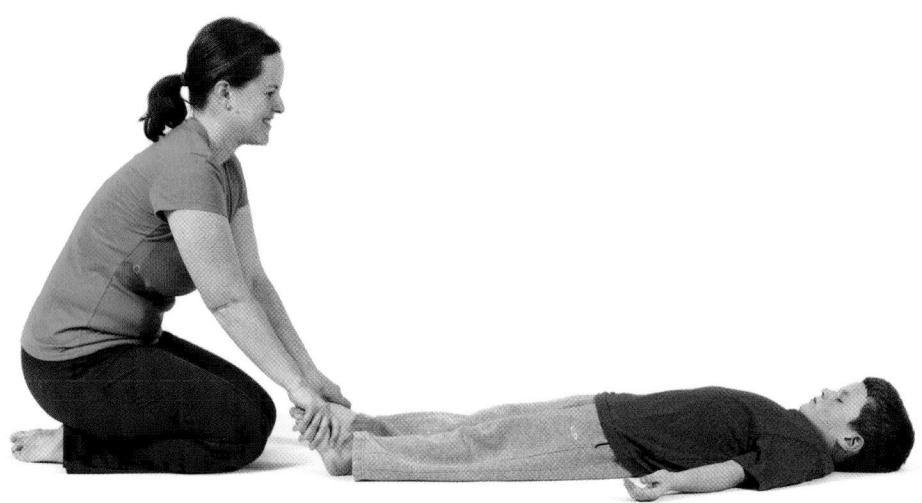

☀ Leg and Foot Massage

LEG AND FOOT MASSAGE

Benefits

Calms and centers

Enhances connection through positive touch

Nurtures

WHAT TO DO

Have your child lie down in *Savasana* Pose (Chapter 6) and play some restful music. First, firmly sweep your hands down from your child's knees to her toes a few times. Next, grasp your child's feet and provide deep pressure to the soles of her feet. Move your grasp down little by little, from the ankle area to the toe area. Finish with a few more slow, firm sweeps from just below the knees down past the feet. This is quite grounding and quieting, especially when done with warm hands and a little lavender-scented foot lotion. On a hot day, using peppermint-infused lotion or just a bit of essential oil on the hands can have a wonderfully cooling effect. After relaxation, encourage your child to return the favor either now or down the road!

WHAT TO SAY

Lie down in *Savasana* Pose. To help your body to calm and relax, I'm going to give you a leg and foot massage using some yummy-smelling lavender essential oil, okay? Your job is to just breathe and relax in *Savasana* Pose.

Benefits

Restores
Calms
Soothes tired legs and lower back

WHAT TO DO

Having the legs elevated during relaxation is restorative. Using bolsters or blankets under the knees works well. If you have an open wall available, have your child lie down with her bottom against the wall and her legs resting up on the wall.

WHAT TO SAY

Pull your yoga mat (or blanket) over to the wall. Lie down with your bottom against the wall and swing your legs up straight to rest on the wall. Good. Allow your arms to rest out at your sides. Feel the weight of your hips, back, shoulders, arms, and head resting on the ground beneath you. Take a deep breath in and let it out with a "Haaaa." Good. Let's do that again two more times.

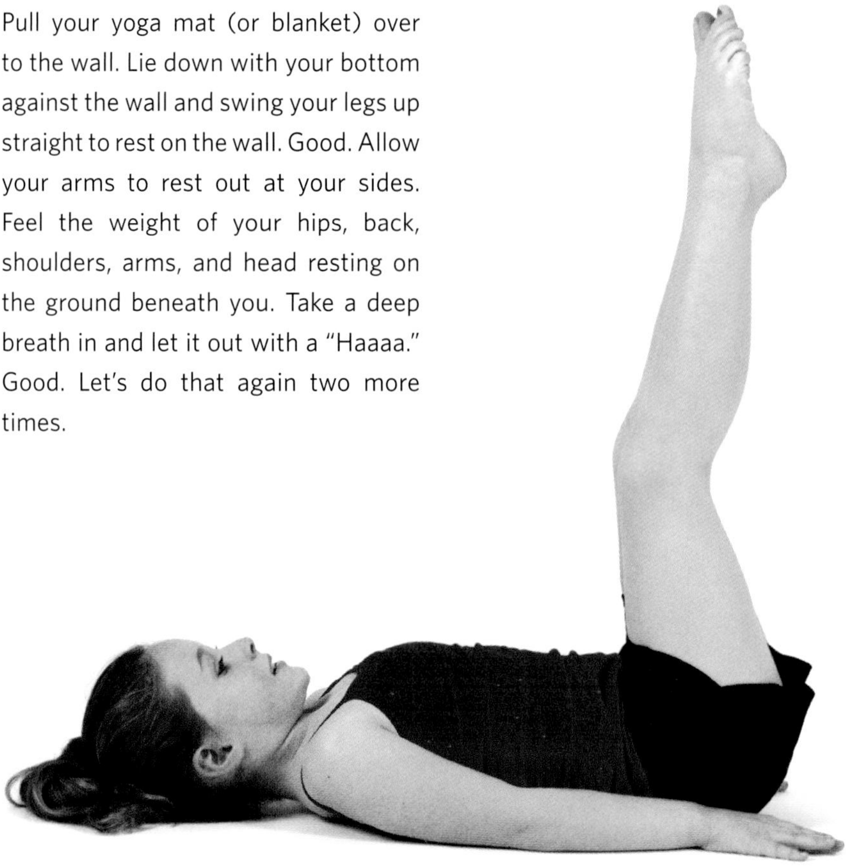

★ Legs Up

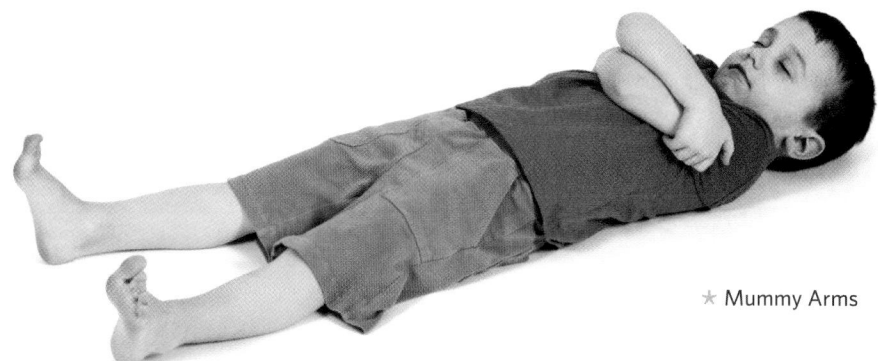

★ Mummy Arms

MUMMY ARMS

Benefits

Calms
Integrates
Encourages self-nurturing
Creates sense of safety

WHAT TO DO

Have your child lie with his arms crossed heavily over his chest as if in a self-hug. Crossing midline with the arms helps to integrate and center. The pressure and weight of the arms over the body is grounding.

WHAT TO SAY

Lie on your back with your arms crossed over your chest. Feel the weight of your arms. Imagine that you are giving yourself a big hug. Take a deep breath in and let it out with a "Haaaa." Let's do that again two more times and then rest and breathe normally.

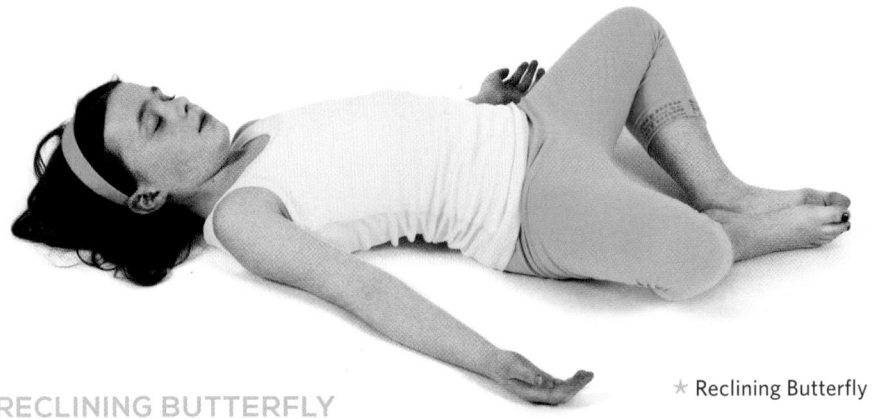

★ Reclining Butterfly

RECLINING BUTTERFLY

Benefits

Stretches the hips and groin

Relieves lower back tension

WHAT TO DO

Have your child come into Butterfly Pose (Chapter 6) and then recline back. This is a comfortable hip opener and feels wonderful on the lower back, and can be especially soothing when combined with Mummy Arms. You can also have your child practice this pose with her legs up against a wall. Should your child feel vulnerable in this position, skip it, or offer a heavy blanket to cover her body.

WHAT TO SAY

Come into Butterfly Pose. Good. Lean back, bringing your lower back to the floor first, supporting yourself with your hands, then your forearms, until you are resting on the floor. Finally, rest your head on the floor gently. Good. Take a few deep breaths in and out, in and out.

CROCODILE POSE

If your child is uncomfortable or challenged to be still while lying on her back, allow her to lie down on her tummy in Crocodile Pose as an alternative (Chapter 6).

CHILD'S POSE

Child's Pose is another alternative relaxation position for a child who may have difficulty lying on his back and/or closing his eyes. See Chapter 6 for a description of Child's Pose.

SEA SCARF

Benefits

WHAT TO DO

This activity requires a large blue, green, or other "sea-colored" chiffon scarf and some peaceful ocean sounds or music. As your child rests in *Savasana* Pose, use visual imagery (see following), to guide your child in imagining what she might see looking up from the ocean floor. Let your child know that you will tap (with your toe) on her shoulder when you see that she is still and ready and that she should open

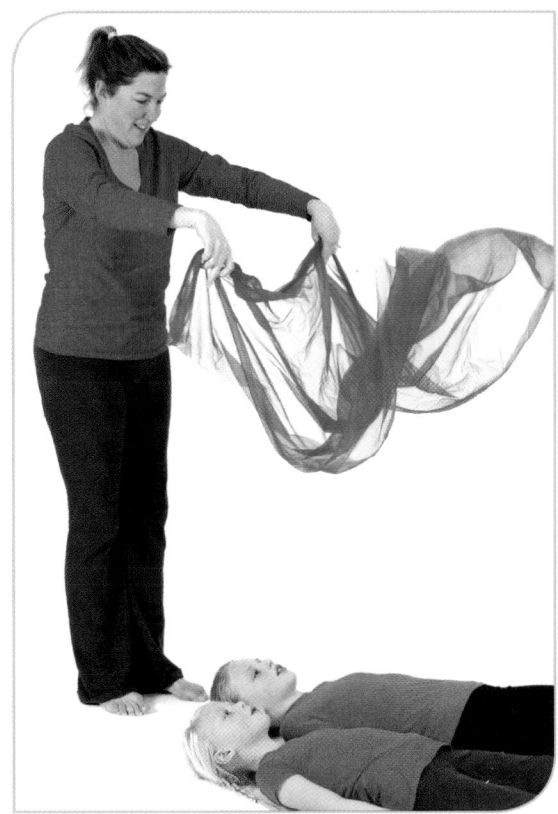

★ Sea Scarf

her eyes to look up when you do so. Stand just behind her head and tap her shoulder with your toe when she is relaxed and peaceful. Flow the scarf up, down, and all around a couple of feet above her head and face (without touching) while listening to ocean music. After 20 seconds or so, pull the scarf away and encourage your child to close her eyes once more to finish out the relaxation. Optionally, you may wish to guide her back to shore to dry off in the sun before coming back into the room.

WHAT TO SAY

Rest in *Savasana*. Imagine you are a sea creature at the bottom of the ocean. What do you see looking up through the blue sea water? Is that a whale passing overhead? What else? Imagine what you might see so that perhaps you might be able to draw a picture of it later on. Good. When I see you are quiet and still, I will come to tap you on the shoulder. When I do, open your eyes and look up for a beautiful surprise . . .

SAVASANA POSE

Savasana Pose is the traditional pose for relaxation in yoga, providing a wonderful opportunity to rest and help the body and mind integrate the benefits of the practice. See Chapter 6 for a full description of *Savasana* Pose.

VISUALIZATIONS

For each visualization activity, guide your child to a deep breathing practice, letting him "Haaaa" as a relaxing extended exhale out through the mouth. Do this a few times, reminding your child to allow his body to sink into the floor a little more with each "Haaaa." Then, begin with the script. Take care to read the scripts slowly with a calm, clear, soothing voice, pausing after each idea to allow your child to process and visualize what you are saying.

AT THE BEACH

Benefits

Brings focus inward

Relaxes

Promotes creativity and imagination

WHAT TO DO

Encourage your child to get out his beach towel for this relaxation, either pretending his yoga mat is his towel or bringing out a real one to rest on. Play ocean sounds softly in the background. These can be found on a sound machine or sound-making app, as well as many CDs. Try an iTunes search for ocean sounds. You might like to have some paper and crayons or pencils ready, or your child's journal, in case you want him to record his experience "at the beach."

WHAT TO SAY

Imagine you are lying on the beach. It is the most beautiful, sunny day. The sand is very warm and you feel your body sink into it as you lie there in the sun. You feel the warmth of the sand soothing and relaxing your head and neck . . . your shoulders . . . and your arms. Your hands feel heavy and relaxed resting in the sand. The soft, dry sand soothes the back of your legs, your feet, and your toes. As the sunlight touches your face, you notice all the muscles in your face and jaw relax. You hear the sounds of waves crashing in and flowing out . . . crashing in and flowing out. Seagulls are calling to each other in the distance. You can smell the salty sea air. You are happy . . . calm . . . peaceful. Let's stay here at the beach for a minute or two. Notice the smells, sounds, and sensations so that if I asked you, you could draw or write about it. (After a minute or two:) When you are ready, take a nice, deep breath in through your nose. Exhale, "Haaaa" through your mouth. Very, very slowly sit up now. Breathe in and out deeply once again before gently opening your eyes. Notice how you feel.

Visualization Resources

There are many wonderful visualization CDs and MP3s for children available to buy or download. The following are some engaging favorites: *Still Quiet Place: Mindfulness for Young Children* or *Mindfulness for Teens* by Amy Saltzman; *Indigo Dreams* (3-CD Set) by Lori Lite; *Discovering Your Special Place* by Charlotte Reznick.

PICTURE IT TREE

Benefits

Promotes positive thinking
Builds confidence
Empowers
Teaches the power of affirmation

WHAT TO DO

What we imagine and think about helps create our reality. This visualization uses the power of positive thought to help bolster confidence while supporting concentration, focus, and ultimately, the means to success. I often use this type of visualization when my students have seemed frustrated with attempts to do a given pose, such as Handstand (Chapter 6). It also works as an empowering exercise to be practiced before testing time at school, a competitive activity, or a performance of any kind.

WHAT TO SAY

Imagine a majestic and beautiful tree ahead of you. It is all alone in the center of an open field. You walk closer to it and see that its branches are spread wide, almost as if to hug you. And its bark seems to be smiling at you. You feel peaceful, warm, and protected standing near this old, wise tree.

Suddenly, you hear the tree whisper to you. You listen very closely and hear it whisper the words, "Picture it and it will be." "Picture it and it will be." You wonder what it means and decide to listen even more closely for a clue. Then the tree says, "Imagine something you'd like to do better. Then, just picture it and it will be."

You sit down with your back against the tree and close your eyes. You think of something that you like to do, but would like to do even better. Maybe it's riding a bike, maybe it's kicking a soccer ball, or maybe it's taking math tests. Or, maybe you'd like to be better at managing your feelings, or being more considerate of others. Whatever it is, picture it now in your mind. And imagine yourself doing it easily and perfectly! Replay in your mind the thing you'd like to do better. Watch yourself doing it absolutely perfectly, over and over again. Notice how you feel as you picture your success. You are so happy and proud! You are doing it! And, now you know you can do it!

You hear the tree whisper, "Now, you can just picture it and it will be." And, suddenly you understand. You now know that if there is ever something you would like to do well, you can take a few moments to close your eyes and imagine yourself doing it perfectly. You can let yourself feel what it would feel like to do it so successfully. And then, you can go out and give it a try, confident that you will succeed because you've practiced and succeeded in your imagination. You can hardly wait to try it!

"Thank you, tree. You are so wise," you say. Listening closely, you hear the tree whisper back, "You are welcome, but know that the wisdom is already inside of you."

(After a minute) It's time to come back into the room now. Take a big, deep breath and start to wiggle your fingers and toes. Stretch your body in any way that feels comfortable, waking up your body slowly and gently. When you are ready, roll to your right side and slowly sit up. Gently open your eyes when you are ready.

Benefits

Inspires creativity

Sparks imagination

Promotes focus and concentration

Enhances sense awareness

WHAT TO DO

This visualization encourages the use of your child's own imagination. First, guide him to choosing a place he'd like to go in his imagination, such as another planet, Candyland, the North Pole, a bear's den, etc. Then tell your child to imagine in his mind what this place might look like, and listen carefully to the details so that he can draw a picture of it later on. Note that there is no right or wrong as our imaginations give us the opportunity to create whatever we'd like! At the end, have your child draw or color what he saw, particularly in his journal, if you are using journals. Note that this open-ended exercise is best suited to your older child, age 7 and up. For younger children, you will want to be more specific with the exercise, presenting it more like the Special Friend Adventures.

WHAT TO SAY

Where shall we go in our imaginations today? You choose. Shall we go to the moon, a mermaid's kingdom under the sea, the Easter Bunny's house? Off to the moon, then! Close your eyes and let's take a few deep breaths together. Ahhh. When I see that your body is relaxed and still, we can begin . . . start to think about the moon. How might you get there? Think about this trip for a minute so that you might be able to describe it to me later . . . now, you've arrived at the moon! Look around. What do you see? Make a mental picture of all that surrounds you, noting each item you see one by one so that you might be able to make a list or draw a picture later on. Can you touch some of the items you see? What do they feel like? What does it sound like on the moon? . . . What does the air smell like? What is your body doing on the moon? Are you floating? How do you get from place to place? Is there someone on the moon to greet you? What does he or she say to you? What do you do together? . . . Let's stay here for a minute as you continue to relax. I will tell you when . . .

Benefits

Promotes new perspective

Releases negativity

Empowers

WHAT TO DO

Change the Channel empowers your child to take control of her emotional responses by learning to pause, breathe, and then react from a more centered state. After practicing this visualization, share with your child some of your own personal examples of occasions when you were reactive and how that felt, and another example of when you were able to pause and breathe before reacting. Encourage your child to share her experiences as well. You might encourage your child (and you can do this, too!) to write in her yoga journal (see Reflection Journaling in Chapter 4) about situations that have or could cause her to feel frustrated or angry. Have her then write about what her first reaction might have been. Then have her write about ways she could "change her channel," whether it be using yoga tools or other methods.

WHAT TO SAY

Can you remember a time when you found yourself feeling or acting negatively? Maybe you had the grumpies or were frustrated about something. Perhaps you had a morning where everything that could go wrong, did. Or maybe someone said something to you that hurt your feelings. Try to recall now what you chose to do. Did you sulk, lash out, or complain to anyone who would listen? If you did act negatively, how did that feel? Was it helpful or harmful? Oftentimes, being and acting angry and negative does not feel good, and can even make a situation worse.

Did you know that we have a *choice* about how we *react* to a bad situation? We have the power to change *our* channel when we don't like our behavior or attitude, just like we change the channel on the TV when we don't like what is on. Let's try it . . .

Imagine you are waiting in line outside at school and someone bumps into you, causing you to drop your backpack into a puddle. Grrr. Naturally, you might feel yourself start to become angry. But then, you remember you can *choose* how to react by simply *changing your channel*. Rather than lashing out, perhaps you use your yoga tools and pause instead to take a deep breath. Of course you are not happy that your backpack is wet. But, you've chosen to turn to a channel of forgiveness, rather than anger. Notice how you feel . . .

When you are ready, take a nice deep breath in through your nose. Exhale, "Haaaa" through your mouth. Very, very slowly sit up now and gently open your eyes.

More Visualizations

For more visualization ideas, I highly recommend those found in any of Maureen Garth's books: *Starbright, Earthlight*, or *Moonbeam*. Other recommendations are *Imaginations*, by Carolyn Clarke, and *Ready . . . Set . . . R.E.L.A.X.* by Jeffrey S. Allen, MEd and Roger J. Klein, PsyD. Eventually, you will be able to create your own on the fly!

BIG WHITE STAR

Benefits

Promotes body awareness

Encourages a sense of connectedness

Inspires a sense of community

WHAT TO DO

This visualization is a progressive relaxation variation that brings awareness to various parts of the body as the light and warmth emanating from the star serves to relax them. As with the other visualizations, dimming the lights, playing soft instrumental music, and using a soothing, calm tone of voice helps set the stage for inner focus.

WHAT TO SAY

Imagine there is a big, beautiful star above your head. It is glowing bright and shimmery, sending light out in every direction. The light is shining in your favorite color . . . maybe it's purple, or blue, or even silver. Imagine what your very own star looks like now . . .

Notice now that one of the biggest rays of light is streaming right down toward the top of your head. You feel the cozy, warm light touch the top of your head and it feels so nice. The light comes into your head and now your face, relaxing all of your face muscles. Now, the light is traveling into your neck . . . shoulders . . . and arms. Feel the light as it moves down into your hands and fingers. The beautiful warm light now travels down from your chest . . . into your belly . . . then down through your legs . . . and finally into your feet and toes, relaxing them and filling them with light.

Notice the light come into your heart now. With each inhale, feel your heart getting bigger and bigger . . . brighter and brighter, filling up with love and warmth for all of the people you love, for all of the people and animals in the world, for everyone you know, and especially for yourself. See the rays of light radiating out from your heart out into the world all around you. Let's stay in this place for a little while, noticing how it feels to be filled with such love and light.

GRATITUDE RELAXATION

Benefits

- Encourages optimism
- Instills appreciation
- Promotes a sense of connectedness
- Prompts mindful reflection
- Lifts mood

WHAT TO DO

Bringing your child's awareness to his blessings is a powerful way to promote positive thinking, a sense of connectedness, and an overall sense of well-being. This visualization can be practiced any time but is ideal for turning around the grumpies! The following script can be simplified for younger children by specifying the types of things for which they may have gratitude. See also the Thoughts of Gratitude exercise in Chapter 4.

WHAT TO SAY

Think about someone or something for which you are very, very grateful. Maybe it is a person in your family or a friend, or maybe it's your cozy warm bed, your bicycle, or even chocolate chip cookies! Whatever it is, imagine it in your mind now, picturing how it looks, how it feels or smells. Think about why you are grateful for this person or thing. How does it make you feel? Do you have pleasant memories with this person or thing?

Take a second now to remember the last time you were with this person or thing and how you felt. Feel the love, warmth, and happiness fill up your heart now. Your heart is expanding with gratitude for this person or thing. Be with this wonderful feeling now for a little while. I will tell you when . . .

Gratitude Rock

Expand and extend the power of gratitude by incorporating a gratitude rock into the visualization. (See Chapter 3 on where to buy.) Set a gratitude rock over your child's heart.

After a minute or two, say: On your chest is a Gratitude Rock. Take this rock in your hands and hold it up to your heart. Feel all of your love and gratitude flow out from your heart and into the rock. You may feel the rock get warm in your hands . . . that is because you've filled it with powerful, positive gratitude energy.

Take a big, deep breath and start to wiggle your fingers and toes. Stretch your body in any way that feels comfortable, waking up your body slowly and gently. When you are ready, roll to your right side and slowly sit up. Gently open your eyes when you are ready.

Look at your special gratitude rock. Imagine you can see it glowing with the light and love you have put into it. Take your rock with you today—maybe you could keep it in your pocket, or in a special compartment of your backpack. When you are having a rough moment, try bringing out your rock and holding it against your heart. Then, remember the relaxation today, and the feelings of love and gratitude you held in your heart. Next time maybe you'll be ready to share your experiences with me!

LIGHT BULB BRAIN

Benefits

Rests and restores the brain

Encourages self-awareness

Promotes self-care

WHAT TO DO

This visualization promotes self-awareness and self-care as it teaches your child to notice when she is tired and take action to nurture herself with a short brain break. Be sure to discuss with your child her experience with this visualization, and help her make the connections to how and why taking care of herself this way is important.

WHAT TO SAY

Imagine your brain has a light bulb inside of it. Your light bulb brain is very hard at work all day, every day. It shines very brightly, filled with energy, thoughts, ideas, and creativity. Sometimes, it can get very, very tired. Think of a time when your light bulb brain can get tired . . . maybe it's right now, or maybe it's after a long day at school. Maybe it gets tired when you've been reading, writing, or concentrating for a long time. What does that feel like? Does that feeling change your behavior or attitude? Here is something you can do to rest and recharge your light bulb brain whenever you need to.

Notice now that your light bulb brain has a dimmer switch. Gently turn the dimmer switch down so that the light from the bulb begins to dim. Feel your light bulb brain begin to relax and settle down. Oh, that feels good! Take a nice deep breath in—when you exhale, see yourself turning the dimmer down even more until your light bulb brain is barely shining at all. You can feel all the muscles in your head begin to shut down . . . your thoughts slow down, your ideas go to rest. Breathe in deeply now, and on the exhale, turn your dimmer all the way to "OFF." Take a moment now and let your light bulb brain recharge and restore itself . . .

When you are ready, find your way back to the dimmer switch and turn your light bulb brain back on. Slowly, slowly, slowly turn the dimmer so that the light in the bulb becomes a little brighter and brighter. Begin to move and stretch your body in any way that feels comfortable, bringing light and energy back into your whole body. Remember that you can use the dimmer switch on your light bulb brain any time your brain needs a rest.

Benefits

Encourages self-knowledge

Promotes trust in innate inner wisdom

Enhances imagination

Instills a sense of safety and support

WHAT TO DO

This visualization is inspired by one of the "9 Tools" provided in one of my favorite books, *The Power of Your Child's Imagination,* by Charlotte Reznick, PhD (2009).

WHAT TO SAY

Imagine you have a very special friend. This is someone who is very wise, someone you can talk to, someone who knows you and loves you, someone you can always trust. Your special friend cares about you and your feelings and helps you any time you need it. Maybe you know someone like this in your life right now. Your special friend might be your parent, grandparent, aunt, or someone else you know and love. Or, maybe you'd like to picture your special friend as a guardian angel or fairy godmother, or even an animal. Whatever it is, picture your very own special friend now in your mind. Feel all the love your special friend has for you.

Know that when you have a question or a problem, your special friend will be there to help you with it. Take a few minutes now to let your friend know what is going on with you. Perhaps you have a problem or there is something you are worried about. Tell your friend all about it in your mind. Feel the warm, caring arms of your friend wrap around you, protecting you and soothing you as you talk. Your friend listens very closely and responds to you with words of wisdom. What are they? What is your friend saying? See if you can listen and hear what your friend's message is to you. Does this message give you a new perspective on the situation?

When you feel a little better, give your special friend a big hug, a thank you, and say goodbye. As you walk away, you hear your special friend reminding you that you can call on her any time you'd like simply by imagining she is there with you. Take a big, deep breath and start to wiggle your fingers and toes. Stretch your body in any way that feels comfortable, waking up your body slowly and gently. When you are ready, roll to your right side and slowly sit up. Gently open your eyes when you are ready.

Benefits

Promotes imagination and creativity

Calms

WHAT TO DO

Once the special friend idea has been introduced, this works wonderfully as a follow-up visualization series. The special friend leads your child to various places where your child inevitably lies down to rest. You can then pick up the next session with your child waking and continuing on with another adventure, again ending with finding a place to rest. These adventures can get very creative! For example, once, in my 6–8-year-old class, we found ourselves following a very long circular staircase making its way up, up, up around a tree and into the clouds. The clouds were made of powdery, fluffy cotton candy. During relaxation at the next class, we started at the clouds, and then took a magic carpet ride over the mountains to land in a meadow of daisies. On the next adventure, we started in the meadow, found the original brick path and followed it into the forest where we came upon a fairy and gnome dance party! The adventures continue during relaxation at each class, and I never know where we might end up next until we get there. Always though, I make it a point to find a cozy place to rest at the end. Following is an example of an adventure to start you off. Remember to pause after each sentence to allow your child an opportunity to process and imagine all you are saying. The younger the child, the slower you should present the imagery.

WHAT TO SAY

(To the Garden)

Your special friend is near and you can hear her come closer until her warm hand reaches for yours. She tells you she has come to take you on an adventure. You walk together down a long brick path until you come to a large black gate. Your special friend is very excited to show you what is behind the gate and tells you that you can open it when you are ready. You take a deep breath and slowly open the gate . . . you cannot believe your eyes! It is the most beautiful, colorful, fragrant garden you have ever seen! There are flowers everywhere, of every kind in every color . . . red roses, purple lilacs, yellow daises, pink petunias, and more. You breathe in deeply and notice that the whole garden smells like a beautiful, welcoming perfume. The grass is lush and green. It looks like rich, thick velvet.

The sky is clear and the most beautiful crystal blue color. You see on the path little animals running here and there—white-tailed bunnies, brown squirrels, and chipmunks. On all of the trees, there are birds of all colors chirping happily. One even comes down to perch on the bench in front of you to say hello.

After wandering around the garden to look at all the sights, you realize you have become very tired. Your special friend suggests that you lie down on the velvety green grass to take a rest. When you do, you feel how soft and lush the grass is. The warmth of the sun feels so nice on your face and body. Your special friend rubs your hair and you find that you are very relaxed and peaceful . . . just rest now for a few moments, enjoying the peace and beauty of your special garden.

Take a big, deep breath and start to wiggle your fingers and toes. Stretch your body in any way that feels comfortable, waking up your body slowly and gently. When you are ready, roll to your right side and slowly sit up. Gently open your eyes when you are ready.

PART III

Putting It All Together

It is wonderful that you want to share yoga with your child. You probably have developed a practice of your own and want to now give him the gift of your one-on-one attention, in the comfort of your home space. Now that you have become familiar with the basic philosophy, benefits, and principles of yoga, and have learned the basic poses, activities, and exercises to build your practice, here is a final chapter on sequencing the elements and some closing words on empowering you and your child in the practice. How do you "create" a practice? In Chapter 10 you'll find some basic sequences that you can use for certain situations and times of the day, and also helpful information on how to create your own sequences. There are no hard and fast rules in sequencing yoga, just what works for you and your child (always with an eye toward safety). This is the special benefit of creating a practice for you and your child alone—you'll learn together what you like to create a truly unique and special practice that's tailored to your needs and enjoyment. By the end of this book, you'll feel empowered and inspired to start practicing!

CHAPTER 10

Sequences

SAMPLE SEQUENCES

So how can you put everything in this book together? The following sequences are provided to help you get started. As you become more familiar with the activities in this book, you may be inspired to create your own sequences that are specifically designed for your child, to suit his special needs and interests. The Creating Your Own Sequences section later in this chapter is full of tips, information, and encouragement to help you do this. The sample sequences are meant for you and your child to do together. (In some cases, you might like to invite other family and friends to participate as well!) Each sequence serves as an example of how a specific plan can be geared toward certain times of day or to address common issues and events that are a part of your child's everyday life, such as test-taking anxiety, bedtime, etc. Feel free to switch out activities as necessary—for example, if your child doesn't like to sing, you may wish to switch out the "Listen to Your Heart" song in the Stress/Anxiety Reduction sequence with a Reclining Twist or another activity you know your child enjoys. As always, pay attention to your child's needs and interests, and have fun!

WARM-UP SEQUENCE
(Sun Salutation, 5–10 minutes, ages 3 and up)

Benefits

Restores
Promotes deep breathing
Enhances circulation
Supports spinal flexibility

WHAT TO DO

Sun Salutation is a popular yoga sequence traditionally used to "greet the sun." Versions of Sun Salutations are often used as the opening sequence for the physical portion of a yoga class. There are several versions of Sun Salutations but all involve movements coordinated with the breath designed to wake up the body and spine, making them a natural choice for a warm-up sequence. The following Sun Salutation sequence is especially fun practiced to music (see sidebar for suggestions). Be sure to encourage your child to breathe in as she opens her chest or lifts her arms, and out as she folds forward. If your child is 4 or under, don't worry so much about the breathing and simply have fun with the movement and music! Have only a couple of minutes? No worries. Just complete the sequence through Step 4, Half Sun Salute, and you and your child will still be gaining the benefits of a beautiful transition into the new day, a warm-up to other yoga poses, or a way to close the day before bedtime.

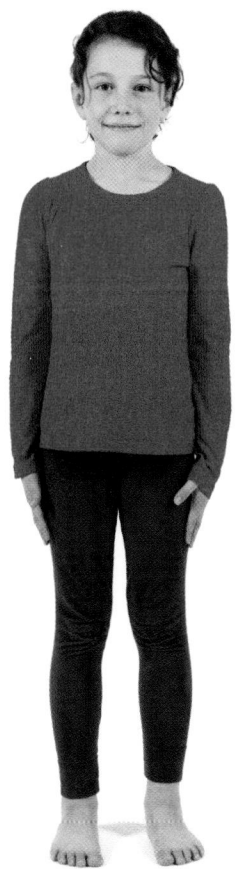

WHAT TO SAY

1 Begin by coming into **Mountain Pose** (Chapter 6). Inhale and exhale deeply a few times as you plant your feet firmly into the earth.

★ Mountain Pose

2 Now come into standing **Crescent Moon** (Chapter 6). Bring your hands over your head and clasp your hands together with your pointer fingers pointing upward. Inhale and stretch up nice and tall. Now exhale and bend to your right, bending from your hips. Inhale to come back up and exhale to bend to the left. Let's flow back and forth two more times.

3 Bring your arms back down to your sides and step your feet out slightly. Relax your knees and begin to turn your upper body from side to side so that your arms begin to swing out and around your body, back and forth in **Washing Machine** (Chapter 6). When the wash cycle is over, return to Mountain Pose and take a deep breath.

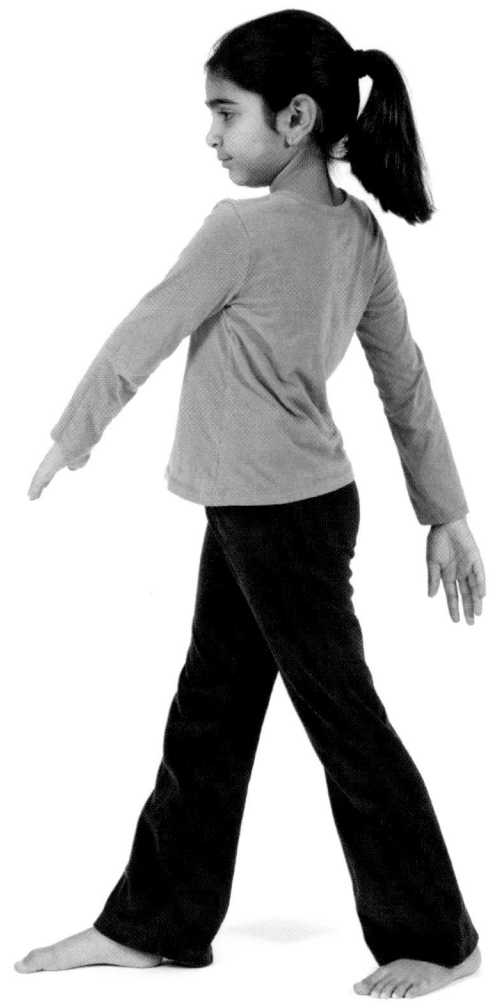

★ Washing Machine

4 Now lets come back to Mountain Pose and do one round of **Half Sun Salute**. Inhale your arms up to the sky to salute the sun. Hello, sun! Exhale and bring your arms straight down in front of you as you fold forward at the hips, keeping your legs and spine straight. Allow your fingers to reach toward the floor near the outer edges of your feet. Now, bring your hands to your shins and inhale and stretch your spine out straight, extending from the top of your head to your tailbone. Exhale and fold forward again, releasing farther into the stretch. Inhale and slowly lift your body as you raise your arms back up to the sun. Hello, sun— we salute you! Exhale your arms down to your sides.

Let's do that again two more times. Up we go to salute the sun! And down we go to bow to the sun.

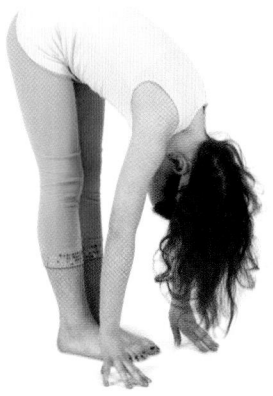

★ Half Sun Salute, forward fold

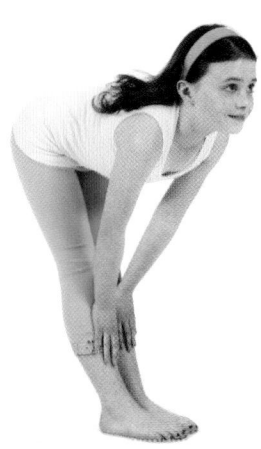

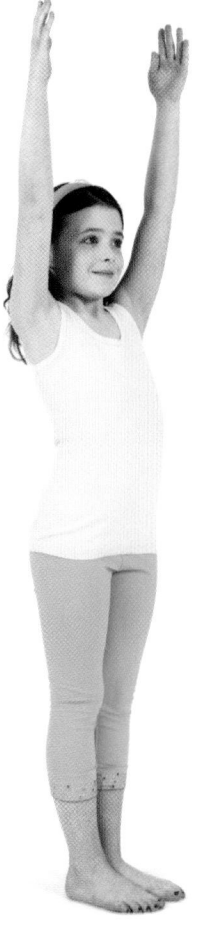

★ Half Sun Salute, reach for the sun   ★ Half Sun Salute, look up

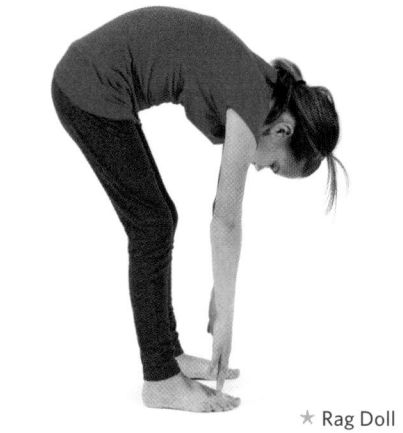
★ Rag Doll

5 Once you are back in Mountain Pose, inhale your arms up to the sun and then exhale them as you fold forward once more to hang in **Rag Doll** (Chapter 6).

6 From Rag Doll, bend your knees and bring your hands to the floor. Take a big step back with your left foot to come into **Roadrunner** (Chapter 6). Adjust to make sure your hands are placed on either side of your front foot. Your back leg should be straight and strong, toes tucked under. Make sure to do a "knee check" (knee should be aligned above or slightly behind the ankle). Good!

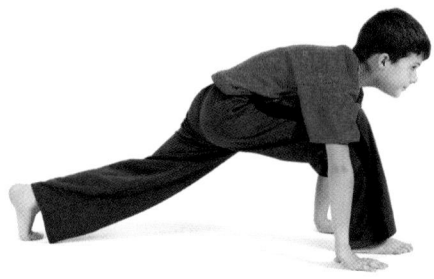
★ Roadrunner

7 Now, step your right foot back to meet your left foot to come into **Plank Pose** (Chapter 6). Remember to keep your back as straight as a plank of wood! Your belly should be tucked up and under and your arms strong and straight. Inhale and as you exhale, bend your elbows to lower yourself to the floor . . . 1, 2, 3.

★ Plank Pose

8 Inhale and rise up into **Upward Facing Dog** (Chapter 6). Look up! Ruff ruff! Shoulder check! Bring your shoulders down away from your ears.

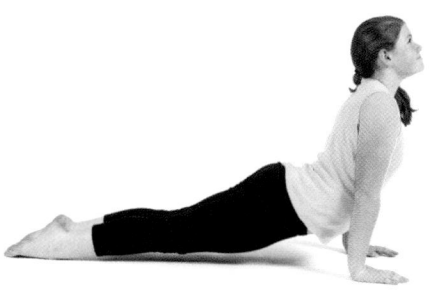
★ Upward Facing Dog

9 Now tuck your toes under and push back into **Down Dog** (Chapter 6). (Optional: Keep barking and don't forget to wag your tail!)

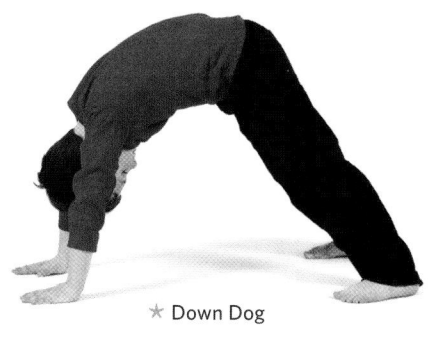

★ Down Dog

10 Now bring your left leg forward to come into **Roadrunner** (Chapter 6) on the other side. Remember, "knee check!"

11 Bring your right foot forward to come into **Rag Doll** (Chapter 6) once again.

12 Bend in your knees slightly and inhale to bring your body back up, arms reaching up high to the sun once again. Hello, sun! Exhale and lower your arms to your sides to return to **Mountain Pose** (Chapter 6). Stand tall, look forward, and feel your strength!

13 Now, that we know the Sun Salutation, let's string it all together and repeat the sequence 2 to 3 times.

Sun Salutation Songs

A wonderfully engaging way to introduce Sun Salutation to children is to incorporate music. Here are a couple of songs with lyrics focused on teaching the sequence:

- The "Sun Dance" from the *Musical Yoga Adventures* CD by Linda Lara is slow paced, perfect for ages 3–6 years. Just follow along with the lyrics and be sure to jam out a bit with the jazzy beats between each verse!

- "Dance for the Sun" from the *Dance for the Sun* CD by Kira Willey is a sweet, whimsical Sun Salutation song, well suited to ages 3–12. This song offers instrumental time at the beginning and end to add in **Washing Machine** and **Crescent Moon,** incorporating the other important movements of the spine.

GOOD MORNING SEQUENCE
(Reach for the Sun Sequence, 10 minutes, ages 2–8 years)

Benefits

Wakes up the body
Promotes parent/child connection
Provides a peaceful, positive transition into the new day
Promotes optimism
Encourages imagination

WHAT TO DO

A positive morning routine = a positive day. Beginning the day with yoga-based movements, breathing, and opportunities for connection and bonding benefits the body, mind, and spirit of both parent and child. It has been said that if you've moved your spine in all five directions, you've done a full yoga practice. Like the Sun Salutation warm-up sequence, the **Reach for the Sun Sequence** encourages those movements: up, forward, back, sideways, and twisting. The script supports the idea of setting an intention for the day and "reaching for our dreams," promoting optimism and a "can do" attitude. You might even consider adding in a discussion of one or more of the Yoga Principles here, such as Be Content or Work Hard (Chapter 3). Note that this sequence can be made calming or energizing depending on the presentation. Let your child decide what she needs and play her favorite calming or energizing music to set the pace. With a group, sit in a circle for Step 1 and continue on as described. As a Good Morning variation for older children, see the Stretch It Out Sequence later in this chapter.

WHAT TO SAY

1 Sit down here across from me in **Easy Pose** (Chapter 6). Inhale your arms up over your head and reach up high to say, "Hello, sun!"

2 Exhale and bring your right hand down to the floor beside you, and reach far over your head to the right side with your left hand to become a

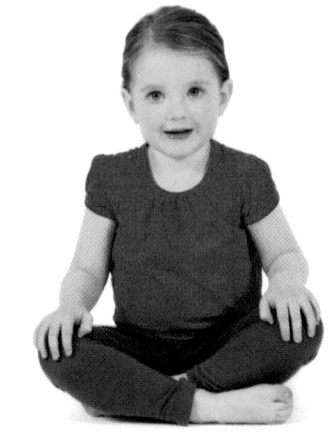

★ Easy Pose

beautiful **Crescent Moon** (Chapter 6). Inhale both arms up overhead again. Now, exhale and switch sides. With another big inhale, reach your arms up to the sun once again. Exhale and bend forward, reaching your arms *way* out in front of you. Use your hands to dig up your dreams and wishes for the day. What are they?

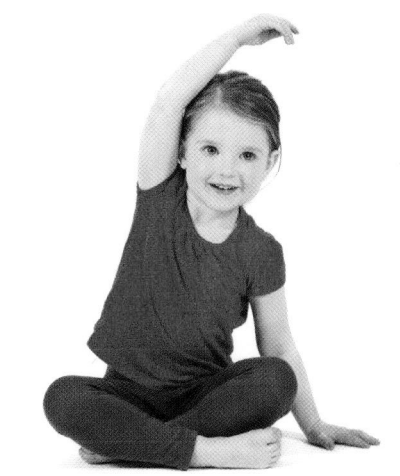

★ Crescent Moon

③ Sit up now and unfold your legs and stretch them out into **V-Sit Pose** (Chapter 6). Let's connect our toes. Good. Inhale to reach up to the sun. Now exhale and fold over to reach for one of your feet. Can you reach to tickle my toes? Inhale your arms back up to he sun . . . and exhale your arms down to the other side to tickle my other foot! Ha!

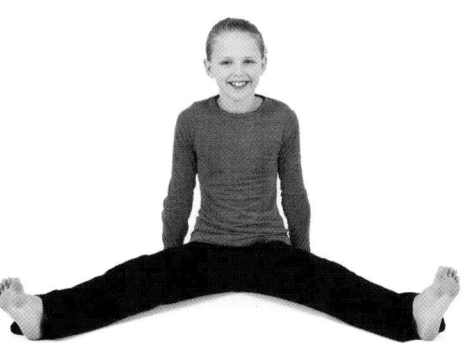

★ V-Sit Pose

④ Sit back up and pull the bottoms of your feet together into **Butterfly Pose** (Chapter 6). Holding your feet with your hands, flap your "wings" (legs) up and down, then press your wings open and rock side to side to soar into the air. Let's sing the "**Butterfly Song**" (Chapter 8). Now sit up tall and inhale deeply (pause), and exhale to fold forward to bring your nose down toward your toes. Breathe in and out here a couple of times . . . how do your toes smell this morning?

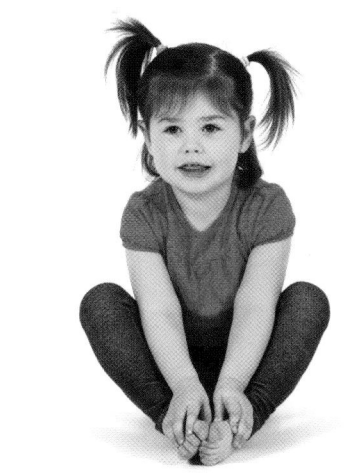

★ Butterfly, flapping wings

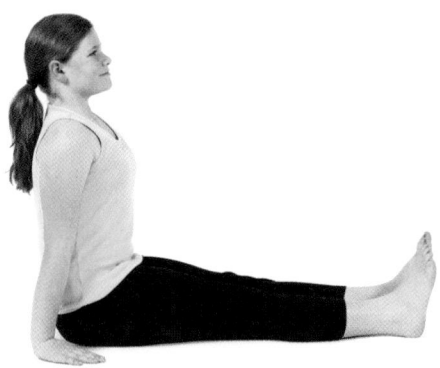

★ Staff Pose

5 Come back upright and stretch your legs straight out to come into **Staff Pose** (Chapter 6). Bring your hands to the floor at your sides and flex your feet so that your toes point up toward the ceiling. Good!

6 Let's make a peanut butter (if allergic, choose otherwise) and jelly **Sandwich** (Chapter 6) for lunch today! From Staff Pose, twist to your left and reach over with both hands to grab a big ol' jar of peanut butter. Unscrew the cover and reach inside with both hands to scoop some out. "Splat!" Pat it on your chest. Now, spread it into your hair, on your face, on your shoulders, and even into your belly button. Now, twist over to your right side to grab a jar of your favorite jelly. What kind is it? Spread it on your bottom slice of bread. Rub it into your hips, thighs, knees, ankles, and even between the toes . . . toe jam! Now, reach up tall and inhale and fold over to press your slices of bread together to make your sandwich.

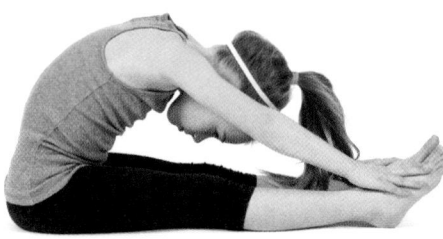

★ Sandwich Pose

7 Create a knife by putting your hands flat together. Cut your sandwich in half by dragging your knife hands between your legs from your feet up to your waist as you sit up. Spread your legs apart to create two sandwich halves (**V-Sit Pose**, Chapter 6). Fold over your legs, one at a time, to nibble your knees to eat both halves of your sandwich. *Yum!* Rub your belly to show you are full!

PLAYTIME SEQUENCE
(10 minutes, ages 2–8 years)

Benefits

Encourages storytelling

Promotes creativity and imagination

Inspires playfulness

Improves mood

WHAT TO DO

Yoga comes alive through story, imagination and play! The **Mouse, Cat, and Dog Story** encourages children to *be* the animals and act out the story as it's being told. Simply use the script to tell the story and demonstrate the poses as you tell it so your child can follow along. It will be very helpful to first teach the individual poses to your child before combining them with the story sequence. This 10-minute sequence can easily be repeated (in fact, your kids will beg you to repeat it!), so if you have the time, you can extend your yoga session simply by telling the story more than once. As this sequence tends to get the blood (and laughter) flowing, it can serve as a fun warm-up to other activities. Once it becomes familiar, encourage your child to lead the story.

WHAT TO SAY

1 Once there was a teensy, tiny little white mouse (**Child's Pose**, Chapter 6). He was a happy little mouse, minding his own business, nibbling at a piece of cheese. "Squeak, squeak, squeak."

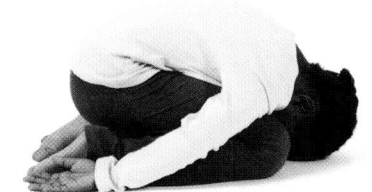

★ Child's Pose

2 But then, along came a cat! The kitty cat was very happy to see this mouse because, as you know, cats *love* to chase mice. "Meeooww!" (**Cat: Happy Cat**, Chapter 6)

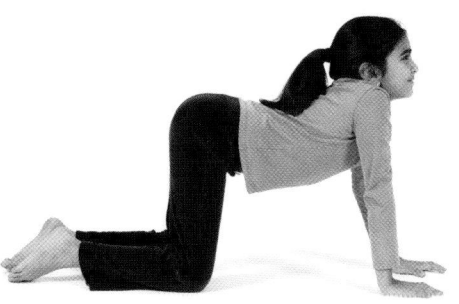

★ Happy Cat

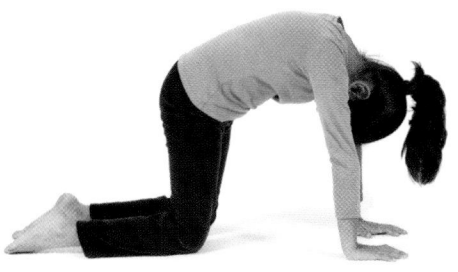

3 Suddenly, though, the cat got very scared. "Hissss!" (**Cat: Scared Cat**, Chapter 6). Show me that again . . . Happy Cat, "Meow!" and Scared Cat, "Hiss!" Good!

★ Scared Cat

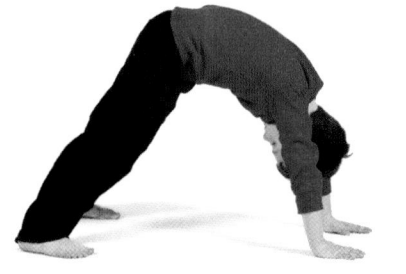

4 Why do you think the kitty got scared? What animal *loves* to chase cats? That's right—a dog! (**Down Dog**, Chapter 6)

5 Dogs love to chase cats and this dog was so excited he barked and wagged his tail (**Down Dog: Wag Your Tail**, Chapter 6). "Woof! Woof! Woof!"

★ Down Dog

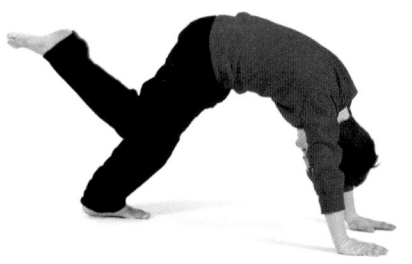

6 The cat's instincts brought her quickly to attention (**Mountain Pose,** Chapter 6).

7 And then, she ran around the neighborhood looking for a place to hide. (**"Walking, Walking Song,"** Chapter 8, pausing between each verse to "look around" for a place to hide.)

★ Down Dog, Wag Your Tail

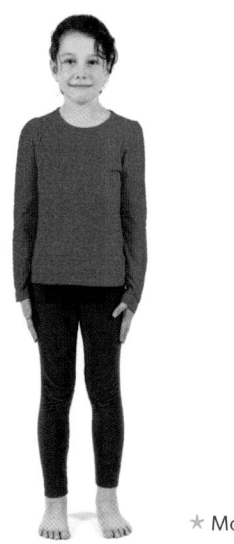

★ Mountain Pose

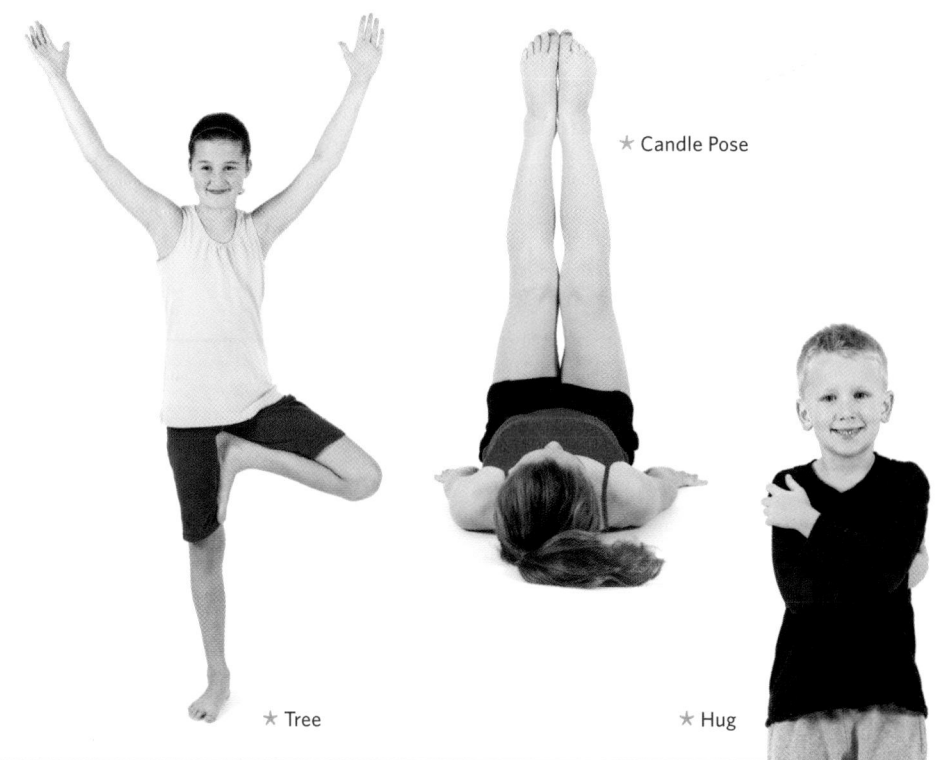

★ Candle Pose

★ Tree

★ Hug

8 Finally, the cat saw the perfect place to hide up ahead . . . it's a tree! (**Tree**, Chapter 6)

9 She quickly climbed the tree, all the way to the very top (climbing motion, reaching one hand as you lift the opposite knee and then switch back and forth).

10 She finally reached the top, looked down, and said, "Uh-oh . . . I've climbed too high and now I'm stuck! Meow!" How can we help the kitty get down from the tree? What can we use to get up there to help her? Yes! A ladder is a great idea (**Candle Pose, Legs Up Variation**, Chapter 6).

11 Rest your ladder up against my tree. Good! (Climb the ladder by lifting your head and shoulders up off the floor and reaching your hands to climb up your legs to the top.) Climb, climb, climb . . . keep climbing! You did it!

12 You made it to the top and the cat is so happy to see you. Give the kitty a big hug (**hug** self tight OR **parent/child hug**). What do you think she says to you? That's right. "Meow!"

STRESS/ANXIETY REDUCTION
(15 minutes, ages 4–12 years)

Benefits

Promotes clear thinking
Builds confidence
Balances and centers

WHAT TO DO

Tests, performances, or new situations can instill anxiety in even the most confident children. This sequence works to reduce feelings of anxiety and provides a physical release of stress and tension, while enhancing memory, promoting clarity, and building confidence.

WHAT TO SAY

1 Lets stand together in **Mountain Pose** (Chapter 6). Inhale your shoulders up and exhale them back and down, "Haaaaaa." Feel the weight of your feet on the floor. Good. Let's do that again two more times. Let me hear you sigh out, "Haaaaaaa." Good.

2 Now, take a big step back with your right foot to come into **Warrior I** (Chapter 6). Let's take a moment to focus on our bodies and get adjusted. Knee check! Is your front knee bent? Leg check! Is your back leg straight with your foot firmly planted flat on the floor? Nice adjustments! Now, inhale your arms up to the sky. Shoulder check! Bring your shoulders down away from your ears. And there you are—a powerful, proud warrior! Say, "I am strong!"

3 Now open to the side to settle into **Warrior II** (Chapter 6). Keep your left leg bent and your back leg straight. Bring your arms straight out to the sides so that they are parallel with the floor. Good! Turn your head to look out over your fingertips. Say: "I am powerful!" Feel your power and show me your muscles!

4 Now, let's move into **Warrior III** (Chapter 6). Turn your body to the front of your mat. With your back toe on the floor, raise your arms straight up to the sky. That's right. Find a focus point either on the floor or out in front of you. Keeping

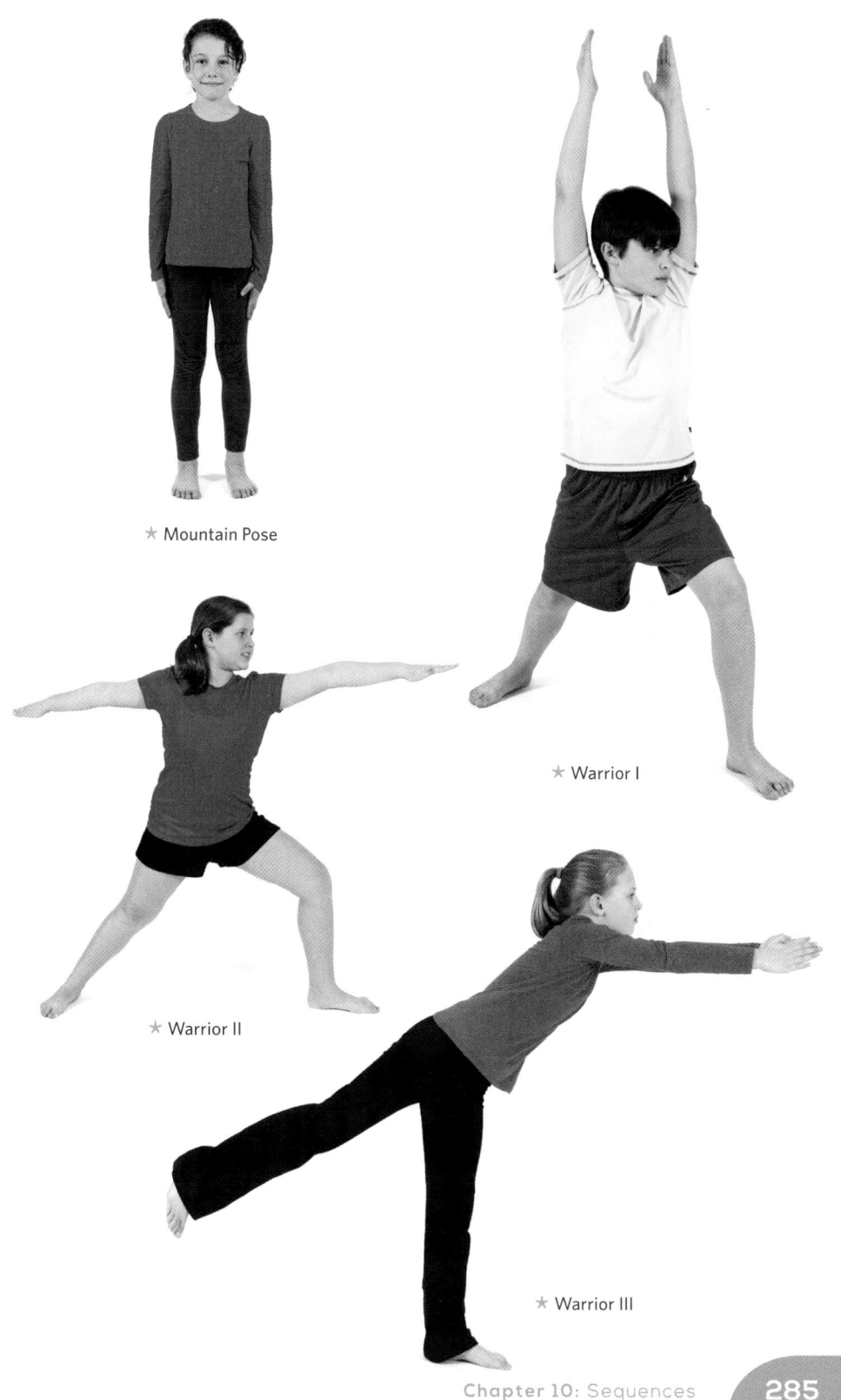

★ Mountain Pose

★ Warrior I

★ Warrior II

★ Warrior III

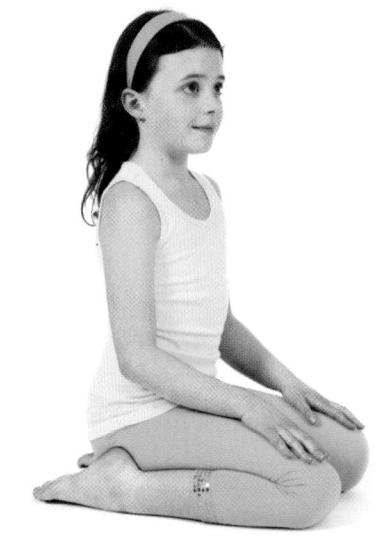

your arms and legs straight, slowly bend forward at your hips as you lift your back toe off the floor. Balance and breathe here. Good! Say "I am brave!" Remember, you are a powerful warrior and can conquer anything! Can you balance here as I count down from 5? 5, 4, 3, 2, 1. Great balance!

5 Return to **Mountain Pose** (Chapter 6) and breathe here for a few moments to rest before we switch sides. (Repeat Steps 2–4 on the other side.)

★ Hero Pose

6 Sit down in **Easy Pose** or **Hero Pose** (Chapter 6), whichever is most comfortable. We're going to sing the "**Listen to Your Heart" song** (Chapter 8) . . . listen, listen to your heart—what does it say? It says "Yes!" to do your best.

7 Come into *Savasana* **Pose** (Chapter 6). Breathe quietly for a few moments. In and out, in and out. Good. I'm going to read to you the **Picture It Tree** visualization (Chapter 9). As I read, try very hard to be quiet and picture in your mind the tree and all the wonderful, wise things it is telling you. The tree wants you to "picture it and it will be!" As you listen, picture yourself (doing well on the test, etc.)—let's begin.

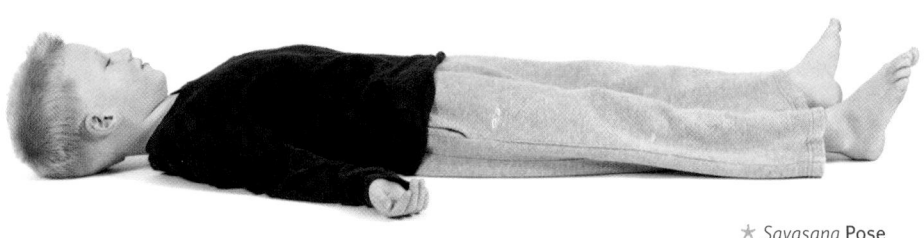

★ *Savasana* **Pose**

FOCUS/CALMING SEQUENCE
(10 minutes, ages 4–12 years)

Benefits

Calms the nervous system
Promotes focus
Balances energy

WHAT TO DO

Kids love moving, laughing, and being noisy, but sometimes your child just needs to calm down and focus—and so do you! Use this sequence to teach your child quick and simple tools for centering and rebalancing when her energy is too high. It's a great way to "clean the slate" before getting homework done or settling down for quiet time.

WHAT TO SAY

1 Sit beside me in **Easy Pose** (Chapter 6). Hmm, is your posture happy or grumpy today? (See Easy Pose sidebar, Chapter 6.) Remember to sit up nice and tall. Good!

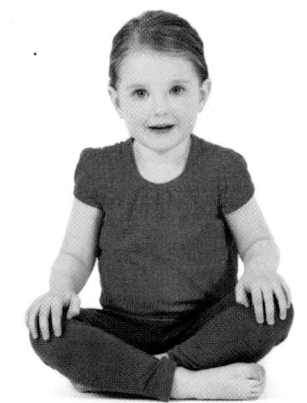

★ Easy Pose

2 What do bumble bees sound like as they swarm their hive? That's right, it's a buzzing, humming sound. We can sound like that too when we do **Bumble Bee Breath** (Chapter 5). Let's try it. Take a slow, deep breath in through your nose before exhaling out to "Hummmmmm" as long as possible. Good. Let's try it again, this time with our eyes closed. Was that a different experience? How so? Now, let's try it one more time but with our eyes closed and our hands over our ears. Where did your focus go? How do you feel? Shall we try that again?

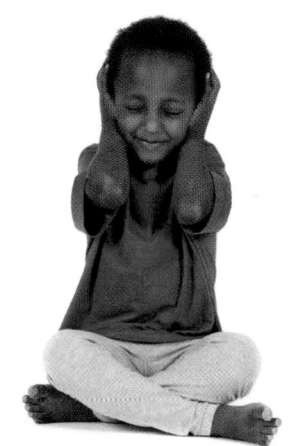

★ Bumble Bee Breath

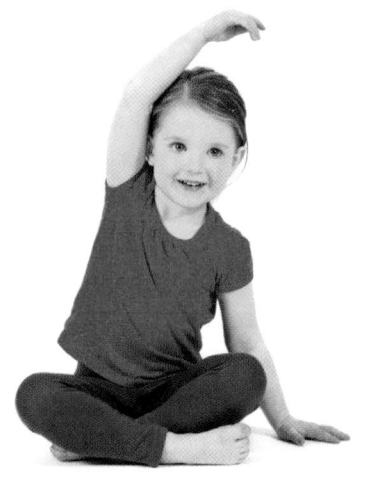

★ Crescent Moon, sitting

3 Let's become a sitting **Crescent Moon** (Chapter 6). Bring your right hand to the floor beside you, and reach your left arm up overhead as you inhale deeply. Now exhale out and bend to your right. Beautiful Crescent Moon! Inhale back up and switch sides. Use your breath to guide your movements to flow back and forth from side to side a few times.

4 Now bring your elbows to your sides with your hands resting on your shoulders. Inhale deeply through your nose. Exhale and swish, swish, swish right and left by turning side to side from your belly (**Sprinkler**, Chapter 6). Let me hear you "pssh," "pssh," "pssh," like a sprinkler. Good! When you run out of water, stop twisting for a moment to fill up your sprinkler hose by taking another deep breath in through your nose. Exhale and twist back and forth, once again. "Pssh, pssh, pssh." Imagine all of your excess energy coming out of your sprinkler hose to help water and grow the grass.

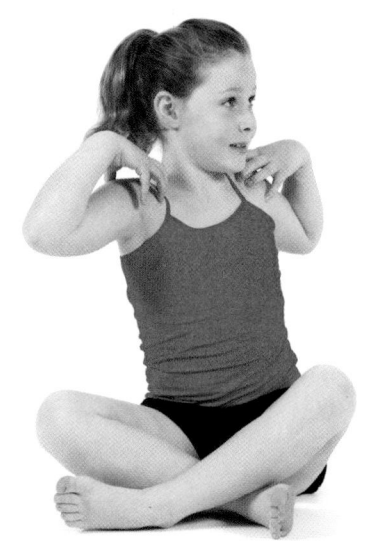

★ Sprinkler

5 Now come into **Sandwich Pose** (Chapter 6). To make the first slice of bread, straighten your legs out in front of you. Point your toes to the sky! Inhale and reach your arms up above your head to create the second slice of bread. Exhale as you fold forward, bending from your hips. Reach your

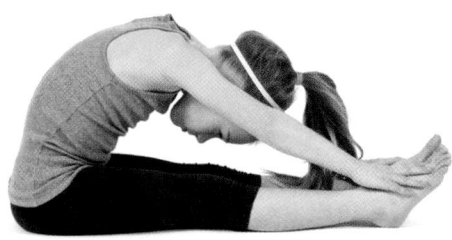

★ Sandwich Pose

hands forward toward your shins or feet. Good. Relax your head and shoulders and breathe in and out here a few times.

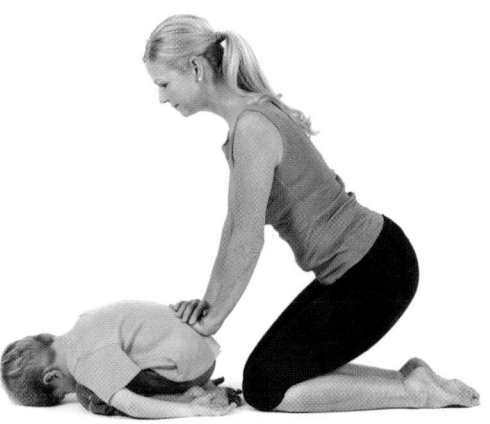

⭐ Rest and Press

6 Come into **Child's Pose** (Chapter 6). We're going to practice relaxing **Rest and Press** (Chapter 4). Is it okay if I press a bit on your lower back? Good. I'll give you a turn and then maybe you can give me one. Go ahead and take a nice deep breath as I rub your back. Just breathe in and out, in and out. (Continue on with instructions, checking in with your child along the way.) All done now. Let's take a nice deep breath in and out together. Very, very slowly come to sit up and gently open your eyes. How do you feel?

STRETCH IT OUT SEQUENCE
(20 minutes, ages 4–12 years)

Benefits

Improves flexibility
Supports spinal alignment
Encourages body awareness

WHAT TO DO

Flexibility is a child's birthright. But in the age of TV, computers, and hours of sitting at a desk at school each day, children can develop tight muscles and joints and poor posture overall. This simple sequence encourages children to flex and stretch their muscles while getting in touch with their bodies. Try it as a helpful way to stretch out before or after athletic practices or as a break from a long car ride or family movie marathon.

WHAT TO SAY

1 Stand tall in **Mountain Pose** (Chapter 6). Find your focus point and take a few deep breaths.

2 From Mountain Pose, come into **King Dancer** (Chapter 6). Shift your weight to your left foot, and raise your left arm for balance. Slowly reach back with your right hand to grab the outside of your right foot. Find your balance and breathe . . . in and out, in and out. Hold King Dancer for at least 3 to 5 breaths. Can you do it? Now switch to the other side.

3 Now come back to **Mountain Pose**. Hop your feet apart and stretch your arms straight out to the side. This is **Star Pose** (Chapter 6), remember? How many points do you have? Count each one with me (point to each extremity as you count with your child): 1, 2, 3 . . . points! Good. Now, stand up tall with your shoulders relaxed. Inhale to open your chest, and then fold forward into **Folded Star** (Chapter 6). Grab the outside edges of your feet or ankles. (For older children: You can grab your big toes with your first two fingers if you like to deepen the stretch.) Breathe in and out. From Folded Star, place your right hand

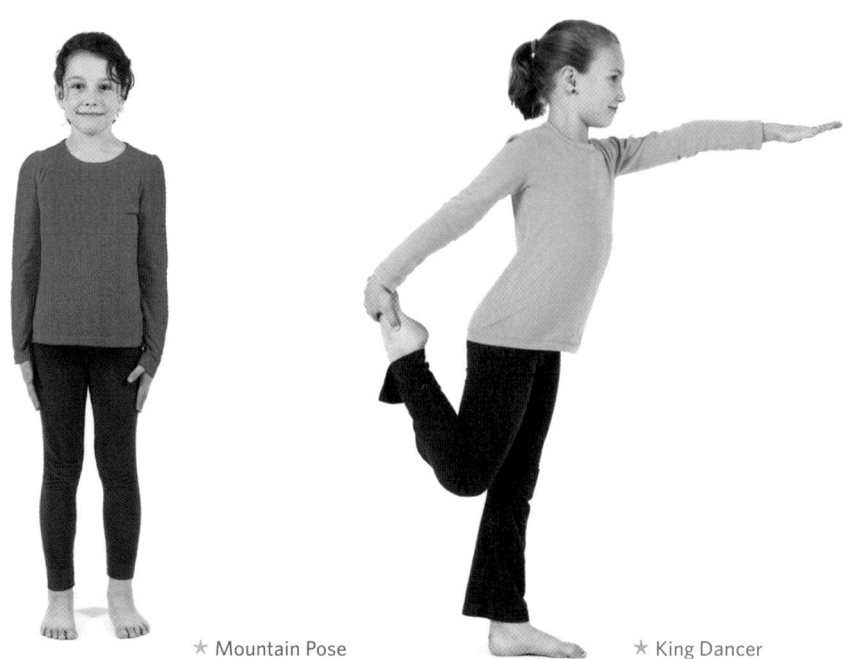

★ Mountain Pose   ★ King Dancer

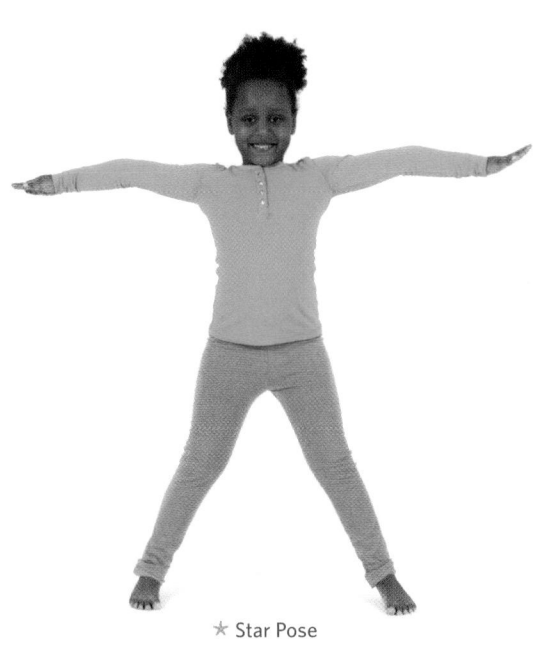

★ Star Pose

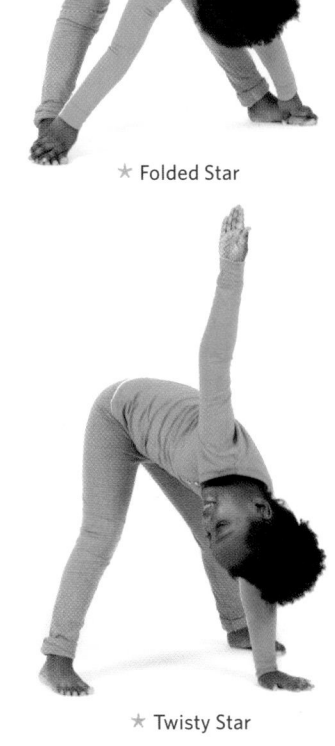

★ Folded Star

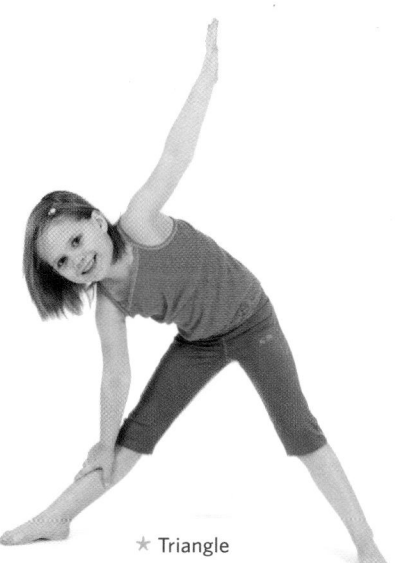

★ Twisty Star

on the floor between your feet. Inhale and lift your left arm to the sky into **Twisty Star** (Chapter 6). Look up toward your other star friends! Breathe here in and out, in and out. Switch sides.

④ Now come back to **Star Pose** again to set up for **Triangle Pose** (Chapter 6). Turn your right foot out to the right. Inhale and reach over to your right. Exhale and bend sideways, reaching your hand to your shin. Reach up to the sky with your left hand. Good. Can you look up and balance for three breaths? . . . Come back to **Star Pose** now and rotate your feet so that you can come into **Triangle Pose** on the other side. When finished, stand back up, shake out your limbs, and return to center in **Mountain Pose.**

★ Triangle

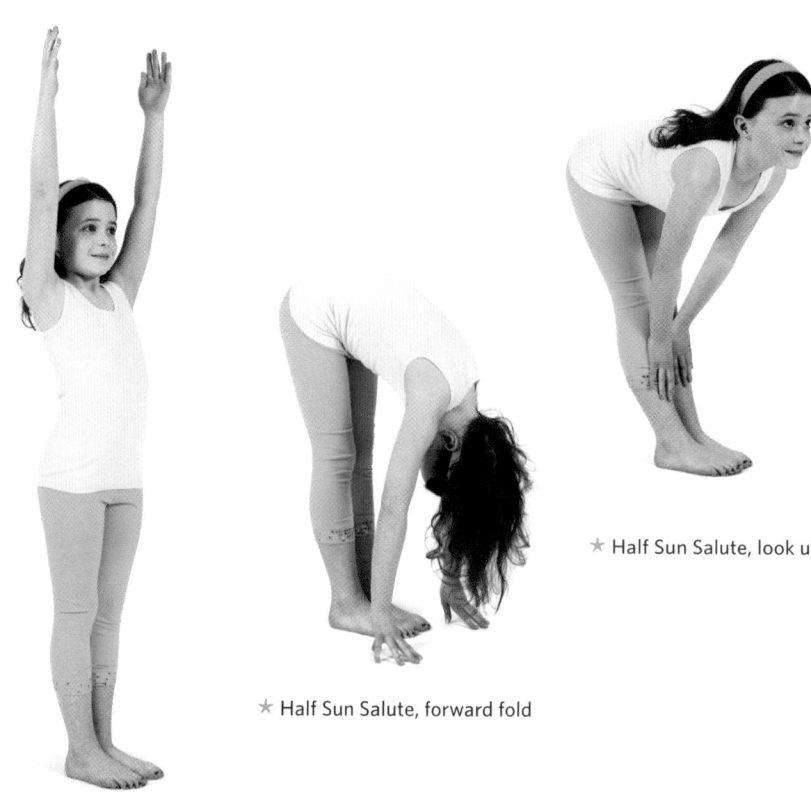

★ Half Sun Salute, look up

★ Half Sun Salute, forward fold

★ Half Sun Salute, reach for the sun

5 Let's do two rounds of **Half Sun Salute** (see Warm-Up Sequence in this chapter). Inhale your arms up to the sky. Exhale and bring your arms straight down in front of you as you fold forward at the hips, keeping your legs and spine straight. Allow your fingers to reach toward the floor near the outer edges of your feet. Now, bring your hands to your shins and inhale and stretch your spine out straight, extending from the top of your head to your tailbone. That's right. Exhale and fold forward again, releasing farther into the stretch. Inhale and slowly lift your body and raise your arms back up to the sun. Exhale your arms down to your sides to return to **Mountain Pose** (Chapter 6). Let's do that again, but this time stay in your forward fold . . .

6 Bend your knees to press your hands into the floor and step both feet back into **Down Dog** (Chapter 6). Breathe here in and out for three breaths.

7 From Down Dog, lift your right leg up and then bend your knee and bring it forward to rest on the floor in **Pigeon Pose** (Chapter 6). Puff out your proud

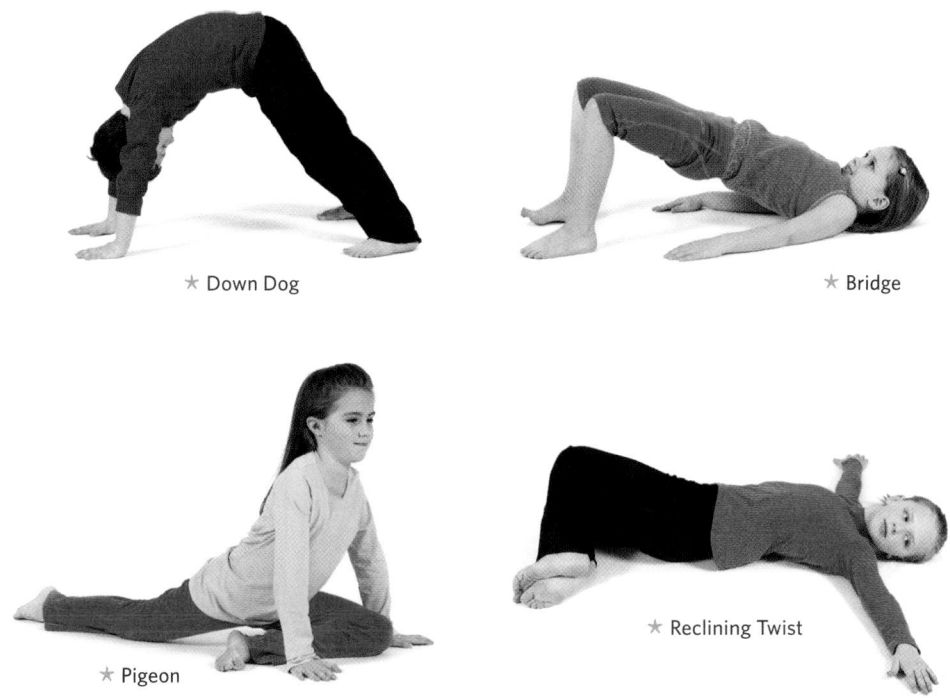

★ Down Dog

★ Bridge

★ Pigeon

★ Reclining Twist

pigeon chest and breathe . . . when you are ready, press into your hands and lift up to bring your right leg back into **Down Dog**. Repeat on the other side.

8 Now lie on your back and get ready for **Bridge Pose** (Chapter 6). Place your feet flat on the floor, hip-distance apart. Here comes the boat! Time to raise the bridge. Keeping your shoulders and feet flat on the floor, lift your hips high into the air. Good! Lift your chest up to arch your spine. (To older children: Shimmy your shoulders back and walk your elbows in to clasp your hands together.) Breathe in and out slowly three times. Now lets lower our bridges. Gently bring your hips back down to the floor, rolling slowly down the spine. Rest and repeat this sequence a few times. When you're finished, pull your knees into your chest and rock from side to side to massage and rest your lower back.

9 Let's wind down now with **Reclining Twist** (Chapter 6). Place your feet flat on the floor, knees bent. Extend your arms wide out to your sides. Breathe in and lift up your feet. Breathe out and drop your knees to your left side as you turn your head to look out over your right shoulder. Shoulder check! Are your shoulders both on the floor? Good. Rest here for a couple of breaths. When you're ready, inhale your knees back up and switch sides.

FAMILY BONDING SEQUENCE

(25 minutes, ages 4–12 years)

Benefits

| Promotes connection |
| Encourages positive touch |
| Promotes teamwork |
| Encourages mindfulness |

WHAT TO DO

A connected family is a healthy family. This sequence encourages physical connection, teamwork, and mindful awareness. If you have multiple members of your family participating, simply double up the partner activities.

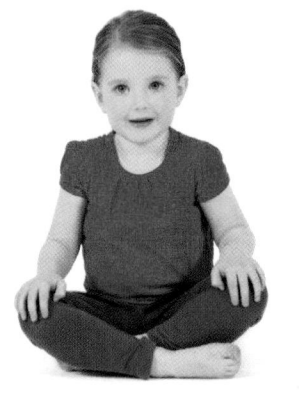

★ Easy Pose

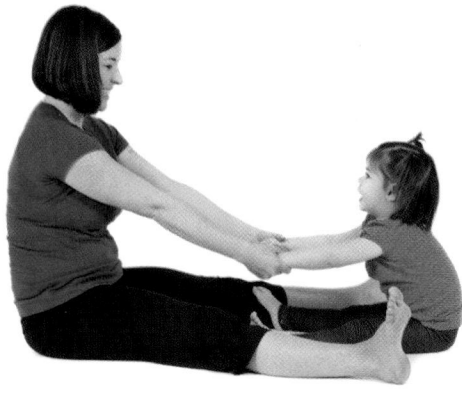

★ Seesaw

WHAT TO SAY

1 Sit with me in **Easy Pose** (Chapter 6) with your hands in your lap. I'm going to ring the chime for our Chime Listening exercise (Chapter 4). Remember to close your eyes and focus on the sound of the chime, raising your hand when you can no longer hear the sound.

2 Now lets **Pass the Chime** (Chapter 4) back and forth, back and forth to each other. Remember to pass the chime mindfully, so that the sound doesn't stop.

3 Sit across from me in **V-Sit Pose** for **Seesaw** (Chapter 6). Let's sit up tall and hold hands. Now, I will gently pull you forward as I lean back. Try to keep your shoulders back and your chest open. Good! Now you pull me by leaning backward. Ahhh. Inhale up and exhale forward. Let's go back and forth, moving with our breath . . . good!

④ Now lets come into **Back-to-Back Twist** (Chapter 6). Let's sit back to back in **Easy Pose** (Chapter 6). Good. Let's breathe in and sit up tall. As we exhale, let's reach our left hand across to our right knee and our right arm out straight to reach around for each other's left knees. We did it! Breathe with me here for three breaths and then we'll switch sides.

⑤ Now let's play **Stick Together** (Chapter 7). Here is the stick. Face me and hold up your right hand. Good. Let's hold the stick between our palms. When I say, "start," let's begin to move to the tempo of the music, slowly and mindfully. The more mindful we are, the more easily we'll keep the stick between us. If we drop it, we'll just pick it up and keep going. Remember that we can't talk, so we'll watch each other carefully. Ready?

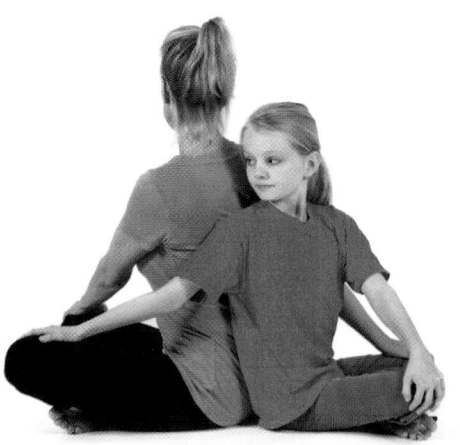

★ Back-to-Back Twist

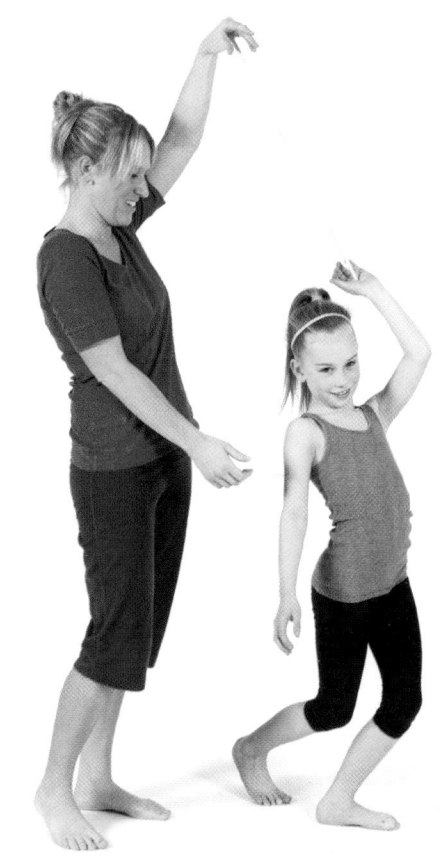

★ Stick Together

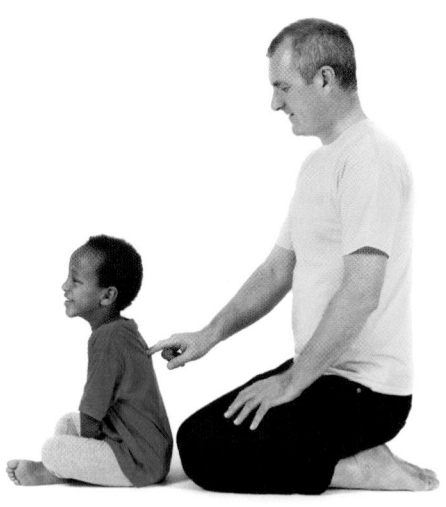

6 Now let's sit together in **Easy Pose** (Chapter 6). I am going to sit behind you for **Back Writing** (Chapter 4). I am going to write or draw something on your back and then you tell me what you think I wrote. Be very quiet and still so that you can feel what I'm writing . . . can you guess what it was? Good. Let's take turns.

★ Back Writing

7 Ahh, it's time to close our yoga session with our favorite part, *Savasana Pose* (Chapter 6)! Breathe in and out, in and out, relaxing your body into the floor.

8 Would you like a **Leg and Foot Massage** (Chapter 9)? Put your palms up if yes, palms down if no . . .

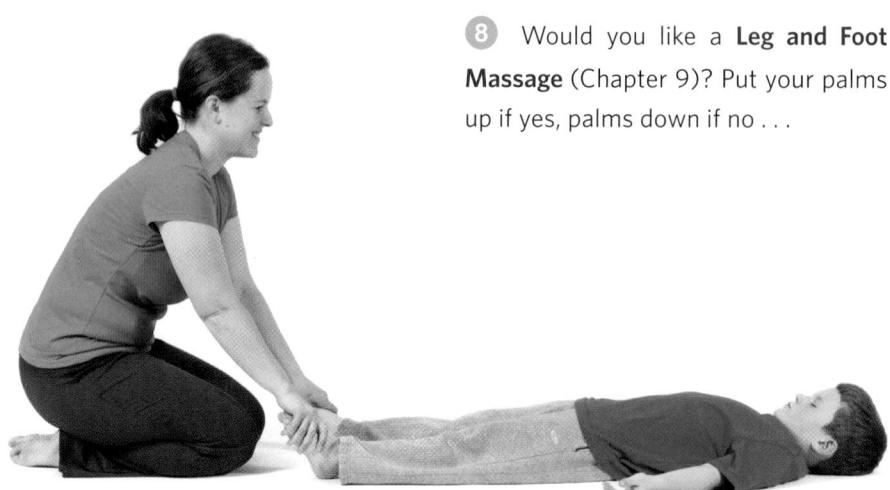

★ Leg and Foot Massage

BEDTIME SEQUENCES
(10 minutes, ages 3–12 years)

Benefits

Calms the nervous system
Encourages gratitude and appreciation
Promotes connectedness and sense of safety

WHAT TO DO

Taking a few minutes to relax with your child at the close of a busy day will help improve her quality of sleep (and yours), while providing an opportunity to reflect and connect. This sequence provides a simple tension-relieving movement flow, a calming, connecting breathing activity, and an opportunity for you and your child to count your blessings before you count your sheep.

WHAT TO SAY

1 Let's do a **Half Sun Salute** (this chapter, Warm-Up Sequence) to say goodbye to the sun, for the day is ending now, and the sun is going to sleep. As you fold forward, say, "Goodnight, sun!"

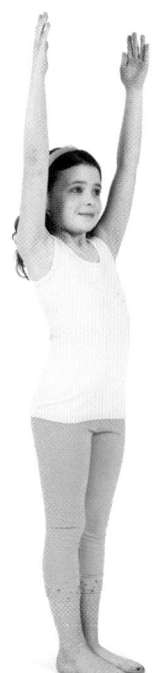

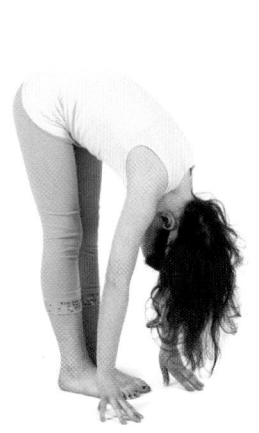

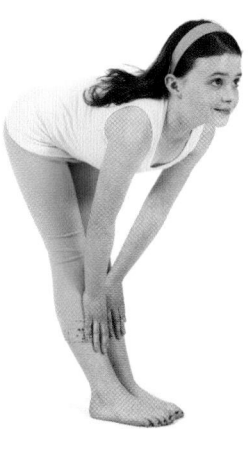

★ Half Sun Salute, look up

★ Half Sun Salute, forward fold

★ Half Sun Salute, reach for the sun

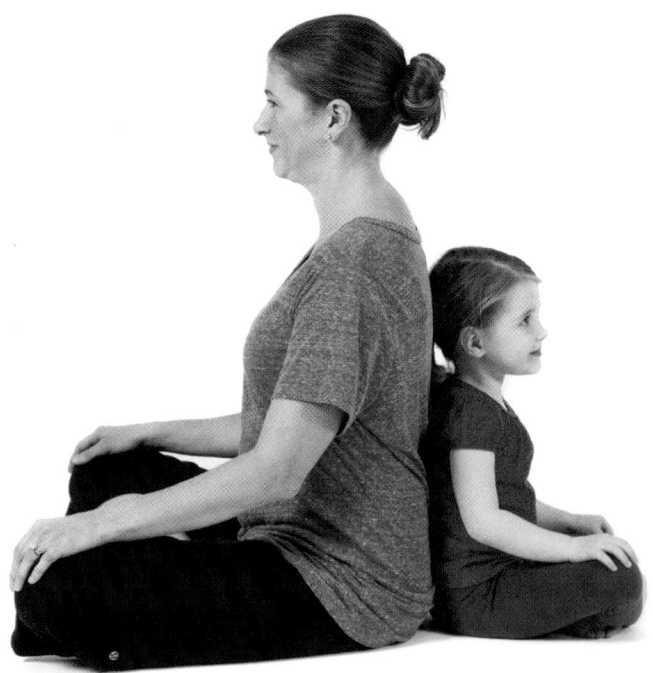

★ Back-to-Back Breathing

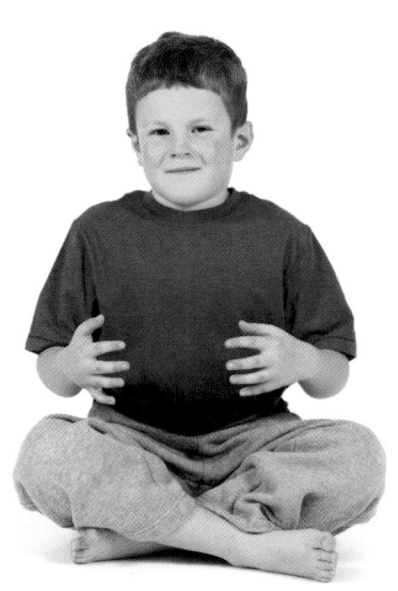

★ Balloon Breath

2 Let's sit down into **Easy Pose** (Chapter 6) to do **Back-to-Back Breathing** (Chapter 5). Let the weight of your body push back against me, and feel the warmth of my back. Let's do **Balloon Breathing** (Chapter 5) together, releasing our day with our exhales. Ahhh . . .

3 As we sit here breathing together, let's think about all the good things about our day (**Thoughts of Gratitude,** Chapter 4). Did someone do something nice for you today? Did something happen today for which you are grateful? Let's say and send a great big *thank you* as we exhale . . .

4 Now give me a *big* hug! Goodnight and sweet dreams . . .

CREATING YOUR OWN SEQUENCES

While it's helpful to have a plan when sharing yoga with your child, there is no rule that says you need to use one! In fact, as you experiment with the various poses, activities, and songs in the book, you and your child will learn what you enjoy and benefit from most and will inevitably make up your own sequences as you go along. That said, it is helpful to keep a few things in mind. Use the following tips for guidance as you develop yoga sequences to practice with your child.

Set an Intention

How much time do you have? What do you and your child need? Bonding time? Time to calm down and focus? Help waking up, or going to bed? A chance to be creative and use your imagination? Or do you just need some time to have fun? Sometimes a simple 1-minute extended breathing exercise is in order—something to calm your child before a game or test. Sometimes you will want a full session—and a plan to go with it.

Consider Using a Theme

When you have the time for a full yoga session, themes are great ways to build sequences and create a playful mood to keep your child's interest. For example, if your younger child likes insects, start with Bumble Bee Breath, then move on to poses such as Cricket and Butterfly. An adventure story can link the poses together (as in the "Mouse, Cat, and Dog Story" described in the Playtime Sequence in this chapter), or use a storybook with insect characters as a guide, doing (or making up) the poses as you read along. For extra fun, add some songs that reference insects, such as the classic "Itsy Bitsy Spider," adding movements to the song, or play Web of Connection (Chapter 7). And for relaxation, you might become the spider, wrapping up her prey in her web until he can't move (Kid Roll-Up, Chapter 9) before sharing a peaceful visualization about an ant family and their busy day (Special Friend Adventures, Chapter 9).

For an older child, consider the intention. Is your fifth grader having trouble sleeping? Your theme could then become "Winding Down to Bedtime." Choose a meditation, a calming breath, restful poses, and a relaxation with a Leg and Foot Massage (Chapter 9). The ideas for themed kids' yoga sessions are endless!

Sequencing Your Session

Again, though there are no hard and fast rules to sequencing, it can be helpful to have a "flow" to the order of poses, songs, and exercises that you put together. The chapters of this book are presented in the *typical* order of presentation that has worked well in my yoga classes. However, it's only a suggestion and works best when you have time to put a full 20–30-minute session together. The chapters are meditation, breath work, poses, family yoga games, songs and chants, and relaxation. In general, a basic kids' yoga sequence would include exercises from most of those chapters, as follows:

- **Opening:** Depending on the age and interest of your child, you might choose to open your yoga session with the short opening song in Chapter 8, perhaps followed by a story about, or a discussion of, one of the Yoga Principles in Chapter 3.
- **Meditation (Chapter 4):** Choose a meditation such as chime listening or candle gazing to help transition your child to yoga time.
- **Breath Work (Chapter 5):** Choose a calming or energizing breath depending on your child's energy or the theme of the session.
- **Warm-Up:** You might choose the Good Morning or Warm-Up Sequence in this chapter or a song and movement sequence from Chapter 8 to serve as a warm-up.
- **Poses and Partner Poses (Chapter 6):** Choose a few poses that align with the intention or theme of the session. Amp up the kid-friendliness by including the fun variations. And don't forget to include a partner pose or two! Don't worry too much about whether the poses "flow" well at first. For the most part, children don't mind (and even enjoy) getting up and down from one pose into the next. It's not until they are older (8+) that they have the attention span and body control to really sustain a flow in a session. At that point, you might consider starting with standing postures, moving to sitting postures, and ending with reclining postures or vice versa.
- **Family Yoga Games (Chapter 7):** It's time to get off the mat. Choose a game or creative movement exercise as an opportunity to play and connect with your child.
- **Songs and Chants (Chapter 8):** Create community by singing a chant or song and doing movement sequence together.

- **Relaxation and Visualization (Chapter 9):** Be sure to include one of the transitions to relaxation as suggested before winding down with a peaceful relaxation and/or visualization.
- **Closing:** End with a closing song (Chapter 8) or a simple *namaste* (Chapter 6).

Important Note about Safety

For safety and to encourage your child to maintain mindful awareness of her movements, it's important to emphasize the finish of one pose or activity before starting another. How we come out of a pose should be practiced just as mindfully as the steps taken to come into a pose. In addition, following each pose and activity, there should be a few moments of grounding in the relevant foundational pose. If standing, that is Mountain Pose. If sitting, that is Easy Pose. If lying down, that is lying flat on our back. This is a safety concern and for the most part is quite intuitive. For example, your child should transition mindfully out of Plow Pose to come up to Mountain Pose before attempting Triangle Pose. She should also come out of Tree Pose back to Mountain Pose before coming into Warrior I.

Recording Your Yoga Sequences

If you decide to plan and write down the sequences you share with your child, you might find it useful to purchase a three-ring binder, a package of dividers, and some clear, protective sheet covers. As you complete your sequences, place them in protective sheet covers and keep them in your "Family Yoga Organizer." Use the dividers to sort your sequence plans by theme, time of day, etc. Then, as you need a sequence, you will be able to just grab one and go on the fly!

Keeping in mind the special importance of each component (poses, breathing exercises, principles, etc.), the time you have, and your child's interests, needs and energy, you should be able to build a sequence that maximizes the benefits of having a practice that is specifically tailored to your child. Don't be afraid to ask for your child's input. As you and your child experiment with putting elements of yoga together, you'll learn much about each other, enhancing your connection, mind, body, and spirit.

Having read through this book, you have probably noticed that sharing yoga with children is, by necessity, an entirely different animal than sharing yoga with adults. A typical adult yoga class is serene and quiet as yogis move their bodies in unison with their breath, while their focus turns inward. Adult participants listen to and follow intently the instruction given by the teacher—they stay firmly on their mats, and then relax peacefully into *Savasana* Pose, without prodding. This is not what a typical kids' yoga session looks like. Though there are beneficial, quieter moments throughout a children's yoga session, they are typically short-lived. And guess what? It's okay!

In his book *Magical Child* (1977, 1992), Joseph Pearce, a renowned child development expert, wrote, "Play is nature's biological plan for learning." Children learn best through play. And play, by definition, is *fun*! Put yourself on a child's yoga mat for a moment—would you rather be told you are going to learn a series of forward bends or play a game called "Peanut Butter and Jelly?" Of course you would much rather play a game!

Yoga for children utilizes storytelling, games, crafts, journaling, creative movement, imagination-building activities, reflective discussions, and more to help kids learn and integrate the practice of yoga and mindfulness. You might wonder if children can still gain the benefits of yoga, and learn how to apply yogic concepts in their daily lives, if they're "just" having fun. If the session is well intentioned, planned, and instructed, you bet they can! Yoga for kids is different because it is designed specifically for them and the unique and wondrous ways they relate to the world.

Yoga provides vital therapeutic benefits for children. And healthy kids make happier human beings. Sharing yoga with children provides them with strategies to build the resilience they need to adapt to the busy, outcome-based world in which they live. Breathing, movement, mindful awareness, and affirmation are some of the many strategies presented in this book that promote adaptability, self-regulation, self-esteem, courage, a healthy body, and a calm, confident, learning-ready mind. This is important, necessary work that can start simply—right now, right at home.

Allow your child's interests and needs to drive your sessions together, thinking of yourself as a partner rather than a teacher. Allow yourself to be drawn into his imaginative world and you'll find yourselves creating, practicing, and growing together. You can't get together time "wrong." No matter what you and your child's yoga practice looks like, if you are honoring your individual needs and that of your relationship, it's automatically "right!" After all, that's what yoga and mindfulness are all about.

Yoga helps children develop the self-awareness to realize how they feel and what they need; teaches them strategies to slow down, unwind, and manage their emotions; guides them through movements that optimize their strength, flexibility, and balance; demonstrates healthy habits; and reminds them to love and forgive themselves. Yoga provides children and families with tools to live a holistically healthy lifestyle. I honor you for sharing this gift with your child and look forward to hearing about your journey using this book.

NOTE FROM THE AUTHOR

I often get asked why I am so passionate about teaching and promoting yoga and mindfulness for children. I could cite supporting research, talk about my teaching experiences, or give a speech on how important it is. Instead, I typically find myself telling a story. Since finding my way to yoga in the 1990s, I can't count the number of times I have wondered to myself, "If I only had had these tools when I was a child, would adolescence, early adulthood, and beyond have been less painful?" To many who practice yoga, this is an all-too-familiar question, because many of us are drawn to the practice as a way to soothe pain, anxiety, and so many other common ailments of modern life. For me, it was a bout of depression and anorexia during my college years that first led me to yoga. Years later, as a newlywed working as a marketing director, I pondered how I might help others avoid, or at least healthfully navigate through, the lingering effects of the types of traumas I had experienced in my early years. And then I thought—better still—how to help *children* navigate the "everyday traumas" of school, homework, broken friendships, and life before they become permanent scars. But how?

Not surprisingly, my own children were my inspiration. As they became toddlers and preschoolers, we began to develop a "language of wellness" in our home. We'd say things like: "When we start to become frustrated, what can we do? We can practice Balloon Breath . . ." and so forth. Looking outside my home for local children or family yoga classes, I came up empty-handed. Then the proverbial "light bulb" came on, and so began my personal journey with yoga for children.

My company, ChildLight Yoga®, has been providing yoga-based classes and programs to children and families in the New England area since 2005 (*www.childlightyoga.com*). The ChildLight Yoga® Teacher Training program was designed to empower adults to bring the practice of yoga to the children in their own communities, now numbered at nearly 1,000 instructors worldwide. In 2007, as a volunteer yoga teacher at my children's elementary school, I realized yoga had an important place in education as well. I saw firsthand the enormous impact even the most basic yoga tools can have on children's learning, teacher morale, and the classroom and school culture as a whole. After several years of piloting, ChildLight Yoga® was expanded to include the Yoga 4 Classrooms® program, which has empowered thousands of educators to integrate yoga and mindfulness into their class day. Now, with the creation of this book, I hope to inspire parents to bring basic yoga and mindfulness tools into the home!

In the article "Healing Power of Yoga," which appeared in a 2010 issue of *Yoga Journal*, Sat Bir Khalsa, PhD, assistant professor of medicine at Brigham and Women's Hospital (Boston) and renowned yoga researcher, stated: "I think of this [yoga] as hygiene. We have dental hygiene, which is a well-accepted part of American culture. Schools teach it, doctors recommend it, parents reinforce it. Imagine if people didn't routinely brush their teeth. That would be unheard of in this country! But what about mind-body hygiene? We have nothing for that."

Khalsa believes if yoga was routinely taught in schools, practiced at home, and written on doctor's prescription pads, we'd be raising a generation that is physically and emotionally healthier, equipped with self-awareness and tools for managing stress. I agree—and as you are reading this book, I'll bet you do, too.

As more and more adult and kids' yoga programs pop up in child-care centers, gyms, classrooms and after-school programs, shelters, jails, and health-care settings, it is obvious we are fast realizing yoga's ability to positively transform lives. And researchers now support that realization with scientific evidence in hopes of driving that point home to policy makers as well. Just imagine a world where yoga and mindfulness are integrated into every classroom and home, and are subsidized by insurance companies. It's coming.

In the meantime, let's keep brushing our teeth . . . and doing yoga! As you breathe, move, connect, and play together, know that you are helping your child practice "mind-body hygiene," supporting a lifetime of health and wellness for the mind, body, and spirit. I wish you and your family the very best in this joyful venture!

Bibliography

Asencia, Teressa. *Playful Family Yoga: For Kids, Parents and Grandparents.* Hightstown, NJ: Princeton Book Company, 2002.

Flynn, Lisa, and Sammie Haynes. *I Grow with Yoga: Yoga Songs for Children*, a CD. 2008. *www.cdbaby.com/cd/sammiehaynes2.*

Freeman, Donna. *Once Upon a Pose: A Guide to Yoga Adventure Stories for Children.* Victoria, BC, Canada: Trafford Publishing, 2010.

Jennings, P. A. "Contemplative education and youth development." New Directions in Youth Development, Special Issue. *Spiritual Development* 118 (2008).

Khalsa, Sat Bir. "Healing Power of Yoga." *Yoga Journal* (2010).

Lite, Lori. *Indigo Dreams: Children's Bedtime Stories Designed to Decrease Stress, Anger, and Anxiety while Increasing Self-Esteem and Self-Awareness*, a 3 CD set. 2007. *www.stressfreekids.com/352/indigo-dreams-3cd-set.*

Pearce, Joseph. *Magical Child.* New York: Penguin Group, 1992.

Reznick, Charlotte. *Discovering Your Special Place: A Soothing Guided Journey to Inner Peace*, a CD. 2004. *www.imageryforkids.com/shop-discspecialplace.html.*

___ *The Power of Your Child's Imagination: How to Transform Stress and Anxiety into Joy and Success.* New York: Penguin Group, 2009.

Saltzman, Amy. *Still Quiet Place: Mindfulness for Teens*, a CD. 2004. *www.stillquietplace.com.*

___ *Still Quiet Place: Mindfulness for Young Children*, a CD. 2004. *www.stillquietplace.com.*

About the Author

Lisa Flynn, E-RYT, RCYT is the founder and director of ChildLight Yoga® and Yoga 4 Classrooms®, organizations providing evidence-based yoga education to children in schools and communities and to professionals whose work supports the well-being of children. It is her mission to teach strategies that help children and youth develop resilience, positive perceptions, good health habits, and mindful awareness. Lisa shares the ChildLight Yoga® Teacher Training and Yoga 4 Classrooms® Professional Development Workshops and Trainer Intensives nationally. She serves as a curriculum consultant and speaks at many education-focused conferences, universities, schools, and yoga centers around the Northeastern United States. She is also a respected leader and collaborator in the school yoga and mindfulness movement and greater kids' yoga community internationally. Lisa has authored several program manuals related to yoga for children and published the *Yoga 4 Classrooms® Card Deck* in 2011. She is an active member of several professional organizations including Yoga Alliance, the International Association of Yoga Therapists (IAYT), Yoga Service Council, and the International Association of School Yoga and Mindfulness (IASYM), in addition to several groups and organizations that are focused on supporting and growing the field of contemplative education.

Most importantly, Lisa is a mom. Admittedly, work, her children's activities, and running a household can become stressful at times. She uses yoga, meditation, gratitude, and positive thinking to bring balance into her life. Her intention is to inspire her young students to do the same, providing them with tools they can use for a lifetime of health and wellness.

Learn more about Lisa Flynn and her work at:
ChildLight Yoga®: *www.childlightyoga.com*
Yoga 4 Classrooms®: *www.yoga4classrooms.com*

INDEX

Note: Page numbers in *italics* indicate exercises, activities, games, or songs/chants. Page numbers in **bold** indicate poses.